"Susan's book is filled with tl experience of cancer. Their wisdom can be utilized to help you fulfill your potential and heal your life while eliminating your disease. Getting well against all odds is not a spontaneous remission. It is self-induced healing. Susan shares what changes you need to make in your life to have that happen. It is about how transformation and harmony in your life gives your body a "live" message and induces a state of healing of your life and curing of your disease."
Bernie Siegel, MD, author of *The Art of Healing* and *Faith, Hope & Healing*

"Physicians cannot hope to fully comprehend, only to be able to empathize with, the unimaginable challenges faced by patients with a new or prolonged diagnosis of cancer. The search for solace and understanding is complex and daunting. *An Inside Job* examines these matters from all angles, and allows all who are confronted with the diagnosis of cancer to explore the myriad of challenges and mechanisms of not just "coping", but coming to a greater understanding, and in the end, making their own peace with the diagnosis.

The book's greatest strength is its diversity, which allows the reader to explore those matters most relevant to themselves, and to read stories of others who may have been similarly challenged. In the end, the recurring theme is that one is never truly alone on their journey. Under the worst of circumstances, such a book can be a wonderful companion."
Kevin R. Fox, MD, Professor of Medicine, University of Pennsylvania Perelman School of Medicine, Medical Director, Rena Rowan Breast Center

"After three decades as a psychologist working in the service of cancer patients, Susan Barbara Apollon has become a wise and seasoned scout. In this wonderful guide, she shows

you how to make the choices and mobilize the energies that will empower you—physically, psychologically, and spiritually—on this journey in ways you never imagined were possible. It is a must-read for patients and practitioners alike."
Donna Eden and David Feinstein, PhD, Co-authors of *Energy Medicine* and *The Energies of Love*

"Life-changing and potentially life-saving. If you have cancer, read this book cover to cover, over and over!"
Susan Silberstein, PhD, Founder and Director, The Center for Advancement in Cancer Education and BeatCancer.org

"This book is a compendium of novel insights and wisdom. By illustrating truths through the literal voices of her patients, Susan Apollon has offered a novel algorithm for both patients and physicians alike. It should accompany every patient on their journey.

The collection of stories is inspirational. Chapter Seven, "Allow Yourself to Grieve" opens up with a guide for those of us who provide medical oncology care. But I particularly like Chapter 22, which discusses what healers want you to know, as this is an essential offering.

The individual subtitles and metaphors for each chapter are well chosen, as are the anecdotes, poems, homilies, and sentiments which are thoroughly explored. All emphasize hope for healing.

To summarize, "hope is not a strategy, but no strategy can work without it. Without hope, every path is uncertain, but with it every journey is inspirational."
Michael Nissenblatt, MD, Regional Cancer Care Associates, Central Jersey Division, Oncology and Internal Medicine, Clinical Professor, UMDNJ-Robert Wood Johnson Medical School

Dear Reader / Dan

May you receive hope,
inspiration and comfort
as you read this book —
with blessings of
love and peace —
Susan

"Susan Apollon has truly captured the essence of the mind-body-spirit therapeutic approach that we all should look to in promoting wellness when challenged with a cancer diagnosis. She presents us with a gift of hope and the reality of survival while sharing her personal stories and the exquisite stories of the many patients she has treated over the years.

She invites all of us, whether or not we are impacted by cancer, on a self-discovery journey leading us to toward emotional, physical, and spiritual healing. She intentionally challenges all of us to explore integrative medicine and apply many of these tenets that will help heal our bodies and our minds.

However, this book is much more than just a repository for relevant clinical resources to be utilized by patients and caregivers. Susan Apollon has created a masterful combination of honesty, empathy, and guidance not only for those living with cancer, but for all of us; in hopes that we abide by her insights and truly prosper in harmony within ourselves in order to live our lives with clarity."
Denah Appelt, PhD, Professor of Neuroscience, Philadelphia College of Osteopathic Medicine

"As a surgeon treating those with breast cancer, I have come to understand that one can be cured, but not necessarily healed. Susan Apollon elegantly explains how healing occurs energetically from the inside. She presents an array of tools and essential techniques to help achieve the self love and energetic balance required for complete healing, coupled with inspiring personal and patient experiences. Anyone diagnosed with cancer or other life threatening illness can benefit greatly from the information contained within Susan's book. I will definitely be recommending this book to my patients to aid in their pathway to healing."
Stacy Krisher, MD, FACS, ABIHM, Comprehensive Breast Cancer Surgeon, Holy Redeemer Hospital and Medical Center, PA

"Susan Apollon, a cancer survivor and psychologist who specializes in oncology, brings her knowledge, experience, and empathy to help those diagnosed with cancer better deal with their feelings, questions, and resultant issues. While she addresses the impact of cancer on physical health, including diet, intimacy, and relationships, she also focuses on one of the least addressed topics: the frequently unappreciated interaction between one's emotions (especially dealing with the stress of the disease) and one's physical self.

Apollon cites numerous heartwarming case studies in which patients muster their emotional strengths to help fight their illness. She also empowers the reader by combining her allopathic training with suggested treatments rooted in Eastern, naturopathic and integrative medicine and introduces the reader to the work of colleagues—including many physicians—whose ideas are meant to help the reader along their journey.

Enormously helpful and educational in both the physical and emotional aspects of living with cancer—and written with unusual warmth and understanding—*An Inside Job* also includes interesting clinical histories—all of which support the author's significant insights. I most highly recommend *An Inside Job*."
Caroline Koblenzer, MD, Dermatology, Psychiatry, Clinical Professor, Cooper Medical School of Rowan University

"Susan Apollon has written a beautiful book that not only underscores the meaning and importance of true healing from a cancer diagnosis, but also creates a path for patients to obtain it. *An Inside Job* is filled with practical advice and interwoven with countless touching patient stories. I highly recommend *An Inside Job* to help navigate the emotional, spiritual, and physical journey of every patient facing the fear and uncertainty of cancer."
Pallav Mehta, MD, Oncology, Hematology, Integrative Medicine, Director of Integrative Oncology, MD Anderson Cancer Center at Cooper

"Susan Apollon's book, *An Inside Job*, gives spiritual and emotional direction to people going through life's journey with cancer. It fills a large gap in treatment that medicine and therapy often miss."
Jeffrey Herman, DO, Psychiatrist, Southampton, PA

"*An Inside Job* is truly a testament to the importance of supporting cancer patients and their caregivers in every way. Additionally, it empowers patients to help themselves. It is a wonderful story about healing for all!"
Neha Vapiwala, MD, Associate Professor, Advisory Dean, University of Pennsylvania Perelman School of Medicine

"I've had the pleasure of referring patients to Susan to help them heal from their breast cancer diagnosis, and also from other adversities they have encountered in their lives. Through this book, Susan has graciously offered her amazing wisdom and insights to those who may not be able to work directly with her. Although the book is dedicated to those who have encountered cancer in their life journey, I found it to be applicable to life adversities in general as well. I look forward to offering it to friends and family members to help them navigate the journey of life, and gain skills and tools to guide them along the way. The most sincere thanks to Susan for this wonderful gift!"
Catherine D. Carruthers, MD, FACS, ABIHM, Comprehensive Breast Cancer Surgeon, Holy Redeemer Hospital and Medical Center, PA

"In her newest book *An Inside Job*, Susan Apollon offers her readers a road map addressing the physical, emotional, and spiritual needs, not only of the cancer patient, but of all of us on this earthly realm.

The paths of those with cancer as well as their caregivers, can be arduous and stressful. Susan shares her Love, Compassion, and

Insight, and like an Angel by your side, offers guidance on the journey to healing."
Robert Sasson, MD, Pediatrician, Newtown, PA, associated with Children's Hospital of Philadelphia

"The inspirational work of Susan Apollon continues in her latest gift of heartfelt sharing. This loving guide on survivorship is filled with hope, compassion, and encouragement. Each page offers insightful pearls as well as stories of courage and healing. Susan provides invaluable techniques to help those on the journey of healing as well as their caregivers and their healers. Once again, Susan's gentle hand and nurturing soul connects us to her timeless wisdom. This is a required reading for all healers and those they touch."
Amy Harvey, MD, Gynecology, Obstetrics, Center for Women's Health, Langhorne, PA

"*An Inside Job* enables the reader to understand the dichotomy of having a choice in whether he perceives his cancer as a looming death sentence or as an opportunity to learn lessons which can improve the quality of his life. Presenting an array of resources in the form of a cornucopia of vital information, legitimate affirmations, valuable tools, and real-life stories, Susan Apollon empowers patients, their loved ones, caregivers, and medical providers to more fully and responsibly take on the physical, psychological, and spiritual challenges imposed by the disease.

Susan's integrative approach to healing and wellness is useful for everyone, everywhere; whether or not they are dealing with cancer or a multiplicity of life's issues. We all need sources of wisdom, warmth, and a wealth of knowledge. Susan Barbara Apollon has provided all of this and more with her new book, *An Inside Job*."
Bonnie Frank-Carter, PhD, Clinical Psychologist, Wayne, PA

"Western medicine, with its ever expanding body of research on the mind-body connection, is finally catching up to what many kinds of healers have been saying for a long time: that energy pervades the mental, physical, and spiritual, and that this energy can be harnessed to heal. An elder stateswoman of the mind-body healing movement, Susan's voice has always been clear and heartfelt. Now, as time and science have marched on, her message is beautifully coalescing with so many others' accounts of healing. *An Inside Job* is her most recent invaluable contribution to the field."
Eric Levin, PhD, Clinical Psychologist, Philadelphia, PA

"When one is confronted with the diagnosis of cancer, it is a life-altering proposition. *An Inside Job* provides thoughtful, useful suggestions in dealing with this difficult situation. It emphasizes that the psychological aspects of the diagnosis can have major impact on how one deals with the illness. It points out that there is an interaction between the mind and body. The physical components are difficult to control but the psychological aspects can be controlled by the patient.

I found this book to be extraordinarily valuable. It makes multiple suggestions on how one can develop a positive outlook despite the fear and concerns created by the diagnosis of cancer. This is an invaluable tool in aiding a patient to control the situation."
Michael Casey, MD, Pennsylvania Pulmonary Medical Associates, Pulmonology, Critical Care, and Internal Medicine, Clinical Professor of Medicine, Penn Medicine, Pennsylvania Hospital

"Cancer has been a long battle for me; although I survived the first diagnosis, the current cancer has made the war more difficult. Susan's book, *An Inside Job*, is an inspiration to all who have had cancer, to those who live with it every day, and to caregivers and

health care workers. This book is a recommendation and reference for all those whose lives are touched by cancer. Thank you, Susan."
Andrea Nora-Tanken, PA-C, MPH, Survivor of T Lymphoblastic Leukemia and presently challenged by Myelodysplastic Syndrome (MDS) with monosomy 7. Assistant Professor, Arcadia University

"As a psychologist and a cancer thriver, Susan teaches us that true healing requires addressing our emotional, mental, and spiritual needs, as well as those that are physical. I have had the honor of seeing Susan as a client and am grateful for her guidance, teachings, commitment, and caring—all of which have helped me with my healing journey.

I smiled as I read *An Inside Job*. I believed my angels were reminding me to continue using the valuable tools that Susan has taught me. I hope those who read this beautiful book will incorporate Susan's guidance and tools to help in overcoming the challenges they may face, as well as to experience peace and healing from the inside out.
Marcy McCaw, breast cancer Survivor and Thriver, Lymphedema Specialist and Physical Therapist, Holy Redeemer Health System, PA

"The body can be cured, but are we healed? Through Susan's evidence-based knowledge and heartfelt stories, she takes us on a journey and teaches us that acceptance of an illness is not a surrender or defeat, but an invitation to more deeply love and heal the self."
Jodi Hutchinson, Director of Integrated Medicine and Wellness, Holy Redeemer Health System, PA

"Finally, someone who encourages you to recognize your inner power! So often we feel that cancer overpowers and controls our destinies. Giving ourselves permission to choose is empowering and gives us back a sense of control over our lives.

Since my first cancer diagnosis nearly 18 years ago, I've learned to focus on my joys, surround myself with love, and relish day-to-day humor. Susan Apollon affirms how these positive actions support healing while giving us permission to put ourselves first and find the ability to be at peace with who we are. She awakens you to your own personal healing power.

Susan looks at healing from all perspectives, giving us the personal ability to make positive choices to impact our recovery. Learn to fight your cancer spiritually, emotionally, and physically, from the inside out."
Jean Shipos, Survivor and Thriver, ovarian, breast, lung, and brain cancers, Executive Director, The Teal Tea Foundation

"*An Inside Job* has helped to validate my feelings, motivate me to take action, and calmed my anxiety and fears. It has given me permission to cry, kick, and scream—and know it is all ok. It has helped me learn to visualize my breathing, enabling me to feel so much calmer. I return frequently to certain chapters which help me to feel more peaceful and which restore my sense of hope for the future. I especially love the stories you share of your patients. Most of all, while it lets me know that all I am experiencing is normal, it teaches me the value of letting go of what does not feel good and holding onto what most benefits me."
Syndi Zinman, Survivor and Thriver of endometrial, ovarian, uterine, and brain cancers; Member of The GyniGirls Cancer Support Group

"Susan Apollon's book, *An Inside Job* is a must-read for cancer patients that want and need to heal their bodies, whether physically, emotionally or spiritually. Without this knowledge, cancer will return and keep returning until all healing is completed … My cancer is greatly diminished and I continue to see Susan and also engage in Eden Energy Medicine …"
Debra Buchanan, a Survivor and Thriver of cancers of the breast, liver, bone, and brain

"Susan's book is palpable, taking the reader inside the heart of a gifted therapist. She invites the reader to tap in, turn on, and tune into a reservoir of experience, education, and expertise; all the Energies of life, love, and light—taking what is needed to facilitate the healing of their own heart.

Susan is the gift that keeps on giving. She has gifted and birthed a most generous and compassionate "care package" that will support, sustain, and serve those who choose to live their best life—to be the best version of themselves."
Josi Feit, Survivor and Thriver of metastatic breast cancer and present cancer challenges

"*An Inside Job* is authentic and wonderful. It immediately pulled me in, making me comfortably feel that someone has my back and that I am not alone. The book offers much for its readers, including exercises which helped me to feel better through my cancer journey, and stories which touched my heart and felt so familiar. Reading *An Inside Job* is like bringing Susan into your home, with her warmth, wisdom, and guidance to help you wherever you may be on your road to healing."
Fiona Havlish, breast cancer Survivor and Thriver, Author of *In Full Voice: Shedding the Labels that Silenced Me*

"This book is an amazing collection of information drawing from the fields of science, medicine, psychology, and spirituality. It offers a way for the person who has been diagnosed with cancer to move from the fear that accompanies such a diagnosis to a place of hope and joy. It does this in a way that is accessible to people of all backgrounds and cultures. *An Inside Job* is truly a treasure."
A GyniGirls Cancer Support Group Member

AN
INSIDE
JOB

A Psychologist Shares
Healing Wisdom for
Your Cancer Journey

SUSAN BARBARA APOLLON

Foreword by Beth Baughman DuPree, M.D.

I dedicate this book to each of you who has ever received the diagnosis of cancer, and to those who lovingly care for you, with the hope that it may ...

Gently shift your perspective of illness and healing;

Guide you safely through the darkness of uncertainty and fear;

Illuminate your path and affirm that you are never alone;

Enable you to forgive and release the past;

Engender feelings of comfort, peace, and hope;

And remind you of how wise, powerful, loved and extraordinary you are.

Table of Contents

Foreword i

Acknowledgments: With Gratitude and Deep Appreciation v

Introduction ix

Part One 1

Chapter One: You Are Energy 3

Chapter Two: The High Cost of Low Vibrations 15

Chapter Three: A Life That Isn't Working 23

Part Two **35**

Chapter Four: Guiding Principles for Your Cancer Journey 37

Chapter Five: Choose to See Cancer as a Gift 55

Chapter Six: What Does It Mean to Heal? 73

Chapter Seven: Allow Yourself to Grieve 87

Chapter Eight: Utilize Crucial Tools for Healing 103

Chapter Nine: Face Your Fear of Death
(Synchronicities and Stories Can Help!) 123

Chapter Ten: Connect with Your Higher
Power and Grow Your Spirit 139

Chapter Eleven: Use the Law of Attraction
to Affirm Better Health 155

Chapter Twelve: Forgive Those Who Need to Be Forgiven . . . 165

Chapter Thirteen: Live in Alignment
with What Is in Your Heart 179

Chapter Fourteen: Breathe Mindfully 197

Chapter Fifteen: Open Yourself to Miracles
and Extraordinary Experiences 205

Chapter Sixteen: Don't Be the Strong, Silent, Solitary Type . . . 217

Chapter Seventeen: Understand the
Healing Value of Intimacy 233

Chapter Eighteen: Do Something Selfless 245

Chapter Nineteen: Nutrition as Medicine 257

Chapter Twenty: Purposefully Care for
Your Mind, Body, and Soul 283

Part Three **303**

Chapter Twenty-One: Be Selective in Creating Your
Medical Team—And Think Integrative Medicine 305

Chapter Twenty-Two: What Your
Healers Want You to Know 311

    Dr. Peter Yi 312

    Dr. Wendy Warner. 317

    Dr. Jingduan Yang 322

    Dr. Scarlet Soriano 332

    Dr. William L. Scarlett 334

    Dr. Bernie Siegel 342

    Dr. Cynthia R. Aks 347

    Dr. William E. Hablitzel 358

    Dr. Amy Harvey O'Keeffe 360

Final Thoughts 365

Appendix: Further Resources for Reading,
Listening, Education, and Support 371

Chapter Notes 391

About the Author 395

Index 397

Foreword

Healing truly is "An Inside Job," and you have the power to heal from the inside out.

Several times a week I sit at my desk, take a deep breath, and pick up the phone to place a call that drastically and completely changes another soul's life. I am a breast cancer surgeon. Having to tell a woman or a man that they have breast cancer is one of the most difficult aspects of my job that has never and will never get easier.

I know that I do not give my patient the cancer, but I also know that I cannot promise that I can take it away, never to return. I cannot guarantee a "cure" from any cancer, even those cancers diagnosed at stage zero. God knows I wish I could guarantee a cure, but I have come to accept that not being able to promise healing doesn't make me a failure as a physician; it makes me a spiritual being having a very human experience. What I *can* guarantee as a healer is the opportunity for "healing" if my patient is open to receive and willing to do their spiritual work. Healing can occur regardless of the outcome to the physical body, just as curing the physical body can occur without healing at the soul's level.

My classical surgical training in the 1980s taught me that "to cut is to cure," and that as a surgeon, my role was to be the technician (albeit a very skilled and caring technician) who removes the malignancy from the body. "Nothing heals like cold steel" was another adage that was thrown around the surgical world, and as a young surgeon in training, I was taught to believe that was my role in the care of a cancer patient.

Through my own journey as a surgeon and healer, I have come to recognize that although my scalpel can cut out the cancer, I cannot cut out the *fear* that a cancer diagnosis brings. I had to look beyond my extensive and excellent Western medical training to find ways to help my patients alleviate fear and find true peace in their hearts.

Fast-forward to 2015. The accreditation organizations for centers of breast care excellence in the United States have recognized what Susan Apollon and I have known for decades; namely, that a "survivorship care plan" is key in the treatment of cancer patients. However, I would prefer to call it a "Thrivership Care Plan," as it is not enough to physically survive the treatment of the cancer. We also need to help our patients truly find healing and begin to thrive in their lives.

I am blessed to be able to refer my patients (and often, caregivers who have lost their loved one to cancer) to Susan for one-on-one counseling and intuitive guidance. I wish every soul who was on their journey could have the gift of Susan in person, but there are not enough hours in the day.

This book is the next best thing. *An Inside Job* shares heartfelt stories of healing, meditation practices, spiritual exercises, and centering techniques. It has been written from the heart of a healer, with the intuition of a woman and the wisdom of a psychologist who has many years of experience in helping patients find healing. In short, Susan has taken her years of grief counseling, her intuitive healing gifts, and the wisdom of her spirit guides and created a healing masterpiece. She has even included a section of guidance from several integrative healers regarding what they want you to know from a physician's perspective. Each of us has to find healing in our own way, and with Susan's expert guidance you will find your way by adopting and practicing the healing techniques that resonate with you.

I often write a message in the cover of my book when I give it to my patients. That message says, "Adversity is the opportunity for spiritual growth." Susan has known this for years, and has even discovered that the Chinese characters for Crisis and Opportunity share a common symbol.

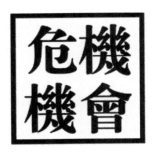

When cancer rocks your world, you have two ways to approach the diagnosis. You can mourn the loss of the life you currently live (which is most likely a fast-paced, over-scheduled, disconnected rat race). Alternatively, you can choose to see cancer as a gift or as the beginning of a new, authentic, hopeful, love-filled journey. If you choose this option, you will realize that every year, every day, every breath, and every moment is the gift, for not one of us is guaranteed tomorrow. Crisis *is* Opportunity. Allow your cancer crisis to guide you to not only survive physically, but also to thrive in your life emotionally, physically, and spiritually.

An Inside Job: Healing Wisdom for Your Cancer Journey should be required reading in medical school, as the concept of healing is palpably absent from current medical education. This book should also be physically handed to every patient when the cancer diagnosis enters their world. I am blessed to have Susan as my friend, my healing mentor, and spiritual guide. She is a gift in my life and in my patients' lives. This book will allow her to be a gift in your life, too, as she accompanies you on a guided tour to finding peace in your heart and healing in your soul.

Much Love and Light,
Beth Baughman DuPree, MD, FACS, ABIHM
December 2014
Medical Director of Integrative Holistic Medicine Holy Redeemer Health System
Adjunct Assistant Professor of Surgery, University of Pennsylvania
Author, *The Healing Consciousness: A Doctor's Journey to Healing*

Acknowledgments: With Gratitude and Deep Appreciation

This book has become a reality due, in major part, to the mindset of three women: Dottie DeHart, Anna Campbell, and Meghan Waters. I thank you all for being so patient with me, and for believing in me. Dottie, you were the first to drop the seed on my plate that a little book of healing wisdom for dealing with the challenge of cancer was needed by the world—and that I should write it. Anna and Meghan, thank you for taking my words and ideas and editing them in just the right formula. Over the years we have worked together, I have come to trust your wisdom and have always felt your genuine caring about the value of the work I do—and about me. Words can't adequately convey the love and appreciation I feel for all of you and my heartfelt gratitude for your loving support. My thanks as well, to you Brad, for your patience and perseverance in working with me to create the most wonderful cover for *An Inside Job*. I appreciate all the time and effort you devoted to creating a cover which would support the truths of this book.

An Inside Job is filled with true stories that validate the healing information I have shared with you, the reader. Thank you, thank you, thank you to each of you beautiful souls who allowed me to write your stories of healing. You are what make this book so interesting, colorful, and fascinating. A special expression of loving gratitude to our GyniGirls, and to my amazing co-leader and dear friend, Amy Harvey O'Keeffe, for allowing me to share your stories and the wisdom you have passed on to me. I can't thank you enough for your contributions. Know that your stories have the power to bring about transformation and healing in those whose names you do not know.

Additionally, I am filled with gratitude for each of the physician healers who said *yes* to my request for participation in this project. Doctors Peter Yi, Scarlet Soriano, Karen Flicker, Donna Angotti, Jingduan Yang, Cynthia Aks, Bill Scarlett, Wendy Warner, Amy Harvey O'Keeffe, Bill Hablitzel, and Bernie Siegel, thank you for choosing to assist the sometimes overwhelmed reader in navigating their cancer journey. You achieved the impossible, carving out time from your overwhelming, full schedules to share your unique perspective and message regarding healing and cancer.

I want every one of you who has ever heard the words, "You have cancer," to know that my heart is, has been, and will always be with you with gratitude, understanding, compassion, and love. I know you are forever changed, made different, wiser, and better, because of your cancer challenge. That is how extraordinary the experience—and you—are! You are all teachers for me, providing me with your thoughts, feelings, and concerns about survival and thriving. I have written this book for you, with the hope that the information provided here will assist you in achieving wholeness, wellness, and ultimately, healing.

Diana Warren, you have been one of my angels during this process. You have been my gracious mentor, guide, teacher, and healer, sharing with me your valuable, intuitive wisdom regarding energy and life—all of which has enabled me to heal my own mind, body and spirit, as well as enhance the healing work I bring to my patients. My heart is filled with overflowing love and gratitude for sustaining me through the journey of writing this book.

Beth DuPree, thank you from my heart for taking your valuable time and energy to read, assess the value of *An Inside Job,* and then write the Foreword for this book. Your support and belief in the value of the work I do and the books I write have always moved and deeply touched me. Know that I am genuinely grateful for you, your loving friendship, and the difference you make in the lives of women everywhere who are challenged by breast cancer and who seek wholeness and well-being. I love you dearly.

An author uses the research and work of those who preceded her or him. There are many to whom I am in debt for their rich, intensive work and research, and on whose shoulders this book rests. My gratitude is extended to Jeanne Achterberg, Deepak Chopra, Larry Dossey, Larry LeShan, Elisabeth Kübler-Ross, Raymond Moody, Marc Ian Barasch and Caryle Hirshberg, Andrew Weil, Brian Weiss, Bruce Lipton, Christiane Northrup, Mona Lisa Schultz, Caroline Myss, Albert Einstein, Gerald Jampolsky, Patrick Quillin, Jane Plant, Louise Hay, Melvin Morse, Kelly Turner, Jon Kabat-Zinn, Joan Borysenko, Belleruth Naparstek, Brené Brown, David Hawkins, Rupert Scheldrake, Donna Eden and David Feinstein, Rachel Naomi Remen, and so many others . . .

Warren, thank you, my love, for your kindness and patience during the writing of this book over the past four years. Your loving understanding and tolerance for so many moments in which I "missed the boat" has repeatedly touched my heart. I could not have pulled this off without your unceasing support and belief in me and the value of this book.

There are many others who will play a significant role in bringing this book to you, the reader. To all of those individuals, know that I feel only sincere appreciation for all your actions, intentions, and desires to make *An Inside Job* a source of hope and guidance for healing. Thank you for your gifts of believing in the message of this book. All of you are contributing to the healing experiences of those who choose to read *An Inside Job*! And may there be many! It is because of you and your efforts that those who have had to confront the unexpected diagnosis of cancer will shift from the vibration of fear to one of empowerment, confidence, healing, and love.

If you have been on a cancer journey, may you find peace and truth in the words: *Cancer has been my wake-up call and a gift in my life.*

With heartfelt gratitude and blessings of peace, love, and well-being,
Susan Barbara Apollon

Introduction

"Although the world is full of suffering, It is also full of the overcoming of it."

HELEN KELLER

"The most beautiful people in the world are those who have known defeat, known suffering, known struggle, known loss, and have found their way out of the depths. These people have an appreciation, a sensitivity, and an understanding of life that fills them with compassion, gentleness, and a deep loving concern. Beautiful people do not just happen."

ELISABETH KÜBLER-ROSS

Nobody wants to receive a cancer diagnosis. In fact, few things are more frightening. But if you are reading this book, it's likely that you or someone you love has just heard those dreaded words: "You have cancer." While I can't remove this experience from your path, it is my hope that the following chapters will help you to find a new way to think about the journey you are on.

I approach the unwelcome visitor called cancer from two different, yet intertwined perspectives. First, I myself am a breast cancer survivor—and breast cancer, unlikely as it may seem, ended up saving my life. In the course of the diagnostic tests required for my radiation and surgeries, my doctors discovered a life-threatening tumor on my adrenal gland. It was removed, and I am here to write these words to you. Cancer is a deeply personal issue for me.

Second, I am a psychologist with nearly three decades of experience. Many of my patients have been diagnosed with cancer. They don't come to me for statistics and conventional medical advice—as is probably the case for you, they are working with capable teams of medical professionals. Instead, they allow me to help them face the very real obstacle called FEAR and receive the gifts of spiritual, emotional, and often physical healing that lie on the other side.

While you and I likely won't speak face-to-face, I am nevertheless honored to share much of the same healing wisdom and hope with you.

Answering Cancer's Wake-Up Call

"No matter what the statistics say,
There's always a way."

BERNIE SIEGEL

In the nearly 30 years I have worked with cancer patients, some have died from this disease. However, more have survived—and with an improved quality of life. Why is this? While there are many potential reasons, I believe my patients' perspectives and attitudes regarding their situations had a huge impact on their healing. In short, my patients chose to view cancer as a wake-up call for life.

Most people, cancer or no cancer, need a wake-up call. We get so caught up in the daily trials, tribulations, and tasks of life that we fail to notice that joy has slipped away. Our physical health blinds us to the fact that many aspects of our lives *aren't* well. (In fact, a deteriorated quality of life can contribute to the development of diseases like cancer.)

It's only after receiving a cancer diagnosis that we suddenly find ourselves noticing the "craziness" and the trade-offs we've been making in order to pursue what we thought was essential. Our perspective changes; we begin to *"live like we are dying,"* and we finally experience life in the fullness we were always meant to. It is this awakening that allows many people to later come to view their cancer diagnosis as a "gift."

Whether you're a patient or a caregiver, cancer enables you to become conscious of what you intuitively know to be healthy, meaningful, and good for you. And if you gravitate toward and focus on those things, I promise, you will make substantial changes in your life. Healing, whether from cancer or anything else, truly *is* an inside job.

While neither I nor anyone else can make promises, there is a very real possibility that you or your loved one could experience physical healing. What I *can* guarantee, for anyone who does the "work" described in this book, is spiritual healing—a restoring of the vibration of *inner* harmony, balance, and peace within you. In fact, the good news about being diagnosed with cancer is that it often becomes the catalyst for "growing" your soul and your spirit, all of which enables you to feel more whole and at peace.

Please believe me: Right now, you have a choice. You can choose to view cancer as a tragedy and a curse. Doing so will only mire you in destructive anxiety, grief, anger, and fear. However, you can also choose to perceive cancer as an opportunity to take a good look at how you're living your life and whether it is working for you. Saying "yes" to this wake-up call will shift you energetically to a place where healing is more likely to occur.

How *An Inside Job: A Psychologist Shares Healing Wisdom for Your Cancer Journey* Helps You Say "Yes" to Healing

You'll find there are three parts to this book.

- Part One explores the energetic aspects of wellness and healing. It will help you understand your body's energetic makeup and how it factors into your healing journey. It will also explain why living with stress, anger, worry, unprocessed grief, and other "low vibration" emotions may suppress your immune system in a way that allows cancer to develop.
- In Part Two, by far the biggest section of this book, you'll discover a wealth of strategies and techniques for embarking on your healing journey. My intention is for you to embrace the tips that resonate with you and leave the rest as you seek to create a life filled with peace, love, positivity, and even joy and fun.
- Part Three is written specifically to provide you with an understanding of how integrative medicine can support your healing journey. To further assist you, a group of highly respected doctors who are known for genuinely caring about their patients offer personal perspectives regarding their own practice of integrative medicine.

Throughout the book, you will find true stories of those who, like yourself, have been challenged by the diagnosis of a life-threatening illness (often cancer). These individuals brought courage, strength, wisdom, and perseverance to their experiences, and were able to find peace and healing within their lives. What an honor it has been for me to share in their healing moments. (In most cases, names and circumstances have been changed to protect their identities, except where I have been given specific permission to use actual names and details.)

If you are a cancer patient, I urge you share this book with your loved ones. It will help them understand the journey you are on, which in turn, will empower them to be as supportive and helpful as possible.

Finally, as you read this book please remember that the Chinese symbol for crisis, difficulty, struggle, and challenge is the same symbol used for opportunity. Ask yourself: Do you want to be a victim or a victor? Will you view cancer as a curse or as a gift? The choice is yours and it will impact every moment of the rest of your life—whether that time is measured in decades, years, months, weeks, or even days.

Cancer saved my life in more ways than one. I firmly believe it can do the same for you. My goal is to help you make choices that enable you to reclaim the tremendous power you've forgotten you have—and to remind you of how extraordinary you really are.

Susan Barbara Apollon

PART ONE

CHAPTER 1

You Are Energy

"*Everything is energy and that's all there is to it. Match the frequency of the reality you want and you cannot help but get that reality. It can be no other way. This is not philosophy. This is physics.*"

ALBERT EINSTEIN

When you have cancer, you tend to spend a lot of time thinking about energy—usually, how much of it you *don't* have. As you read this book and apply it to your own life, I want you to continue to think about energy, but in a whole new way.

When I use the term "energy," I'm generally not referring to how much pep you have in your step. Instead, I'm referring to something totally different: something that can translate into very good news for your cancer journey—and may even help to explain how this disease developed in your body in the first place.

To put it simply, you—as well as everything you see, touch, or feel—are comprised of energy. Yes, *you* are energy, and as such you vibrate at many different levels. In this chapter, I'll explain this concept further. And after tracing the history of energy as it relates to science, I'll explain how you have a say in the kind of energy you experience and how it can influence the quality of your life (and your cancer journey in particular).

Energy: A Surprising Science Lesson

Describing living beings and inanimate objects as "energy" might sound strange to you. Most of us are accustomed to thinking of ourselves and the world around us in other terms. We were taught in school that everything is made of matter, atoms, molecules, elements, and/or compounds. And as far as it goes, that information is accurate. But who's to say that all of the universe's matter, whether it's living or not, doesn't have energy?

In fact, that's *exactly* what many respected scientific thinkers teach. Here's a brief overview of what science has helped us to understand about energy:

- Albert Einstein and his colleagues, all quantum physicists, demonstrated in the laboratory that *everything can be broken down into particles and waves of light energy.*

Their work also revealed that this energy vibrates at many levels.

- Thanks to another scientist, David R. Hawkins, we know that the *highest levels of this energy are those of Love and Enlightenment (or Divine Energy)*.

- Since the mid to late 20th century, scientists and physicians, including Marilyn Schlitz, Dean Radin, Larry Dossey, Bruce Lipton, Russell Targ, Candace Pert, Joyce Hawkes, and many others, have shared their research, theories, and awareness regarding energy. They agree that *your beliefs are energy*, and that when you're aware of this fact, *you can harness the thoughts you create and direct them to vibrate at a higher level*. In this way, you can control how good you feel, and you can also experience an improved sense of being. These scientists' work validates the mind, body, and spirit connection!

- Research on consciousness conducted by eminent scientists such as Lawrence LeShan, Bernard Grad, and others has validated and supported the theories put forth by quantum physics. These theories explain what yogis have known for thousands of years: *We have the power to use the energy of our thoughts to create a reality that connects us with everyone and everything.*

  Specifically, this energy allows us to know what we could not have otherwise known. It has also been demonstrated to have the ability, when focused as intentions of healing and mixed with the energy of love, to contribute to an improvement in—or even heal—plants, animals, and people.

- Einstein, Schrödinger, and, more recently, Rupert Sheldrake all recognized that *the Mind is actually part of a larger field of energy* that can be called many things, including God or the Universe. Because we are part of a larger Mind, we have the ability to tap into, receive, and give back information that can aid our growth or improve our situation. (In this way we are much like radio transmitters.)

The more you "practice" energetically tapping into this extraordinary universal field of knowing, the more your awareness will expand. Furthermore, our connection to a larger energy field means that we are a part of Divine Energy and that it is within us. And because we can tap into Divine Energy to know and experience Love, Wisdom and Love become who and what we are.

Especially if you've never encountered this view of energy before, much of the information above probably seems strange to you. If you're skeptical or confused, I encourage you to do some research on your own. You can learn more about all of the concepts and people I've mentioned by searching online. If you prefer to read good old-fashioned books, I recommend the following:

- *A Practical Guide to Vibrational Medicine: Energy Healing and Spiritual Transformation* by Richard Gerber, MD
- *Power vs. Force* by David R. Hawkins, MD, PhD
- *Reinventing Medicine: Beyond Mind-Body to a New Era of Healing* by Larry Dossey, MD
- *Messages from Water* by Masaru Emoto, PhD
- *The Biology of Belief: Unleashing the Power of Consciousness, Matter and Miracles* by Bruce Lipton, PhD
- *The Field: The Quest for the Secret Force of the Universe* and *The Intention Experiment: Using Your Thoughts to Change Your Life and the World*, both by Lynne McTaggart

You'll also gain a greater familiarity with vibrational energy as you continue reading this book.

Using Energy in Your Cancer Journey

As I explained in the introduction, a diagnosis of cancer often inspires us to understand who and what we are in a much deeper, richer way. Personally, it is my wish that every cancer patient and caregiver might come to understand that everything—including your thoughts—is energy ... and that you have the power to shift this energy in your favor. Without a doubt, this knowledge is the most powerful tool I have in helping my patients.

I stated earlier in this chapter that quantum physics has demonstrated in a laboratory setting that everything in the universe can be broken down to particles and waves of light. Furthermore, each of those particles and waves vibrates—but at different levels and speeds. As a human being, what you think about and focus on influences your vibrational energy. That's important, because energy attracts like energy. (You may be familiar with this concept as the Law of Attraction.)

Essentially, wherever you are vibrationally, you'll attract experiences of a similar level of vibration (much as a tuning fork causes corresponding strings on musical instruments to resonate).

Here's what that means: *As you face cancer, the quality of your life depends on the choices you make about what you are going to focus on.* That is, you get to choose whether or not you will spend time contemplating, ruminating on, or just plain thinking about things that feel good—or not.

Feel-good thoughts will cause you to vibrate at a high level, one that promotes health and healing, and that allows you to manifest your hopes and dreams. (Many of the tactics I'll teach you throughout this book are based on this principle.) However, non-feel-good thoughts, the kind that cause you to experience suffering and pain, attract similar vibrational experiences. In fact, they may suppress your immune system and promote cancer's spread. (We'll look at this specific topic in the next chapter.)

Now, I would like to share a true story with you. It was written by a woman I greatly admire about her cancer journey. Lauren's story strongly demonstrates the power of positive energy and the importance of consciously focusing on high-level vibrations.

Lauren's Story: Positive Energy Promotes Against-the-Odds Healing

The story of my cancer began when I was 34 years old, in my last week of pregnancy with my first child. I had worked full-time as a radiologist (with no symptoms) until five days before my diagnosis. I was on maternity leave eagerly awaiting the birth of my child, hoping for a girl. I had a grand mal seizure in the middle of the night, and was raced to the hospital by ambulance where my two best friends, Amy Harvey and Beth DuPree, were waiting for me.

After an MRI and CT scans, it was determined that I'd had a pregnancy-related stroke and was transferred by helicopter to the University of Pennsylvania Hospital's stroke center. Upon arrival, a neurologist informed me that the abnormality in my brain was actually a tumor, not a stroke, but that it was probably benign. After intravenous medications to protect me from more seizures, I delivered my wonderful daughter and named her Francesca. She was the most beautiful thing I had ever seen.

I then had to deal with the brain tumor issue. When a matter-of-fact, cold, insensitive neurosurgeon spoke to me at the University of Pennsylvania and raised the possibility of cancer, I made a vow that I was not going to let him cut into my precious brain, the organ that I used for my livelihood. I felt that if he was so careless about giving such terrible news to a patient, how could I be sure he would be careful in doing my brain surgery? I was so frightened at the prospect of some surgeon cutting into my brain and me waking up not being able to speak, think, or move my arms and legs.

Since I had a few weeks to make this monumental decision, I began a countrywide search to find the best neurosurgeon to perform my surgery. I asked my physician friends for recommendations and sent my films and story to several neurosurgeons who specialized in brain and spinal cord tumors. Then I waited for their replies. I was looking for a neurosurgeon who would treat me as a human being, not as just another interesting case.

I ended up choosing the chief of neurosurgery at Memorial Sloan Kettering Hospital in New York City (MSK) because I felt that he treated me and my baby with respect and he inspired confidence. After having the surgery at MSK, I emerged with my brain intact, speaking and moving all extremities! First hurdle over!

Several days later, I was given the diagnosis of a Grade Three multicellular tumor, which was classified as cancer. Brain tumors are classified Grade One through Four, with Grade Four being the worst (yet most common, and almost universally fatal). Grade Three tumors are treated the same as Grade Four tumors since they are quite likely to recur and become Grade Four. My tumor was in the frontal lobe on the left side, and was about the size of a ping-pong ball. Fortunately, that part of the brain is rather silent, meaning that it can be removed with minimal effects. I was shocked. How can a woman age 34 have cancer? And at the birth of her first baby? It seemed unreal.

I was offered a treatment plan at MSK that terrified me. It involved life-threatening chemotherapy to completely obliterate the bone marrow, followed by a high-risk stem cell transplant. This was very dangerous because during the four to six weeks of treatment, the body is exposed to every pathogen and can get quite sick very quickly. It also meant I would only have limited time with my family, especially my newborn baby. I decided I would do that only if I had no other options.

I sought a second opinion, and chose the University of Pennsylvania where I was very comfortable, having spent time there as a medical student. I met with a wonderful neuro-oncologist, Dr. Peter Phillips, whom I chose as my doctor. Together we created a treatment plan that we could both live with. The new plan included radiation to the brain, followed by a course of easier chemotherapy to last about a year or until my body could not tolerate any more. Since this was much more palatable, I then began focused brain radiation for six weeks, Monday through Friday.

However, another hurdle came up during the second week of radiation. I noticed pus coming from an area of my scalp incision in a spot that previously would not heal. Given my medical knowledge, I knew this had to be an infection. I was treated first with oral antibiotics, and when it returned two weeks later, with IV antibiotics. I was told that if the infection came back one more time, I would have to go back to MSK to have the incision opened up and cleaned out under anesthesia.

My radiation treatments were accelerated in case I needed to go back to the OR. There is nothing creepier than undergoing radiation on the weekend when the entire department is deserted. I finally finished the radiation and got ready to start the chemotherapy. That night, my incision once again starting oozing and I knew I'd have to endure a second brain surgery. I was devastated, so I held Francesca tight, sobbing until no tears were left.

After the second surgery, the piece of bone that had been taken out to do the initial surgery was removed because my medical team thought it might be the source of infection. To allow the infection to completely heal, a metal plate could not be put in its place until the infection was completely gone. That left me with a dent the shape and size of an egg half on my forehead, extending into my hairline. If I styled my remaining hair just right and the wind didn't blow, it wasn't too obvious to anyone else, but I knew it was there. I felt very vulnerable whenever there were flying balls in the air; if one hit me I was sure it would hit my brain tissue directly, and that was terribly scary!

Because it was a bone infection, I had to be treated with six weeks of IV antibiotics before any chemotherapy could begin. Thankfully I was allowed to have this at home with a long-term indwelling catheter so I could still be a mom.

We had intended to have a nanny who came to care for Francesca every day while I went back to work. When I was diagnosed with the brain tumor, it was clear that she would need to be a live-in nanny. We were fortunate to find a lovely Italian woman who came with great recommendations. My husband and I took a Reiki course because we heard wonderful things about it, and our nanny took it as well because she also found it fascinating. From then on, while Francesca was napping, our nanny would perform Reiki on me to help the healing process.

My husband and I also began to attend church every Sunday and we joined a prayer group. We went to every healing service the church offered, and I felt peaceful whenever I attended. The church community was so kind and supportive. I know that there were people praying for me across the country through various prayer chains, and that helped me to fight this cancer. Plus, I had my little girl to live for, and I was determined not to leave her without a mother.

Eventually I started my chemotherapy, and the side effects were minimal. However, at my daughter's first birthday party, I noticed tiny red dots on my thighs that hadn't been there before. I had read about this in medical school. It could only mean that my platelet count was dangerously low from the chemotherapy, leaving my body at high risk for bleeding. I really didn't want a platelet transfusion. I'd never had any kind of blood transfusion before and I wasn't ready to start now. I was fearful of blood-transmitted diseases even though I knew they were rare. But the cancer nurses convinced me to do it, and I embarked on a series of platelet transfusions to maintain my blood counts so I could continue my chemotherapy. Just a few months later I had to stop the chemo because my blood counts were staying too low for too long.

So there I was, in limbo. No treatment, and no idea how long I would live. I never asked about my prognosis, because being a physician, I know that nothing is ever 100 percent. I knew the likelihood of me having a normal lifespan and living to a ripe old age were slim, but I also knew that somebody has to be in that small percentage that survives, and I was determined to be that person. My baby was my reason to live.

I had a schedule of MRI checkups every three months. I went back to work just a little to feel normal again. My hair grew back, and I really felt fine. I was enjoying watching my daughter grow into toddlerhood. But I still had that dent in my skull. Since it appeared I was going to live, at least for a while, I decided to have another surgery to put a plate in my head and get rid of that awful dent. In the interim, there was a small questionable area on the MRI. We wondered if it was residual tumor, or just some scar from the radiation. It was decided that during the surgery that area would be removed and checked to see if it was a tumor. It turned out to be an area of inactive cancer, which in a way was a relief because at least I knew what we were dealing with. As a result, I had another year of different chemotherapy.

Since then, I have been healthy and have defied the odds for this type of brain cancer. I do feel that my diagnosis of cancer has enabled me to do what I always wanted—to raise my child myself and have enough money to do it. I have a generous disability policy that allows me to do so. I also found that reading other people's successful cancer stories gave me inspiration that I could beat this dreadful disease. I spent so much time waiting in doctors' offices for appointments that I was able to read many books. I always found someone who was worse off than me, and that encouraged me when I was starting to become discouraged.

I have given myself permission to spend time and money on non-traditional treatments and therapies that were not taught in medical school. These include acupuncture, Reiki, massage, tapping, nutrition counseling, and lifestyle coaching. I enjoy helping patients with cancer navigate the complex world of cancer treatment, because I know from experience that their lives have been turned upside down and they cannot think clearly. I have also become much more appreciative of living in the moment and finding joy in the myriad aspects of life, both good and bad. All in all, having cancer was a blessing in disguise.

What I Want You to Take Away

There is no doubt in my mind that Lauren's choices shifted energy in her favor. You'll notice that she had a strong will to live, for herself and for her daughter. She participated in integrative treatments, read uplifting material, grew spiritually, helped others, and always made decisions that felt intuitively right to her—even when these choices did not align with a physician's recommendations. All of these things helped her to vibrate at a high level, which she and I feel contributed to her healing. In Section II of this book, we will look at many of the energetic tools Lauren used in more detail.

Here's what I want you to take away right now: Your life, like Lauren's, is shaped by the thoughts and experiences you choose—and make no mistake, the decision is always yours. I promise, when you learn to be conscious and in control of what you are focusing on, you can begin to create high vibrational experiences, which will transform and heal your life.

CHAPTER 2

The High Cost of Low Vibrations

"When I was in that state of clarity ... [during her near-death experience] I instinctively understood that I was dying because of all my fears. I wasn't expressing my true self because my worries were preventing me from doing so. I understood that the cancer wasn't a punishment ... It was just my own energy, manifesting as cancer because my fears weren't allowing me to express myself as the magnificent force I was meant to be."

ANITA MOORJANI, IN *DYING TO BE ME*

In the scientific community, the study of the mind-body connection is called Psychoneuroimmunology. Yes, it's a big word. But its implications are pretty simple: What you think and feel has the ability to impact how your immune system functions, whether that happens in a healthy or unhealthy way. Many scientists and medical professionals believe this and so do I. And if you're facing cancer, I feel it's especially important for you to understand how your mental focus can have a very real effect on your body's processes.

As I explained in Chapter One, focusing on thoughts or images that make you feel good will enable you to be at a higher level energetically and, consequently, will draw to you a higher level of vibrational experience. In other words, positive thoughts will attract positive experiences. The reverse is also true. If you've fallen into the habit of negative obsessing and/or fear-based thinking, you need to know that you *can* shift to a healthier, happier mindset—and cancer might be just the impetus you need to make the change.

Low Vibrations and Cancer

Not surprisingly, a cancer diagnosis can cause you to vibrate at a very *low* level. You're filled with pain, grief, despair, resentment, and/or anger. As you look toward the future, you undoubtedly feel apprehension and fear. Anxiety and stress are never far away. It's normal to have thoughts like, *I'm afraid of what will happen. I'm afraid cancer might kill me. And if it doesn't, how will I ever get out from under all of these medical bills?*

You wouldn't be human if you didn't consider these possibilities. Nevertheless, all of these negative feelings weigh you down and can keep you from experiencing healing, as surely as stones might weigh you down if you were trying to swim. Let me explain.

The Science of Negativity

Candace Pert, PhD, was the author of *Molecules of Emotion: The Science Behind Mind-Body Medicine* and a molecular bioscientist, as well as former chief of brain biochemistry at the National Institute of Mental Health (NIMH). Pert was the first scientist to demonstrate that the brain secretes chemicals called peptides, neuropeptides, neurotransmitters, and hormones, and that these chemicals have the ability to mediate mood and emotions.

Furthermore, Pert's research shows that the surfaces of cells found in the brain and throughout the body (including the immune, endocrine, and nervous systems) contain molecules made of energetic particles. These particles vibrate in response to the information that they send and receive. In particular, the information they *receive* can actually change the makeup of the cell, causing mutations and metastasis.

Specifically, when you experience fear, stress, danger in your environment, or any other conditions that your body's wisdom determines to be negative, you vibrate at a lower energetic level, creating an imbalance of chemicals (if you're curious, they include various neuropeptides and neurotransmitters, as well as hormones like cortisol and adrenaline). This imbalance causes cancer cells to grow and multiply in number.

To put it less scientifically, Pert's research has shown that the "molecules of emotion" secreted by the brain are related to the development of cancer cells, which can circulate from their point of origin to different parts of the body. The mind-body connection between our emotions and the development of illnesses (such as cancer) is no longer in any doubt.

Given this information, it doesn't surprise me that many of my patients tended to dwell on their fears, regrets, and hardships long before being diagnosed with cancer. In addition to the illness-encouraging properties of negative emotions, low vibrational energy also disables the immune system, and like many other diseases, cancer finds it easier to flourish in an environment where it doesn't encounter much resistance. (Interestingly, cancer often emerges in cancer patients' caregivers, whose responsibilities tend to drain them of physical and emotional energy.)

Please don't misunderstand—I do not blame my patients for "causing" their cancer, nor do I think that your own diagnosis is "your fault." (One of the central tenets of my philosophy is that we are all doing the best we can, based on where we are on our individual spiritual journeys.) I'm simply pointing out that your body may not have been as effective in warding off this disease if its power was compromised by low vibrational energy in the past, and I want to make sure that you understand that your current attitude and outlook will have a measurable impact on how your cancer progresses.

Enough theory. I believe that this concept is best illustrated through real-life examples, and to that end, I'd like to share the story of one my patients with you. (Indeed, I will be sharing many stories illustrating the cost of negative emotions—and the healing power of high vibrations—throughout this book.)

Maya's Story: The Cost of Grief

For more than a year, Maya and her family lovingly cared for her mom who had been diagnosed with ovarian cancer. A strong and intelligent woman with an exceptional work ethic, Maya's mom, Annette, fought diligently and defiantly for her life. Yet over the months, she began to deteriorate. Annette's husband, daughters, and grandchildren stayed close, honoring her wishes about what to do with the assets she had worked so hard to gather over her lifetime. Annette eventually lost her challenge with cancer, leaving her family deeply grieving—and responsible for their father!

Within a year of Annette's death, Maya came to me. She had been recently diagnosed with lung cancer and wanted to do all she could to meet the demands of this challenge. She also hoped to experience emotional, mental, and spiritual healing. She was weary from such an extended period of anticipatory grief for and subsequent mourning of her mom. She experienced many of the feelings that accompany the loss of a loved one, including guilt (because she could have done more), frustration (because she had not done enough) and anger (at herself and the situation). Maya was also aware of the fatigue her lung cancer was taking on her body, and how it was impacting her work and her roles as a mom, daughter, sister, wife, and professional.

Since her mother's death, Maya had been worried about her father. She knew he felt lost, and that she and her sister needed to continue to care for him because he had been totally dependent on their mom for just about everything—including managing their assets and running the family's home. Maya felt especially anxious about taking on the responsibility of managing her father's finances.

Maya knew she was doing all she energetically could to work, care for her family, and fight her cancer. She often shared with me her thoughts and feelings about what the future might hold for both her husband and her daughter. *How would they manage without me?* she would wonder. These worries and concerns added to the low vibrations Maya experienced while she was grieving her mom. None of them supported a healthy immune system, which she needed for healing. While Maya knew this, it was nevertheless difficult for her to not focus on her concerns.

Little by little, Maya began to experience a greater sense of peace as we worked on issues related to grieving her mother and her identity as her mom's daughter and caretaker. She also addressed and processed her need to forgive herself for not adhering to her mom's extremely demanding work ethic, which had worked for her mom but not for Maya.

Additionally, Maya engaged in learning energy techniques that enabled her to replenish her strength, energy, and motivation. In particular, Maya worked with an energy practitioner who helped her to better deal with the effects of her chemotherapy treatments. This practitioner would also assess any imbalanced energy Maya might have and then replenish her energy by correcting whatever was out of balance.

Maya shared with me that she left her energy sessions feeling more calm and relaxed. In fact, she often had unexpected energy to make dinner for her family and even attend school functions for her children after work. Though she was not well, she enjoyed doing things for her daughter and husband (such as vacuuming, cooking a meal, or doing the laundry) because they enabled her to feel that she had improved her quality of life.

As the months passed, Maya began noticing a greater lack of energy, an increased need to sleep, and intense pain spreading throughout her body. Despite traditional and integrative treatments, Maya's illness seemed to move more quickly than anticipated. I believe that this was partially due to the extended period in which Maya had been grieving—for her mom and then, in time, for herself. She knew she was dying (which, in itself, is often a powerful lower vibration), and she was able to prepare herself and her family.

What is important to note here is that while she had not experienced physical healing, Maya *had* experienced spiritual healing. When I visited with her in the hospital, I felt her peace. I will always keep Maya in my heart, partly because of the dignity she brought to the dying process and partly because of the dignity with which she lived her life. She was and is a beautiful soul.

Choose to Shift Up.

Here's the good news: Your health, your experiences, and your life do not have to be at the mercy of your negative emotions. When you consciously choose to focus on a thought or belief that is positive, comforting, or hopeful, you're clearing out that emotional clutter that's weighing you down. You're energetically shifting yourself to a better place.

When you shift the energy of your thoughts up, you can literally fight your cancer by prompting your immune system to produce those cells needed for healing cancer, such as T-cells, natural killer cells, and macrophage cells. If you would like to tap into the power of the mind-body connection, all you have to do is find something, whether it's a story, a thought, a memory, or a hope, that fills you with joy, excitement, and passion—all of which are high vibratory experiences. This will unlock your brain's production of healing chemicals, including feel-good endorphins and immune system-boosting hormones like DHEA.

Section II of this book provides a wealth of ways to make this shift. For now, I urge you to start being more conscious of what you are feeling and thinking. Notice how often you experience negative and low-vibratory emotions and thoughts as well as what triggers them. In some cases, patterns of negative thinking may be the result of bad "thought habits" you've developed over the years. (By that I mean you generally like your life but need to do a bit of mental spring cleaning.) In other cases, they may indicate a life that's seriously out of balance—a subject we'll explore in the next chapter.

CHAPTER 3

A Life That Isn't Working

"There are only two kinds of people in the world: those who are alive and those who are afraid."

RACHEL NAOMI REMEN, MD

As we've just discussed, your thoughts and focus have an impact on your health; one that you may not have known about or considered before. But while your mental processes *are* significant, they aren't the only thing that influences the way your body functions.

In this chapter, I want to review some *non*-psychological lifestyle factors that can lead to a lack of physical balance and make it easier for cancer to exist. Much of what we'll cover probably won't be "news" to you. In fact, you've probably heard most of it before. But bear with me. If you want to heal, you first have to be honest about your life, and what *isn't* working in your favor.

As you read, try to identify habits and choices that may be compromising your health. Then, I urge you to commit to changing them. (You'll find concrete tactics to help you do just that in Section Two of this book.)

A Lost Sense of Balance

Well-being is all about balance. Unfortunately, the "normal" modern lifestyle (which actually isn't "normal" at all) often pushes us away from what's healthy and manageable, and prompts us to make decisions that overload our bodies and minds. As a society, we are just too busy, too stressed, too consumed with so-called "success," too worried about our looks and our image, and *not* plugged in at all to our spiritual and emotional roots.

On an individual level, the lack of balance I've just described can weaken your immune system while depriving you of the physical and mental nourishment you need to remain healthy. Here, I'll point out some of the specific ways in which your life may be out of balance. While Section Two will include much more detail on how you can heal your life, I'll also share a few thoughts here on how balance can be restored in each area:

- **Your diet consists of too many unhealthful foods.** As a society, we eat too many processed foods devoid of nutrients. Yes, fast food drive-thrus and frozen prepared meals are convenient. Salty chips and sweet candy bars give us a few moments of pleasure while helping us to manage stress. And sugary caffeinated beverages provide the pick-me-up we need to keep working just a little longer. But overall, these foods and drinks leave us feeling sluggish, make us overweight, and contribute to numerous health problems, including high blood pressure and heart disease … and yes, maybe even cancer.

  We need to choose more fresh, natural foods like vegetables, fruits, whole grains, fish, and lean meats in moderation—all organic, when possible. These are foods our bodies crave and deserve.

  Specifically, try to adhere to an alkaline diet (which is high in fruits, vegetables, nuts, and legumes) rather than an acidic diet (which is heavier on meat, eggs, dairy, grains, and processed foods). That's because cancer has more difficulty surviving in an alkaline diet! (You can learn more about alkaline diets and find numerous recipes with a simple online search.)

  No, it's not easy to bypass the easy, plentiful foods and choose the more labor intensive (and often more expensive) ones. Yet, eating more healthfully, at least part of the time, is doable. Most of us *could* make better choices with advanced meal planning, better budgeting, more careful shopping, and a willingness to exercise reasonable portion control. We simply need to honor ourselves enough to do so.

- **You live a sedentary life.** Many of us have good intentions regarding exercise. But when push comes to shove, we elect to stay in bed instead of getting up early, or we collapse on the couch after work instead of changing into gym clothes. Our routines are so engrained that the mere thought of reordering them to include regular walks, bike rides, or fitness classes is overwhelming. As a result, our bodies lack conditioning and strength, and we miss out on an important outlet for stress, anxiety, frustration, and other low-vibration emotions.

It may not be effortless, but you *can* fold exercise into your life. You don't have to become a marathon runner overnight (and no one is expecting you to!). Simply walking outside for 30 minutes every other day can make a world of difference in your physical health, plus it gets you outside in nature, helps you connect with neighbors, and gives your mind valuable time to recharge while your body is working hard—all of which raise your vibrational energy.

- **You don't allow yourself any quiet time.** We live in a world that's full of noise, distractions, and stimulation. Any time we have a free minute (which, as we rush from place to place, doesn't happen often), we flip on the television, check email, shoot off a text, or scroll through the latest social media news. Our inner voices are totally drowned out, and as a result, we rarely (if ever) stop to examine how fulfilled and happy we are, what is and isn't working in our lives, and which direction our intuition is pointing.

You don't have to live a monastic lifestyle to experience regular quiet time and reap its centering, clarifying benefits. Take a hot bath to relax your body, for example, and allow your mind to relax too. Or set aside ten minutes to pray or meditate at the beginning and end of each day. Drive to work or to the store *without* turning on the radio. When you allow your thoughts to speak to you without having to compete with outside distractions, you will feel more at peace and will be better equipped to make healthy decisions.

- **Your primary relationships are unhappy ones.** For many of us, dysfunction rules the day when it comes to our relationships. We are living in marriages that aren't working. We struggle to improve unhappy parent-child relationships. Instead of affirmation and support, we get competition and criticism from our so-called friends. All of these dynamics (and many more) drain us of positive energy while harming our self-worth and miring us in unfulfilling social ruts that don't allow us to grow.

   Many people never take action to heal unhealthy relationships because they take these dysfunctional dynamics for granted. Don't compromise your health and happiness by telling yourself that things can never change, and the best you can do is to simply endure. For the sake of your body, your mind, and your spirit, you *can* and *should* take action. That might mean working with a counselor, backing away from toxic individuals who refuse to change, or simply admitting that your own behaviors need to change. Sometimes it may mean ending a marriage. None of this is easy. It *is* worthwhile.

- **You have no social network.** As life goes on, responsibilities and obligations tend to mount. Many of us get so wrapped up in the needs of family, home, and career that we drift away from and lose touch with friends. (This happens to women, who are natural caregivers, in particular.) While we tell ourselves that we don't "need" active social lives, the truth is that we become isolated without them. We also deprive ourselves of an important outlet for stress relief, rejuvenation, and self-actualization when we don't spend time with friends.

   It's important to cultivate friendships. Whether you are an extrovert or an introvert, as a human you are a social being. For the sake of your mental and emotional health, it's important to be honest about and honor your need for meaningful connections. Don't forget that having a companion to laugh with and a caring shoulder to lean on are much more important than keeping a spotless house or spearheading every PTA campaign, for instance. Make social time a priority when scheduling your life.

- **You've lost touch with your Source.** While religion is not a part of my counseling, spirituality most definitely is. No matter what my patients believe or which (if any) religious tradition those beliefs fit into, I have noticed that many of them are disconnected from Divine Energy. Like my patients, many people make their way through life acting as though they are "alone." They never progress beyond the lower realms of vibrational energy—and thus experience more discord, fear, stress, and ill health—because they don't allow intuition, higher wisdom, and unconditional (Divine) love to enter into their lives and guide their decisions.

  The truth is, we are all connected to the universe in meaningful ways. We all have the power to tap into Divine Energy, whether we call it God, Buddha, Nature, Mind, Mother, or something else. Connecting with our Source takes practice, but it's something we are all capable of— and something that is necessary in order to maintain holistic health. You can take the first steps toward your Source simply by finding a place of worship that works for you (be it a church, synagogue, mosque, or Mother Nature), by meditating or praying, or by focusing on high-vibration emotions like love and gratitude.

- **There's no fun in your life.** As I've stated before, it's all too easy to allow work, responsibilities, and "have-to" tasks (as opposed to "want-to" tasks) to dominate your life. As a result, many of us simply survive each day instead of enjoying the time we've been given. This sends the Universe the message that we don't *want* to thrive, and that we don't believe we deserve enjoyable experiences. Though it may not be our intention, a low-fun lifestyle attracts more burdens and negative experiences into our orbit.

Give yourself permission to stop existing and start growing. We all need more than work for self-actualization. Remember that interests and hobbies aren't frivolous; they're necessary for fulfillment and health. If you find it difficult to "unclench," start by simply watching a funny movie, relaxing in a bubble bath, playing with your pet, or drinking a glass of wine.

- **You're disconnected from Nature.** Many people don't see anything wrong with living their lives within human-made and human-controlled enclaves. In fact, many of us are only outside for the time it takes to get in and out of our cars, or to take out the garbage. This breeds a lack of respect for the Earth that supports us, causes us to think and operate *only* within manmade limits, dulls our senses and instincts, and has a documented ill effect on health. (For instance, hospital patients heal more quickly when they have a view of nature from their windows!)

  Fortunately, it's not difficult to make time for walks outside, to look out the window instead of at a television screen, to plant flowers, and to pursue activities with others that take us out into Nature's wonderful world.

It All Comes from a Lack of Self-Love.

The balance-damaging circumstances I have discussed so far are common—and in most cases, correctable. What I mean is, most of us *can* control what we eat, how we spend our free time, and to some extent, even how much of it we have in the first place.

We can make positive changes and re-order our priorities without totally upending our lives. We simply choose not to make decisions that work toward our well-being. Why is that? The answer is simple: We don't love ourselves enough to make healthy choices.

Unfortunately, a lack of self-love has even forced some of us into situations so unsustainable that correcting the balance really would mean reordering the fundamentals, and in some areas, starting from scratch.

Think about it: When you read my words about "choice," do you believe that they don't apply to you? Are you working 12-hour days, feeling constantly exhausted, overwhelmed, and trapped? Are you driving yourself into the ground just to keep your head above water? Do you feel only fear and anxiety when you look to the future? Even before your cancer diagnosis, were you burdened by a lack of energy and consistent health problems? If so, you haven't loved and respected yourself enough to craft a life that works.

Ask yourself how your life got to this point. Did you buy a too-big house? Did you feel that you *needed* a newer, more stylish car? Are you in career that stifles and stresses you? Have you put yourself in serious debt so that you can send your kids to the "right" schools? Did you marry someone who "looked good on paper" rather than someone who inspires genuine love, compassion, and laughter? Do you feel that in order to be "worthy," you must present a false face to the world?

If you answered "yes" to these questions, you're not alone. While I am, of course, not familiar with the details of your unique situation, I *can* confirm that many of my patients (and probably you, too) have bought into society's claims that our lives need to look a certain way; that "success" can only be defined by a specific, narrow set of criteria.

As a result of these beliefs, we willfully deny ourselves love. We focus on accumulating "stuff" (i.e., status symbols ranging from homes to cars to clothes to gadgets) while forcing ourselves to perform jobs we hate and that take up all of our time. And because we're disconnected from our Source and surrounded by low-vibrational energy, we lack confidence, are fearful of the future, and experience less-than-optimal health. This is exactly the sort of environment in which cancer, and many other diseases, thrive.

Fortunately, there is no reason why you can't downsize, simplify, reinvent yourself. (Yes, that's possible *and* advisable even at this stage of your life, as you're facing cancer.) Bricklayers, groundskeepers and store clerks can be as fulfilled and happy as physicians, stockbrokers and attorneys—and often, they're far more so.

Life should not be an endurance event. No prestigious job, well-appointed house, or luxury vacation is worth your emotional, mental and, yes, physical health. In fact, the abrupt loss of all of these things through a cancer diagnosis can be the wake-up call that forces you to identify and begin correcting the things that aren't working in your life.

As you continue reading this book, you will learn multiple ways to take advantage of all of the gifts (yes, that's right: gifts!) that cancer can give you. You will also read the stories of individuals who used their cancer diagnoses as the catalyst to finally build fulfilling, nourishing, and health-affirming lives.

For now, here is what I want you to understand: In order to create a balanced life that excites you and that allows enough time for healthy habits to flourish, you *must* love yourself. Even then, it probably won't be realistic to make one big, drastic sweeping change—*especially* since overcoming cancer will necessarily be occupying much of your energy. That's fine; "baby steps" are a lot better than nothing. As long as you're working toward a better life you're on the right path.

The Art of Letting Go

Understandably, you may be thinking right now that while you "get" the importance of being able to love yourself unconditionally, this is easier said than done. And while you "get" that it isn't good for you to beat yourself up with self-criticism, self-judgment, and worries about what others will think about you (all low vibrational experiences), you just can't help yourself because you have been thinking this way all your life and do not know how to release this way of being, existing and thinking.

Many times, I have found (and still continue to find) myself exactly where you are. That's why, to close this chapter, I'd like to share a poem that one of my oldest, dearest friends sent me. It validates everything that you and I struggle with, but nevertheless demonstrates that it's up to us to let go of all the habitual mental thoughts and criticisms that do not feel loving, kind and compassionate to us.

If it feels right to you, consider making a copy or two of this poem. Post the poem where it will motivate and remind you of your power to release whatever it is that is no longer serving you.

"She Let Go"

by Ernest Holmes

Without a thought or a word, she let go.
She let go of fear. She let go of judgments.
She let go of the confluence of opinions swarming around her head.
She let go of the committee of indecision within her.
She let go of all the 'right' reasons.
Wholly and completely, without hesitation or worry,
She just let go.

She didn't ask anyone for advice.
She didn't read a book on how to let go.
She just let go.
She just let go of all the memories that held her back. She let go
of all the anxiety that kept her from moving forward.
She let go of the planning and all the calculations about
how to do it just right.
She didn't promise to let go. She didn't journal about it.
She didn't write the projected date in her Day-Timer.
She made no public announcement.
She didn't check the weather report or read her daily horoscope.
She just let go.
She didn't analyze whether she should let go.
She didn't call her friends to discuss the matter.
She didn't utter one word.
She just let go.
No one was around when it happened. There was no applause or
congratulations.
No one thanked her or praised her. No one noticed a thing.
Like a leaf falling from a tree, she just let go.
There was no effort. There was no struggle.
It wasn't good. It wasn't bad.
It was what it was, and it is just that.
In the space of letting go, she let it all be. A small smile came over
her face.
A light breeze blew through her.
And the sun and the moon shone forevermore.

*"Love is not something we give or get; it is something that we nurture
and grow, a connection that can only be cultivated between two people
when it exists within each one of them—we can only love others as
much as we love ourselves."*

BRENÉ BROWN, PHD, IN *THE GIFTS OF IMPERFECTION*

PART TWO

CHAPTER 4

Guiding Principles for Your Cancer Journey

"Thoughts, the mind's energy, directly influences how the physical brain controls the body's physiology … Buried in exceptional cases (in medicine) are the roots of a more powerful understanding of the nature of life … The fact is that harnessing the power of your mind can be more effective than the drugs you have been programmed to believe you need."

BRUCE LIPTON, PhD, IN *THE BIOLOGY OF BELIEF*

One of the gifts of having lived a good number of years is the wisdom you manage to collect over time. Regardless of your age, I'm sure that you have learned lessons simply by engaging with life itself, rather than from books you have read and classes you have taken. This type of acquired wisdom provides you with a grounding of truth on which you can safely base the difficult and not-so-difficult choices you need to make in your life.

The same is true of your cancer journey specifically. You can, and should, learn as much as possible about what you're facing from your doctors, from books, and from any other resources you may have. But there are some things about cancer that *only* those who experience it understand. I have gathered thirteen of those cancer-related truths—which I call guiding principles—here. (Some I learned during my own cancer journey; others from my patients; still others I acquired both ways.)

I encourage you to read through these guiding principles and embrace them as truths passed down from those who have walked a similar path. Many of them, I think, will provide you solace, peace, healing, understanding, and direction. (And that being the case, we'll look at a number of these guiding principles in greater depth throughout this book.)

Keep in mind, though, that each person's journey is different. If something—anything—does not feel right to you, then you alone get to decide whether you will honor it or not. The choice of how to respond to your situation is yours—and will always be yours!

1. **Guiding Principle: Healing Is about Wholeness and Harmony.**

   I define healing as anything that contributes to you feeling greater balance, harmony, wholeness, and well-being. In other words, you experience healing when you feel good, relatively in control of your circumstances, and peaceful.

Here's another way to look at it: Healing is what you need any time you feel that you are out of balance—be it tired, stressed, fearful, or worried—or when you sense a disconnection between your mind, body, and spirit. Boiled down to its simplest state, "healing" is anything that restores your inner sense that all is well, and that returns you to a healthy state of empowerment.

2. **Guiding Principle: There Are Different Aspects of Healing.**

It's important to understand that healing is not simply about *physical* healing, although as a cancer patient, that will be a large part of your focus. Healing can and must be applied to your mind and your soul if you are to achieve wholeness and balance, tap into your own resources and gifts, and fully live your hopes and dreams. In fact, you can have a healing experience without experiencing physical healing at all.

Given that healing is about the restoration of balance, harmony, and wholeness, by resolving what has caused you emotional, mental, and spiritual pain, and by connecting with your Higher Power, you are relieved in many ways, allowing you to vibrate energetically at a higher level.

3. **Guiding Principle: You Can Choose Your Own Healing Medicine.**

We are privileged to live in the 21st century—privileged because we have access to some of the finest and most advanced technological advances in the history of medicine. But that doesn't mean that those of us in the West should discount traditional therapeutic medicines and the ancient wisdom of various cultures around the world.

While modern Western medicine can do great things, it isn't perfect. For instance, my own patients are often frustrated because they need to take medicine for the problems created by their previous medications. As you encounter frustrations of your own, remember that you get to choose the kind of medicine you wish to experience, as well as the doctors and kinds of medical establishments that will provide you with your treatment. That list might include the integrated methods and techniques of Eastern medicine, such as energy medicine, acupuncture, Reiki, Therapeutic Touch, and more. It might also include the world of Native American Medicine and other tribal cultures. Personally, I have chosen to practice integrative psychology because this allows me the freedom to integrate the best tools and wisdom from Eastern and Western medicine and psychology.

The guiding principle here is that you are born with your own resources, including your intuition. If you can come to recognize yourself as a being who is not separate from but very much connected to your Source (whoever and whatever that may be), your sense of confidence will grow, along with the trust that you are being intuitively guided to receive what is needed for healing. You can, and should, use your own wisdom and knowledge to listen to the needs of your body so that you can make the best use of both traditional and integrative medicine. The same holds true for your choice of foods, thoughts, and lifestyle. Each is a piece of your healing equation.

4. **Guiding Principle: It's All about Energy.**

We've already covered the basic "hows" and "whys" of vibrational energy, but it's worth repeating here: When you think about whatever is disturbing or distressing you, you vibrate at very low levels. On the other hand, when you think about what is positive, kind, and compassionate, as well as what you appreciate and are grateful for, then you vibrate at a very healthy, high level. And when you choose thoughts that feel good to you, your brain responds by producing chemicals that enhance your immune's system ability to keep you healthy. Fear is an especially low vibrational form of energy.

It is natural to feel fear at the time of diagnosis, but if you stay focused on your fears (especially the fear of not getting well and of the possibility of dying), you are making it difficult for your body to enlist its resources to enable healing to occur. You have the power to feel good—or not—just by being conscious of what you choose to think. Choose to focus on hope and healing.

5. **Guiding Principle: Being Love Is the Key.**

When you think about your most precious memories, how many of them feature feelings of great love, be it for your puppy, kitten, child, friend, parent, grandparent, or even (especially!) yourself? Chances are, the majority do. That's because experiencing unconditional love enables us to experience joy, which is one of our highest purposes in life.

Being love is a state of being ... It is a state in which you exist as the vibration of love—every thought, action, intention and feeling stems from and is unconditional love. Those who have had NDEs (near-death experiences) have described being on the receiving end of such love—which takes place when in the presence of the Light. Such love, they report, is something they have never before felt. This love has the power to change or transform you as it has for those with NDEs. They return feeling great love and compassion for family members, society, and strangers. Their love touches everyone with whom they come into contact.

While there are many kinds of love, it is the choice to be love—meaning that you choose to be in a state of loving energy which you direct toward yourself in the most compassionate, unconditionally accepting manner possible—that most acutely influences the quality of your journey through life. Being love allows you to accept yourself unconditionally, and enables you to love and accept others unconditionally—and receive their love in return.

Bear in mind, too, that self-love often involves being courageous enough to choose and do what is right for you—even if it means failing to please someone else. (Remember, illness often occurs when you excessively put another's needs, wants, and energy before your own. Illness also manifests when you become a victim of measuring yourself against others or their belief systems, causing yourself to feel that you are either not measuring up or are doing "the wrong thing.") When you choose self-love, though, you are reclaiming your awareness of your own power, which raises your vibrational energy and contributes to your healing!

6. **Guiding Principle: There Will Always Be Things You Can't Change. (And, That's Okay.)**

Like it or not, there are aspects of life over which you have no control: the weather, politics, aging, birth and death, pain that accompanies illness and trauma, or the painful, unfair, and unkind thoughts and actions of others, to name just a few. Your task is to accept that life can't be controlled, and to recognize that your happiness is totally dependent on how you choose to respond to this truth. In other words, your happiness—and your healing—are a function of how you choose to respond on the inside to that which is taking place on the outside.

It is when you stop resisting and choose an attitude of acceptance and positivity that you are able to shift your energetic experience to a higher plane and thereby attract and allow in experiences that are more in alignment with your hopes and dreams. Yes, it may seem paradoxical, but you really do experience greater happiness when you choose to stop trying to control everything. And on a spiritual level, you evolve by learning the power of surrender and of love.

7. **Guiding Principle: You Can Choose to Live Consciously.**

You are always breathing, thinking, feeling, responding, and communicating. But how often do you take the time to notice what you are feeling and thinking before you speak and act? If you practice the art of becoming aware of how you are feeling from moment to moment, you can learn to tweak the thoughts that cause you pain. This allows you to modify your actions and reactions in order to experience less hurt—and more healing—as you shift energetically upward.

Here's a tool to apply when something is said or done that feels upsetting: Look at the individual you are with (your boss, a friend, a family member) and, before responding, consider how you would feel if the other person were not in your life. Let yourself experience the love or genuine caring you have for this person. Then, consciously choose to fill your heart with compassion and formulate a more loving and kinder response than the one that immediately flew to mind. In addition to preserving and improving the relationship, you will feel better about yourself.

One more thing to consider: The problems presented by difficult individuals contribute to your growth and evolution—another reason for filling yourself with gratitude, appreciation, and love! By choosing the following perspective, you expedite your own healing: The people in your life who have caused you the greatest resistance (or problems) are those who have enabled you to make the choices responsible for you becoming the person you are right now. I have always thanked those against whom

I have had to push because without them, I would not be who I am today. Today, I send those people my love and my gratitude.

8. **Guiding Principle: Three of Your Most Powerful Gifts Are Breath, Imagination, and Intuition.**

Many years ago, it became apparent to me that you and I are born with three precious gifts—gifts that when acknowledged and harnessed, allow us to experience more joy, increased peace, and real healing. These gifts are your breath, your imagination, and your intuition.

If you need proof that these are powerful resources, consider the following: How many times have you taken huge sighs to release your tension? How often do you escape the stress of the moment by choosing to lose yourself in a daydream or two? Have you ever known who was at the front door or calling on the phone before you answered either one?

When you learn to live your life by consciously breathing, imagining what you need for your health, and intuitively responding to the needs of your body's wisdom, you experience what you need for healing!

There is much to say about these gifts and they will be further described and explained throughout this book.

9. **Guiding Principle: Like Energy Attracts and Allows Like Energy.**

"In a universe where 'like goes to like' and 'birds of a feather fly together,' we attract to us that which we emanate."

DAVID R. HAWKINS, MD, PHD

Remember that since you are vibrational energy and everything, including your thoughts, is energy, *your thoughts determine your level of energy—and how well you are!* In order for your immune system to work at its best, your goal should be to always be in what I call "a feel good place."

When you focus on things that are negative and upsetting, you probably won't experience much improvement in how you feel, or in the events that take place in your life. That's because the experiences you attract and allow to come to you match the level at which you vibrate. So, as often as possible, focus on thoughts that feel good when you put your hand on your heart. Experiencing a sense of unconditional love, well-being, or peacefulness at the level of your heart helps you to attract and allow to come your way like-energy situations and people. (In this instance, you will be attracting and allowing to come your way wonderful, peaceful energy.) I use the words *allow to come your way* because you are responsible for your own experience; in other words, you allow your world to be created via the choices you make in your thoughts, feelings, and actions.

"Like energy attracts and allows like energy" is simply a statement about how energy works. When you honor it, you have the power to enhance the quality of your life and your health.

To see how quickly attraction works, close your eyes and think of someone you dearly love. Put your hand on your heart, and notice you good you feel. Now, think of someone who has been problematic for you, causing you distress. Put your hand on your heart again, and notice the difference. Where you place your mental focus determines whether or not your brain produces life-enhancing chemicals that enable your immune system to keep you healthy. Like energy attracts and allows like energy, both internally and externally.

10. Guiding Principle: It's Crucial to Live in Alignment with Your Values.

By now, you have a sense of the healing power of the energy of love—and of your thoughts. If you choose to make the most of these tools, you need to be clear about what your values are as you journey through this lifetime. Your values define you and provide you with a measuring stick of whether or not you are living in a state of grace, being true to who you really are, and what you are really about. They are a significant part of the foundation of your purpose ... even if you do not know just yet what your purpose is.

I am willing to bet that you know your values but have not actually verbalized them or written them down, thereby concretizing them. Just stop for a moment, grab either your journal or a notepad and, at the top, write, "What I Value Most in This Lifetime." You'll want to consider the non-tangibles, like honesty, loyalty, compassion, kindness, wisdom, presence, consideration, and practicality. Knowing—and living in alignment with—these core values enables you to vibrationally and energetically produce the chemicals needed for health and healing.

11. Guiding Principle: Yes, You Can Shift the Gears of Perspective.

The lovely thing about being a soul in a physical body is that you get to choose how you are going to think, perceive, or look at a situation. You can choose to see it positively by focusing on good aspects of the person or event, or you can focus on the negative qualities. Choosing positive aspects helps you feel better (and vibrate at a higher level), while focusing on the negative causes you to feel more poorly).

One of the most valuable and healing perspectives to adopt is that everything in life is a teacher for you, and that the lessons you learn have the power to enable physical and spiritual healing. Whether or not you are genetically predisposed to developing cancer, this disease still speaks to you about being energetically out of balance on a variety of levels. If you look at cancer as a plea from your body to take better care of it, you'll become more aware of better choices you can make regarding your thoughts, actions, lifestyle, and so much more. Choosing this perspective enables energy to begin rebalancing your body and spirit, which in turn, begins the healing process.

Ultimately, perspective is an individual matter. The way you see a situation may be the antithesis of the way someone near and dear to you sees the same thing. That's okay. The bottom line is that a positive perspective, no matter how personal it may be, will expedite healing within your body.

12. Guiding Principle: You Grow and Change with Each Moment.

The way you think and feel at this moment is different from the way you thought and felt a moment ago, and is also different from how you will think and feel a moment from now. That's a great thing for you and your healing potential, because it means that you are in a perpetual state of development. Your cells are repetitively dying and being reborn, and often expanding in the nature of their function. In other words, what your cells "understand" and the manner in which they respond to a problematic situation now is very different than might have been the case several years ago.

Being in a constant state of developmental flux enables you to evolve, change, and grow on all levels—emotionally, mentally, physically, and spiritually. This type of personal evolution doesn't mean that you will outgrow pain, loss, and grief—but it *does* mean that you can learn to process them at a more advanced, vibrationally higher level of development.

Practically every one of the patients with whom I have been honored to work over nearly thirty years has experienced an awareness of personal growth. This change began the moment they first learned of their loss, whether it was health or a loved one. My patients' identities and consciousness continued to evolve, enabling them to recognize that they are more than simply human beings having a spiritual experience—they are, in fact, spiritual beings. This has contributed to a heightened sense of trusting their own intuitive wisdom, as well as empowering them and helping them to realize that they are not alone. My hope is that you will experience the same type of growth.

13. Guiding Principle: Even Grief Needs to Be Balanced.

You have most likely encountered your share of significant losses—most recently, the loss of your health (not to mention the loss of your peace of mind and sense of security). The problem is that grief and loss can be so overwhelmingly painful that it's tough to think about anything except what you have lost and how difficult it is to go on living. As a result, your vibrational energy is low, and you attract similarly negative experiences into your life. That's why it's so important to intentionally choose something to focus on that makes you feel joyful and peaceful.

To balance grief, I suggest thinking about something that makes you laugh or smile, and allows your heart to sing: a special person, memory, event, joke, uplifting movie, dream, funny story, etc. You can also exercise, which releases the endorphins and hormones that your body needs in order to function at an optimal level. And, as I'll explain later in this book energy medicine (e.g., Reiki, qigong, tai chi, acupuncture and other similar energetic methods) allows you to balance and repair blocked and imbalanced patterns of energy that have been caused by your grief, thus enabling your body to better care for you. Finally, you can engage in something about which you are extremely passionate (enabling you to vibrate highly) so that, again, your brain produces needed chemicals to energetically balance your grief.

14. **Guiding Principle: Consciously Tap into the Will to Live.**

I have a 15 × 12 inch metal plaque that I look at every morning because I want it to set the tone for my day and for my life. The plaque has the following quote by Coach Vince Lombardi: "*The difference between a successful person and others is not a lack of strength, not a lack of knowledge, but rather a lack of will.*"

That is especially true when it comes to meeting your cancer challenge. If healing is to occur, you *must* have the will to live. Yes, having hope and cultivating high-level vibrations is important, but these things do no replace wanting, deep down in your soul, to live. Verbalize this wish to yourself, to your loved ones, to your doctors, and to anyone else supporting you on our journey. The will to live is energetically known to the body. Your cells know what is in your heart; they know when you wish for something and when you don't. Your life force can be strengthened or weakened by your inner desires.

In my practice, I have seen time and time again just how important the will to live is. I have known an amazing number of patients who have experienced physical healing despite a prognosis that suggested otherwise. And yes, I have had a few patients who shared that they did not want to pursue treatment (usually, against the wishes of their families). They did not live. Remember, the choice—and the will—must be yours.

Guiding Principles Sustain Mary Ellen.

To conclude this chapter, I would like to share the story of Mary Ellen. As you'll read, many of the guiding principles I have shared in this chapter helped Mary Ellen navigate her cancer journey.

Mary Ellen had survived the breakup of her 18-year marriage in 1996 and the loss of her mother in January 2000. A single mom with three children, she was working in her first year of teaching gifted second graders in Pennsylvania.

In early February of 2000, Mary Ellen noticed that her back pain was becoming much more severe and that she was losing weight. She was also dealing with an unusual rash on her body. Mary Ellen began consulting with doctors who provided diagnoses including shingles, anxiety, and muscular problems. The doctors wanted to provide medications, but Mary Ellen intuitively knew they were not what she needed. From October to February she went for numerous scans, but nothing was noted. Her pain continued to worsen.

Finally, a friend who was also a doctor advised Mary Ellen to go to a different hospital. He met her there and saw to it that she was given a CAT scan with dye, a test that hadn't been performed before. During the procedure, the doctor saw something suspicious in Mary Ellen's lung. She was told to come in for a biopsy of her lung, which resulted in a diagnosis of non-Hodgkin lymphoma.

Mary Ellen was stunned. She had never really considered the possibility that she was dealing with cancer. Fortunately, though, her doctor couched this news in soothing, reassuring language: "Don't worry, Mary Ellen. This is a treatable form of the disease." This doctor gave Mary Ellen the hope she needed at that moment. Interestingly, when Mary Ellen sought a second opinion, the findings were the same—but the news was presented in a completely different way. This medical team chose to accentuate the negative, removing the suggestion of much hope: "You have Stage 1V B

Cell non-Hodgkin lymphoma, with only a 50 percent chance of survival!"

Immediately aware of the difference in how the findings were presented to her, Mary Ellen listened to what her intuition was telling her and chose to focus on the positive, hopeful news of the first doctor. Remember, our beliefs have the power to affect our physiology and our biology. Mary Ellen knew that what she need-ed for her body to heal were positive, affirmative words of hope. Going into her treatment, Mary Ellen's attitude remained posi-tive. Her conviction that she intended to get better was demon-strated in the manner in which she arranged her life. For instance, worried about the possibility of losing her new teaching position, she quickly arranged to have her treatments on Fridays so that she would not have to take sick leave.

As in every one of the stories of survival that my patients and others have shared with me, the experience of cancer led to Mary Ellen receiving extraordinary, heartfelt, unexpected gifts of love from her community. In particular, her friends formed a group called "Angels for Mary Ellen." The name says it all. This group enabled Mary Ellen to survive on a day to day basis. They made dinner for her and her children, ensuring that a dinner was deliv-ered to her home each night of the week. They drove her to work, helped her with her lesson plans, and also prayed for her.

And thank goodness for humor, another important strategy Mary Ellen used to heal. Actually, Mary Ellen shared with me that she had thought of writing a book titled *A Thousand Reasons You Can Be Happy You Have Lymphoma*. Some of her reasons would have included the following: Kids get home cooked meals, and you don't have to blow dry your hair. Mary Ellen's humor saw her through the loss of her hair, eyebrows, and eyelashes which took place by the third treatment.

Mary Ellen's cancer journey also facilitated her spiritual growth. During her treatment, she wrote letters to the Virgin Mary. She told me that she felt she was speaking directly to Mary and, given that by her fourth chemo treatment she was in remission, she felt that she was being heard.

Furthermore, when she prayed to Mary, Mary Ellen received signs she interpreted as indications that she was would experience healing. Shortly after requesting such a sign, Mary Ellen noticed a cardinal flying directly in front of her car during her commute. The following day, also on the way to work, Mary Ellen experienced the same thing. And on the third day, she noticed a cardinal on her deck. Cardinals had never before been in her life, and their sudden consistent appearance, she believed, was Mary's way of giving Mary Ellen the sign she desperately needed that she was going to be okay. She felt unbelievably grateful for this gift. Even now, Mary Ellen stops, prays, and gives thanks to Mary each time a cardinal comes into her path. Cardinals have come to be representative of something special, extraordinary, and even sacred in her life.

On the very day she had learned that she was in remission Mary Ellen received a call from her school principal, informing her that she was to be given a teaching contract, which assured her of having a job. Mary Ellen was able to finish her treatments and rest over the summer, so that she could return to teaching the following fall, feeling replenished.

Mary Ellen continues to receive regular CAT scans. And although she has had several scares, she remains resilient, wise, and strong. Mary Ellen reached her five-year remission anniversary mark around the time of her 50th birthday, and treated herself to a brand new convertible. Cardinal red, of course!

I asked Mary Ellen if she would share the lessons she learned from her experience with cancer, and she graciously agreed. Here's her list:

- Never, ever give up.
- Ask for help.
- It is ok to have a messy house and not be perfect.

- Enjoy myself more and appreciate the small things.
- I live my life so that if it were my last day, it would be a great day.
- I appreciate my family and friends so much more.
- It made me realize what is NOT important. So, I do not complain or talk about people.
- I try not to have fear.
- I feel like I am a new person, stronger, though I have always had to be strong.
- Rather than asking why I got cancer, I ask, why not me?

In Conclusion

As you continue reading this book, you will see evidence of these guiding principles woven through the advice and additional stories I share. I hope that you'll revisit them from time to time as you read this book and throughout your journey. I believe they sum up everything you need to know to experience hope, healing and happiness even as you meet the challenge of this unwelcome visitor called cancer.

CHAPTER 5

Choose to See
Cancer as a Gift

*"The disease is the teacher. It's not a curse. It's not bad luck. We're
not victims. God hasn't singled us out for more pain than anyone else.
The disease is there to teach us something about ourselves that we need
to change."*

RENE CAISSE, RN AND AUTHOR

Perhaps the title of this chapter upsets you, or at the very least, baffles you. I understand. When you get the diagnosis of cancer the last thing you feel is gratitude. Fear, anger, confusion, and disbelief are probably more accurate. The truth is, it's impossible to be told that your body has been invaded by an aggressive disease—one with the potential to kill you—and *not* be viscerally and psychologically affected as you contemplate the loss of control, the treatments, the pain, and the decline that *might* be in your future. Those sorts of "what ifs" are the definition of scary.

But, as I've said before, you have a choice in how you view everything that happens to you. Once the initial shock wears off and you've had time to process your diagnosis, it's time to make your choice. You can lock into that fear and negativity and spiral into despair, *or* you can decide to view cancer as a gift (or at least a wake-up call) and let it be a catalyst for learning how to focus on what makes you feel good.

This mental shift may not happen overnight. You may have to make the choice again and again; the times you spend in gratitude and joy interspersed with times of sadness, anger, and despair. Life is a journey and sometimes there are detours. But I promise that you *can* come to see the positives in cancer. In fact, the meaning you choose to give your experience will powerfully influence your body's response to the cancer. When you view cancer as a challenge that will enhance the quality of your life in some way, you are choosing a response that stems from self-love, rather than from fear, which is self-destructive.

For example, many times I've seen a cancer diagnosis enhance my patients' sense of purpose and encourage them to focus more on the things and people they love and are passionate about. And yes, I have experienced this myself.

Cancer Opens Our Eyes.

Here's what often occurs: In the years before cancer "happens," we let the stream of life move us along. We go where it sends us; we deal with the problems and obstacles that it washes into our paths. We *don't* make much of an effort to chart our own course. And because we're so used to this state of affairs, we fail to notice that we've been swept into a dull, diminished existence, far from the destination we had once hoped to reach.

But then, we hear those words: "You have cancer." The time we've spent—and the time we might no longer have—on earth is suddenly thrown into harsh perspective. When seen against the backdrop of our own mortality, the choices, compromises, stress, and responsibilities that have dominated our lives suddenly don't seem "worth it." And guess what? They aren't.

When we understand that truth, we're finally free to take the wheel and steer our lives in the direction our intuition tells us they *should* be headed. In this way, cancer paradoxically enhances our quality of life and shifts us energetically to a place where health is supported and affirmed.

For some people, it's an amazing revelation that they don't *have* to worry, obsess, and live under constant pressure—there is another richer, healthier, and more joyful way to live, even while battling a disease like cancer. I know, because that very thing happened to me. I chose to view cancer as an experience that would enhance my life, and received many gifts as a result. Allow me to tell you about them.

My Cancer Journey—and the Gifts I Received

First and foremost, my own cancer journey gifted me with the ability to be here to write this book. If it had not been for my cancer, I would have died. Let me explain.

Nineteen years ago, I was diagnosed with breast cancer. I needed to undergo not only a lumpectomy, but also a surgery to have all of the nodes in my right arm removed. Additionally, I underwent several diagnostic scans of my entire body.

Both of my surgeries resulted in my blood pressure rising far above normal limits. My scans also revealed the possibility of a tumor called a pheochromocytoma on my adrenal gland, which was soon confirmed by my surgeon and my endocrinologist. I underwent a dangerous surgery, called an adrenalectomy, to remove the tumor.

Had my breast cancer not required those scans, the adrenal tumor might not have been found, and would probably have been fatal. So you see: I am here, able to tell my story, thanks to the gift of my cancer. It is largely due to these circumstances that my perspective on cancer is positive and filled with gratitude.

Additionally, cancer gave me other gifts, which I'd like to briefly share here:

- **Cancer gave me the gift of a wake-up call regarding my lifestyle ...** Meeting the challenge of cancer showed me that the pace I had been keeping was unsustainable, and that I needed to stop always putting others before myself. At the time, I had been working long hours five to six days a week. I strongly and intuitively felt that I was being given the opportunity to see my life from a higher vantage point, and that it was imperative that I value and love myself enough to take better care of my health. I knew I had to change the focus of my practice (which had been highly stressful and time consuming) to one that would allow me to reduce the number of days I worked each week, thus providing me with a better quality of life.
- **... the gift of loving support ...** Cancer also validated the strength of my friends' love for me. I felt so cared about, so loved, and so valued that these feelings became

powerful sources of healing for me. I will never forget the day I came home from the hospital and welcomed my dearest friends into my house. As I lay stretched out on our living room couch with everyone around me, my friends said, "Susan, you have to let us give back to you now. It is time for you to receive. You are always giving, and now it is your turn to let us give back to you." I will never forget those words, and I will always treasure the love I felt radiating from them.

- **... the gift of time with my mother ...** Until my diagnosis of cancer, I would never have considered the possibility of taking so much time off from work. But I was told that I would have to take at least six weeks off when I had my pheochromocytoma surgery. This was a gift from heaven because my mom, an angel in her own right, came to take care of me. I treasured those days, especially as we would sit out in our backyard, enjoying the beauty of the birds, nature, and the ability to connect with all that represented love for me—especially my mom. Mom died four weeks after I finished my radiation. My cancer enabled us to have so much more time together than we would have had otherwise. This was a beautiful gift that was due specifically to my cancer journey.

- **... the gift of time with myself ...** Following my radiation treatments, I often treated myself to an outdoor lunch on Palmer Square in Princeton. I still recall the luxurious feelings I had while I ate a leisurely lunch and enjoyed the weather, watching those who were passing by and knowing that my good feelings were assisting my immune system as it healed my body. I do not usually give myself time for such treats, but cancer made this possible, and I was extremely grateful.

- **... and the gifts of perspective and gratitude.** During my cancer journey, I developed the awareness that I had the resources and resiliency to come through a major health challenge—meaning that I could perhaps handle more challenges like this if necessary. I also came to realize that my situation was not as severe as that of others who were receiving treatment with me. I felt exceptional gratitude, knowing that I could have faced a much more difficult challenge. Now I could better connect with my cancer patients, having an inside view and perspective of their journeys. As a psychologist who specializes in helping those with cancer heal, having walked the walk enabled my patients to feel more comfortable sharing their stories and feelings with me.

So, yes, for me, cancer provided me with an abundance of good things. I do not fill with fear, anger, pain, or resentment when I think of my cancer challenge. I fill with heartfelt gratitude and a sense of having received numerous blessings. And I'm not alone.

Gifts for the GyniGirls Support Group

"We acquire the strength of that which we have overcome."
RALPH WALDO EMERSON

I am a member of a gynecological cancer support group, The GyniGirls, where I have often heard women speak of the surprise gifts that have come out of their challenges with cancer. You've read about some of the ways in which cancer gifted me, personally. Now I'd like to share how it has enhanced the lives these women, too.

- **Cancer gave the women of the GyniGirls the gift of "taking their power"** ... The majority of the women in GyniGirls have acknowledged that the group has enabled them to learn to "take their power." In other words, the group has empowered them to focus on what they have control of, rather than what they do not. They have learned to share their feelings with their family members and doctors if they do not completely agree with what is being recommended or ordered for them. They report that they are not as timid as they once were, and that they feel more confident about listening to their own intuitive guidance regarding their treatment, choice of doctors, lifestyle choices and relationships.

- **... the gift of clear priorities ...** Many of the women have frequently commented that facing the challenge of their illness has taught them to reprioritize what is really important to them. They now prioritize activities that enable them to spend time with their loved ones, including their family and good friends. Everything else begins to take a back seat.

- **... the gift of unexpected kindness ...** Their illness, these women tell you, has taught them who their true friends are. So often, they have shared disappointment that those whom they have known for years seemed to have abandoned them. They have also spoken of unexpected surprises and gifts coming from colleagues, neighbors, and friends who have showered them with expressions of concern and kindness. Life is interesting and full of surprises ... and cancer has a way of demonstrating this.

- **... the gift of spiritual growth ...** The women in our group have shared that cancer has enriched their spiritual growth—an especially valuable gift. Receiving the diagnosis of cancer traditionally fills you with fear; yet, over the months and years during which we have come together, members of our wonderful group have frequently spoken of the awareness that they are not alone.

Synchronicities have reassured them that life is filled with small miracles. They are more aware than ever that they are more than they had previously believed themselves to be. Their shared stories of synchronicities, miracles, angels, and signs received from the Universe and/or their loved ones have inspired all of us, and have helped to reinforce our sense of empowerment.

- **… and the gift of fellowship.** The GyniGirls group itself is a gift that is the result of having cancer—and each of us in the group is aware of this. We value the strength of our community, and its help in enabling us to meet our challenges. Every woman feels safe, not judged, unconditionally accepted, and loved—and consequently, every woman knows that there is nothing to fear when we come together. We have all been "there," to some extent, and have come to feel the power of love. We know we are blessed, and that if it were not for the cancer experience, this loving, supportive opportunity to help one another grow our souls would not be part of our lives.

A Rabbi Experiences Cancer's Gifts.

I would like to share one more story with you; this time, about a person of the cloth. As Andy's story demonstrates, even a rabbi can face a crisis of faith when confronted with cancer—and can receive numerous unexpected gifts as a result of journeying through treatment and recovery.

Life was going well for Rabbi Andrew (Andy) R. Sklarz. At 42, he was married to a wonderful woman, Susan, with whom he had two children: six-year-old Dani and baby Alex. But at his yearly physical in 2001, everything changed. An abnormality had showed up in Andy's bloodwork, and a few weeks later the truth was revealed: Andy had chronic myelogenous leukemia (CML).

Shortly after his diagnosis, Andy was referred to me. Admittedly, he came to our first session feeling that his life "was truly coming to an end and looking for a miracle." So began our joint healing journey—a journey of reclaiming his inherent power and well-being.

Our early sessions were truly difficult for Andy. When he first came to see me, he was extremely "resistant" and filled with anger at the unjustness and unfairness about his situation. Like so many, when first informed of a cancer diagnosis, Andy felt as though he was being punished and that he was being betrayed by God. (Yes, even rabbis are human and experience these normal feelings!)

But probably the greatest emotion Andy dealt with was fear—the fear of dying and not being able to see and share in the joys of his children growing into their potential, as well as the fear of not having opportunities to experience his own life's journey.

Throughout our time together, Andy and I used many of the healing tools I'm going to share with you in this book, including the power of intention and affirmation, the Law of Attraction, breathing techniques, meditation, the value of following his passion, integrative medicine, and more. And along the way, something amazing happened: Andy received a number of gifts that were directly tied to his experience with leukemia. Here is a summary of those gifts, as Andy described them to me:

- **Cancer gave Andy permission to really have fun.** Andy had always loved to laugh deeply and enjoyed just being silly at times; however, prior to his diagnosis he had felt that he had to hold back because others were somewhat disapproving. But one of the gifts of cancer is that it allows us to discover and honor who we really are. Andy realized that in fact, his laughter, joy, creativity, and silliness are part of what make him such a great rabbi who is dearly loved by many.

- **Cancer gave Andy new eyes.** Andy says that cancer brought him to—and then out of—a dark tunnel. In other words, being diagnosed with CML, and then finding his way back to health and well-being, has broadened and shifted his perspective. For example, rather than seeing life's "warts and blemishes" as defects, he has learned to view them as challenges and opportunities to learn valuable lessons. Best of all, Andy now looks at the future through the lens of hope; a perspective he admits eluded him before his diagnosis.

- **Cancer helped Andy learn the value of gratitude.** He now spends time being conscious of and giving heartfelt thanks for all his blessings. He is particularly grateful for CML because it has brought this rabbi closer to God. Rabbis are people, just like the rest of us (which is easy to forget!). They too, have their own challenges and dark nights of the soul.

- **Cancer sparked spiritual growth.** Leukemia has brought Andy face to face with his God, the one who lives within and without. Even his concept of life and death has been expanded to include more possibilities. In his own words, "I believe in—and I accept—possibilities now." Andy has shared with me that he now recognizes that each of us experiences what we need to experience in order to learn and to heal—*not* because we are being punished. Furthermore, Andy recognizes that part of his job is to assist others in finding and making a connection with their own higher wisdom, or soul. When he gives a powerful sermon, he always thanks God for helping him. Andy says, "I don't feel quite as alone," and acknowledges that his cancer journey has strengthened his faith.

- **Cancer taught him to be more compassionate and loving—to himself and others.** Andy admits that this is not always easy for him, but that he is working on it.

- **Cancer has helped Andy detach from the past and forgive others.** According to Andy, there are times when someone won't agree with your decisions or let go of their need to be "right." He says, "Then I have to say, 'Okay, that is their misfortune; that is their loss,' and then simply move on because you need to do what feels good for you."

- **Cancer gave Andy the power of choice.** For Andy, having cancer was the ultimate empowering experience. He recognizes that when faced with something dreadful (such as a leukemia diagnosis!), he has a choice: He can choose to focus on something over which he has no control, or on something that feels genuinely good and wonderful to him. Focusing on his faith (and in particular, his belief that God is with him) enables him to feel good and contributes to his healing.

- **Cancer helped Andy learn that healing encompasses the mind, body, and spirit.** Andy is gradually learning that his healing is not a function of his medication alone, but also of his own innate power, and of his amazing will to survive. He continues to nurture his connection with the sacred (both within and without) and to work at unconditionally loving himself and others, all while striving to live fully in the present.

Today, Andy is in remission and is monitored on a regular basis. He continues to enjoy life, especially time with his wife, Susan, and his children. He bikes daily, plays the guitar and piano, and is involved in the Leukemia & Lymphoma Society. He serves as the rabbi of a synagogue in Greenwich, Connecticut.

Andy's story is important because it teaches us that meeting the challenge of illness can help everyone—even men and women of the cloth—to grow personally, emotionally, and spiritually, as long as we are open to receiving these gifts. Andy says that in his life, cancer was analogous to Jonah being stuck within the whale.

Cancer forced him to come to a standstill and to re-examine everything he thought he knew, which ultimately enabled him to identify what was getting in the way of fully living his purpose. Just as the whale turned out to be a gift in disguise for Jonah, cancer turned out to be a gift in disguise for Andy. I hope you'll keep his story in mind as you grapple with your own diagnosis.

What Can Cancer Teach *Me*?

Based on my own experiences as a patient and as a psychologist, I feel it serves each of us to ask, in the midst of our difficulty, *What can this teach me? What am I learning from this experience that can serve my journey through the rest of life?* Identifying these lessons will "open" the gifts that cancer can give you and will provide access to powerful, high-vibrational healing tools.

You have just read about the gifts that others have received from cancer—but it's important to realize that cancer's gifts vary from person to person. Sometimes they have to do with the quality of our relationships. Other times, the lessons teach us that we must let go of whatever we have been holding onto: beliefs, habits, and fears that have depleted our immune systems and contributed to our illness. Cancer's lessons might also clarify how we can fulfill our hopes and dreams. Cancer can even reveal to us the truth that we are resilient; that we have the power to heal ourselves and get through our darkest days.

Here are some gifts I encourage you to look for during your cancer journey. As you read through this list, ask yourself what cancer may be trying to teach you. We'll discuss many of them further in other parts of this book.

- **Cancer teaches you to love yourself.** Before your diagnosis, you may have habitually put the needs of others before your own. (In fact, many of my cancer patients are diagnosed after acting as a caregiver for another for a prolonged period of time.) Now though, taking care of yourself—in other words, self-love—must become your priority.

When you love yourself enough to fight for survival, you will find that you have the strength to push through pain and treatments. And knowing that you have that deep reserve of inherent power will bolster your resiliency and your appreciation of who you are. In the future, your strengthened sense of self-love may enable you to say "no," to more confidently speak the truth, and to unashamedly seek out the things that make you happy and healthy.

- **Cancer teaches forgiveness.** Part of loving yourself is accepting yourself unconditionally. And that means forgiving yourself and others for grievances and other issues you have been carrying with you, perhaps for a lifetime. For instance, if you have blamed yourself for not achieving a certain dream or goal, cancer might be the catalyst for making peace with the past, along with putting an end to viewing yourself as a "failure."

- **Cancer teaches you to clarify and value your relationships.** So often, patients tell me that the people they thought might be there for them in their time of need weren't, but that other unexpected individuals stepped up to support, help, and assist them in numerous ways. Similarly, you can expect cancer to help you determine who your true, most committed friends are.

  Due to your inner guidance, you'll probably feel the desire to gravitate toward these people who believe in you and are working with you toward survival. And as you'll no doubt understand, you will realize that the individuals in whose energy field you feel safe and wonderful, are truly invaluable.

- **Cancer teaches you what is and isn't important.** As I have alluded to before, cancer causes you to evaluate what's working in your life and what isn't. (That includes your relationships, your living environment, your work-life balance, your activities, your priorities, and more.) Because cancer is such an overwhelming foe, you will instinctively want to clear out unnecessary debris that is no longer necessary or that is preventing you from finding a healthy balance.

- **Cancer teaches you to be responsible for yourself (and only yourself).** Except for the very young and the very old, most of us should claim responsibility for ourselves. If you feel that others' well-being and circumstances depend on you, it's likely that cancer will alter this mindset. Since you're embarking on a full-time job of loving and caring for yourself, you may be required to pull back from adult family members and friends who expect you to care for them. In reality, you have been allowing them to draw your life-force away from you, and cancer will be the catalyst for pushing them to reclaim their own lives as well.

  Over the years, I have observed that pulling back from those for whom you feel responsible is initially difficult and stressful. However, in time, it becomes a gift for you because you feel liberated and free: two feelings that feel wonderful to your cells, which have been burdened by your feelings of responsibility. This choice of self-love empowers the working of your body's immune system in meeting the challenge of cancer.

- **Cancer teaches you that each moment is precious.** This concept might be somewhat clichéd, but that's because it's true! Cancer lights a fire underneath you, because suddenly you are aware that you may not have all the time you'd once thought you did. I encourage you to act on each impulse to spend time with a loved one, to pursue a heart-felt desire, and to live out all the dreams you can.

By choosing to make the most of each moment—and to not focus on the list of passionless obligations you have imposed on yourself—you'll feel happy and your brain will produce the chemicals your immune system needs to fight your cancer. You'll find that the state of *being* in the moment is a state of peace, involving an awareness of your connection to the earth and to "all there is." In this type of *being* you are not seeking, desiring, or striving for something or someone you do not have. Rather, you feel delight and peace, and are conscious of having all you need, as well as a sense of connection to your own essence and to your Higher Power.

- **Cancer teaches you lessons that enable you to heal spiritually and psychologically.** You learn unequivocally what you have control over and what you don't. More specifically, cancer teaches you that while you may not have control over what happens to you, you do have control over how you handle those circumstances. If you choose to live lovingly and passionately in the moment, without resistance (in other words, without fear, anxiety, and the need to be in control), and to maintain a positive perspective, you'll increase your body's ability to heal, as well as restore balance to your mind, body, and soul.

Always, always look for the lessons in the midst of pain and hardship. They have the power to change the course of your soul's journey—and the direction of your life.

Stop Resisting.

At this point, you may be thinking something along these lines: *I certainly wouldn't mind absorbing some of the lessons above. But what I absolutely can't do is bring myself to view cancer as a gift. I don't want to accept that this disease is in my life, period, much less that it has the power to influence so many things beyond my physical health.*

Once again, I understand. It is human nature to rail against destructive forces that come uninvited into our lives. But this is the truth: You cannot change what's past. You can't travel back in time to change lifestyle factors that may have contributed to your cancer, or to cause it to be detected earlier. You are right here, right now. So is cancer. If you want to make the best of the future's unlimited potential, you must stop fighting against what *is*. Accept that cancer is part of your life, stop resisting, and move forward. Acknowledging that you have an unwelcome visitor does not mean that you must buy into whatever prognosis that may accompany it! Those of us who try desperately to resist what we can't control soon discover that it is we ourselves who suffer.

One of my favorite quotes comes from the wisdom of Esther and Jerry Hicks' teacher, Abraham: "The path of least resistance is the path of greatest allowing." Think about it. When you are relaxed and in peace, you vibrate at a higher level, your body is able to produce the chemicals needed for your healing, and you are allowing in what you need for healing to occur. You are also better able to hear your own intuitive wisdom, especially if you take the time to meditate and/or quiet yourself.

Here's what I can promise you: When you choose to allow in, rather than resist what comes to you, and to be flexible and adaptable, you'll find that the very things you most want (even if you didn't consciously know you wanted them) tend to manifest. You'll experience greater happiness and increased well-being when you choose to stop trying to control everything. Spiritually, you'll evolve by learning the power of allowing, surrendering, and of loving.

I experienced this recently during a hospitalization. After four days, I was so eager to get home that I found myself resisting (being aggravated, disappointed, and annoyed by anything and everything that was getting in the way of my own healing). It took a doctor to remind me of what I usually practice and teach my own patients: to be patient! As soon as my doctor said those words, I realized that I needed to allow in all that was occurring and to stop resisting the process. The path of least resistance would be my path to greatest healing. As soon as I became conscious of what I was doing, my perspective changed and the healing moved along beautifully. I was able to leave the hospital the next day.

Once again, the choice is yours. In your life, will cancer be a lesson and a gift, or will it be a curse, a punishment, and a burden? Know this: The perspective you choose will have a powerful impact on your life.

CHAPTER 6

What Does It Mean to Heal?

"*Healing may not be so much about getting better, as about letting go of everything that isn't you—all of the expectations, all of the beliefs—and becoming who you are ...*"

RACHEL NAOMI REMEN, MD

"*... Loving and accepting their imperfections (of my children and my husband) is much easier than turning that light of loving-kindness on myself ... Practicing self-love means learning how to trust ourselves, to treat ourselves with respect, and to be kind and affectionate toward ourselves.*"

BRENÉ BROWN, PhD

If you've been diagnosed with cancer, the word "healing" probably means one thing to you above all others: the restoration of your body and the eradication of your disease. It's synonymous with remission, or better yet, *cured.* In short, you want your cancer to go away and your body to return to normal.

And yes—physical wellness *is* one aspect of healing. But, as I pointed out in Chapter Four (Guiding Principles for Your Cancer Journey) it's not the only one. Healing can be mental, emotional, and spiritual, too. If you take to heart and apply the truths I share in this book, you increase the odds of healing occurring on all of these levels.

Maybe this isn't what you want to hear. *All I want is to be rid of this illness,* you might think. *I really don't care what happens spiritually if I still have cancer.* If you've read every chapter up to this point, though, what I'm going to say next won't surprise you: It's very likely that spiritual and emotional healing *need to* occur in order to pave the way for physical wellness.

Healing is such a different experience for each of us. There is no one prescribed formula that "works" for everyone, given that we are all born with unique qualities and that our journeys differ from one another's. That said, my research dealing with cancer patients who have recovered partially or fully, as well my work with cancer patients in my private practice, have demonstrated to me that a significant factor in the healing process is self-love. That self-love is often expressed through commitment to making the changes required for surviving and thriving, and leads to spiritual and emotional evolution. What I'm saying is, in so many cases I've observed, physical healing was preceded by emotional and spiritual healing.

As you read this chapter, remember that genuine and lasting healing happens holistically. When you shift yourself energetically to a higher place, you help your body to overcome disease— and you also experience more love, joy, and peace than you ever thought possible.

Here, I'd like to offer a fuller definition of healing, and help you to understand why you need to focus on healing more than "just" your body throughout your cancer journey.

A Holistic View of Healing

So what is healing, exactly? First, healing is something you need when you are not feeling your inherent sense of physical power. It is the restoration of balance and harmony after you have been feeling "off" or out of balance. This definition of healing is probably the one with which you're most familiar. It certainly applies to your cancer, and can also come into play when you are dealing with various kinds of emotionally and mentally challenging circumstances that may not always have physical roots.

For instance, perhaps your fear and anxiety after receiving your cancer diagnosis resulted in frequent stomachaches. Maybe learning that you were laid off from a former position, combined with the subsequent job search and financial worries, caused you to experience debilitating stress headaches. Or finding out that a previous girlfriend or boyfriend wanted to end the relationship contributed to weeks of grinding exhaustion. Essentially, learning of the loss of anyone or anything near and dear to you (including your home, your pet, a person, and certainly your health) has the power to create imbalance within you—and to disempower you physically.

Secondly, healing is what you need any time your mind and spirit are out of balance (be it tired, stressed, excessively worried, and/or panicky), on a small or large scale. In this type of situation, emotional or spiritual healing is needed to restore your internal sense that all is well so that you can return to a healthy state of empowerment. When healing occurs, you have a sense of being energetically aligned with your heart. You feel a wonderful sense of increased peace, which can also include passion and joy.

Often, these different types of healing—physical, emotional, spiritual—happen in concert. With the vast majority of my cancer patients, I have found that what needs to be healed is *more* than just the body. Not only are you dealing with a physical disease; you're also feeling overwhelmed by the many fears, stresses, and anxieties that disease has introduced. In addition, you may need to address long-entrenched dysfunctions that have caused you to vibrate at a low energetic level and that may be making it easier for disease to flourish. For example, these dysfunctions might include unhealthy habitual ways of responding to personal relationships with loved ones, or long-standing fears and concerns about your health, job, future, or finances.

In order to truly heal, then, you need to repair *all* of these breaks, tears, and fragmentations. Focusing only on the physical aspect of healing would be like repairing your home's broken air conditioner while ignoring the leaky roof, sagging floorboards, and mold-infested basement.

To give you a better idea of what I mean, I'd like to share the story of an incredible and inspiring woman with you.

Josey's Story: Lessons of Healing

Josey is an extremely positive and energetic wife, mother, and grandmother whose appearance and manner belie her age of 60-plus years. More than a decade ago, Josey was stunned to receive a diagnosis of breast cancer. However, she lost no time in making the decision to have her breasts removed, followed by a regimen of chemotherapy and radiation.

According to Josey, this was an extremely "scary" time in her life—and no wonder! Nights were especially difficult. She often felt terrified and could not sleep. It was during this time that Josey began working with me after being referred by her rabbi so that she could regain a sense of control—which she did.

Through the discomfort of dealing with chemo and the grief of losing a treasured part of her identity (her hair), Josey strove to remain resilient. She told me that although she cried uncontrollably while shaving off what remained of her hair after it began to fall out in clumps, she took out the wig she'd had made and went to the market with her husband John. She was amazed that the same people who normally said "Hello" to her continued to do so, not indicating that anything was out of the ordinary. *Maybe life can be almost normal*, she thought to herself. And for a while it was, thanks to Josey's positive approach and determined efforts to focus on what felt good to her.

But Josey's cancer journey wasn't finished yet. Three years later, she underwent an echocardiogram to be sure that her heart had not been affected by her chemotherapy. Imagine her shock and horror when her cardiologist called to inform her that a tumor had been noted on her left chest wall, and that another had been found in her right lung!

Again, Josey, who is a take-charge gal, acted quickly. Both tumors were excised. A few months later, two more tumors were found in the middle lobe of her lung, which was then removed. At this point Josey had no breasts, one full lung, and a small piece of the other lung left. She received radiation and medications for the cancer, which further took their toll on her health and comfort. Ultimately, though, I'm so happy to report that Josey's committed work with her doctors, with me, and most of all with herself, paid off. She has been free of cancer for several years.

When you consider Josey's arduous, ongoing journey with cancer, her physical healing alone is cause for great celebration. But as a supporter, teacher, and friend, I was also privileged to witness Josey's healing on several other levels as well.

Josey has always been a positive person, but (like many of us) she is also prone to worry and anxiety. The tools she used in her journey (many of which I will share with you in this book) facilitated emotional healing and growth. Josey says that she's more aware and conscious than ever before. She has become extremely adept at noticing low-vibrational thoughts and feelings, and replacing them with ones that make her feel good. Josey's fear no longer controls her.

Cancer also prompted Josey to heal relationships that had previously been unhealthy and dysfunctional. Josey had always lived her life worrying about making others happy, and often sacrificing her own well-being for their benefit. While loving and prioritizing herself sounded selfish to Josey when I initially suggested it to her, she also intuitively knew that this was needed for her healing. She learned to become more conscious of others' energetic vibrations; specifically, of whether they were raising or lowering her own. Without being hurtful, Josey learned to let others know exactly what she did and didn't need from them. Of course, all of Josey's loved ones supported her decision to focus first on her needs, experiences, and happiness. Today, Josey says that even with all of her scars and physical limitations, she knows that she is deeply loved by her husband, children, and friends.

Finally, I would like to mention Josey's spiritual healing and growth. When she was diagnosed with cancer, her relationship with God was somewhat fear-based. In particular, after her first encounter with breast cancer Josey made a "deal" with God while visiting her parents' graves. "Let me be well enough to get my children to the point where they can take care of themselves before I die," she told her Higher Power. Not surprisingly, when Josey's cancer returned she was terribly worried that God would hold her to that deal! In my heart, I knew that God would want what Josey wanted for herself: to be here, healthy and happy, for herself and her family. I encouraged her to make a new deal with God, which she did.

Josey now takes a new approach to spirituality and believes in the power of All That Is. She feels the presence of loving energy, especially in trying times. For example, during the most difficult parts of her surgeries and treatments, she has experienced signs that her deceased loved ones (her mom, in particular) are present. Josey feels strongly that there is something higher helping her to be whole and balanced. This soothes and comforts her, and inspires her to love and serve others.

Today, Josey continues to enjoy her life, especially spending time with family and friends. Josey recognizes the transformative power of healing emotionally, mentally, and spiritually, as well as physically.

The Elephant in the Room: Spiritual Healing Without Physical Healing

Now, I'd like to write a few words about what you are probably thinking—let's be honest, *fearing*—right now. Your body might not heal. Your cancer might not go into remission or go away for good. Your disease might end your life.

This is the elephant in the room that I feel we must address. It's also the part that is incredibly difficult for many people to accept: No one—not your doctor, not me, and not you—can *guarantee* physical healing. We're all going to die at some point, and when you have cancer, it may happen sooner than you had imagined.

However, as I've said already in this book and as I want to reiterate here, the odds of experiencing physical healing increase when you choose to fill your life with positive, high-vibrational experiences. In fact, a relatively small number of my cancer patients have died from this disease. This is one reason spiritual healing is so important: It may save your life.

The other reason, paradoxically, is that spiritual healing helps you experience a better death. Personally, I have a deep knowing that the Divine spark we call "life" does not wink out when the body dies. I have spent my life studying extraordinary experiences and I am 100 percent convinced that the spirit, the soul, the essence that makes you *you,* goes on to greater and more glorious levels of existence after the "machine" that houses it has stopped functioning. Spiritual healing will almost certainly help you realize this truth and may even completely alleviate your fear of death—which, in turn, can enable you to respond to your challenge with greater calm and a release of resistance. (I will talk more about this subject later in the book.)

Here, I want to share the stories of two patients who *did* die as a result of cancer. (Their names have been changed here.) My intention is not to discourage or frighten you. Rather, I want to highlight just how powerful and transformative emotional and spiritual healing can be, even when they aren't accompanied by physical wellness. I also want to show you that healing doesn't look the same to everyone; its definition is always incredibly personal.

Anita, a nurse, was one of my earliest cancer patients. At only 30 years of age, she, learned that she had an advanced case of melanoma. To the surprise of many who knew her, Anita chose only palliative treatment, because she wished to enjoy her life with her husband for as long as possible. Anita was one of my greatest teachers. She was one of the first who showed me that healing does not have to be physical. For her, it had everything to do with healing emotionally, mentally, and spiritually. Anita came to therapy terribly troubled by unresolved issues with her family. Over time, she was able to heal the strained relationships she'd previously had with her parents and siblings. Anita was completely at peace when she died.

After being diagnosed with an aggressive form of cancer, Sue, who was only in her early fifties, experienced true healing by taking responsibility for and control of her life. Having lived in a family and marriage where there had been years of significant stress and discord, Sue chose to release all resistance, to forgive those with whom she had unfinished business, and to begin living with love and peace. She died fully on her terms, thankful to be experiencing one of the very highest vibrational levels. Throughout her experience, Sue was very much aware that she was not only dearly loved, but that she, too, was a being of love. Her love of self and others actually empowered her. She experienced a healing of her spirit, her soul, and her life. I was honored to be a part of her journey, both while alive and while dying.

The bottom line is, healing can occur on many levels. For some, there is complete physical healing. For others, there is the ability to continue living a relatively high-quality physical life, despite the need for treatments, with the hope for remission. And for others, there is the increased experience of peace, growth, and well-being, despite the recognition that cancer is present and may never disappear.

The nature of the challenge of cancer is that everything becomes relative. While you, of course, wish to experience a full cure, many—including my patients—make peace with the idea that a complete healing or cure may not occur, but are grateful for the treatments that enable them to continue to live a quality-filled life.

Wherever you are on your cancer journey, it is my hope and prayer that you seek and experience the healing you most need. It may help to embrace the perspective that all of us are exactly where we are "meant" to be in our souls' journeys—and that the choices we make (wherever we are) contribute to the quality of our healing experience. I find that this thought by itself yields immense amounts of comfort and reassurance.

To close this chapter, I would like to share a simple exercise to help you realize your healing intentions.

Write Down Your Healing Intentions and Affirmations.

I often recommend that my patients write down their vision for themselves. Committing your intentions to paper, even more than speaking or thinking them, gives them energy. My own intentions (provided also in the form of affirmations) include the following. Use whichever format (intention or affirmation) feels right to you. I have left some of the intentions unfinished to show that they can (and should!) be tweaked to fit your feelings, needs, and goals.

I intend to allow in …
I am allowing in all that I need for well-being, balance, and harmony.

I intend to focus on breath to quiet myself …
I am focusing on my breath to quiet myself, go within, find peace, and shift to a higher vibration.

I intend to love life …
I love life and life loves me.

I intend to be here in joy …
I am here for joy and am allowing in all that brings me pleasure.

I intend to love myself unconditionally …
I am learning to love myself unconditionally.

I intend to empower myself …
I am empowering myself by releasing my fears, guilt, and pain.

I intend to be thankful for …
I am so thankful for all my blessings and choose to live in a state of gratitude.

I intend to be aware of how I feel …
I am choosing to be aware of how I feel and, if not good, to tweak my thoughts to feel better.

I intend to choose to release …
I choose now to release and detach from anything and everything that does not serve me.

I intend to strengthen my immune system by …
I allow in the people and circumstances that feed my immune system with life-enhancing vibrations.

I intend to be love …
I am love, I am loving, and I am loved.

I intend to look in the mirror and …
Each time I see myself in the mirror, I say, "Hi" and "I love you!"

I intend to remind myself that I am …
I am resilient and resourceful and capable of getting to the light from here.

I intend to feed my cells thoughts …
I feel my body's cells thoughts that vibrate highly so they can care for me.

I intend to choose to live …
I am choosing to live consciously, noticing all negativity, and choosing to release it immediately.

I intend to focus on …
I am focusing on what makes my heart sing!

I intend to know my connection …
I am discovering my connection to my Higher Power.

I intend to view my challenges as opportunities …
I am shifting my perspective to view challenges and problems as opportunities for healing.

I intend to go with the flow …
I am fluid, flexible, and going with the flow.

I intend to learn to listen …
I am learning to listen to my own inner guidance.

I intend to ask, moment to moment, what I can learn …
I am asking, moment to moment, "What lesson is this teaching me?"

I intend to be aware that I am …
I am aware I am never alone, and am always watched over and protected.

I intend to be aware that …
I am aware that everything is perfect.

I intend to focus on and affirm only what feels …
I am focusing on and affirming what feels uplifting, positive, and joyful.

I intend to get to know …
I am getting to know who I really am.

Each morning and evening, whether they've changed or not, take a few minutes to write out your intentions. Read them aloud while visualizing them in your mind's eye. Then, put your pen or pencil down. Close your eyes and follow your breath in and out, breathing deeply, for a few minutes. This will quiet your mind and indeed, your whole being. Now, see yourself manifesting your heart's desires—living what you have imagined are your hopes and dreams. Feel your joy, enthusiasm, passion, and excitement as you do this, using all of your senses.

This powerful little exercise lends wonderful energy to your healing intentions and shifts you energetically to a higher level, making it easier for the Guiding Principle of "Like Energy Attracts Like Energy" to work for you.

"I believe we are here on earth to become complete, and anything that helps us to do that is a blessing. The problem is that some blessings do not feel very good when they happen. What you may define as a curse can become a blessing if you let it become your teacher and show you that not all of the side effects of cancer are bad."

BERNIE SIEGEL, MD, IN *FAITH, HOPE AND HEALING*

CHAPTER 7

Allow Yourself to Grieve

"Don't cry because it's over. Smile because it happened."

Dr. Seuss

"We can endure much more than we think we can; all human experience testifies to that. All we need to do is learn not to be afraid of pain. Grit your teeth and let it hurt. Don't deny it, don't be overwhelmed by it. It will not last forever. One day, the pain will be gone and you will still be there."

Harold Kushner,
in *When All You've Ever Wanted Isn't Enough*

Many of us associate grief, first and foremost, with death. If that's you, you may be thinking, "I'm not dead yet, and I'm certainly not finished fighting, so grief has no place in my life." Let me gently assure you that it *does*. Grief has a much wider definition than many people realize. It can also manifest and affect you in unexpected ways. And anyone who has been touched by cancer—whether you're a patient, a survivor, a caregiver, or a loved one—needs to grieve.

The good news is, grief isn't *just* an expression of unpleasant, painful emotions. It's also a powerful vehicle for healing and spiritual growth.

First, Understand What Grief Is.

Grief—which is both a feeling and a process—stems from loss. And anytime you're separated from someone or something you love, that's loss. It doesn't have to mean death. It can be the loss of your youth or a job or a dream or your house. It can certainly be the loss of your health to cancer, and possibly the long life span you had anticipated.

Any time you experience loss, and for any reason, you've lost a part of your identity, a piece of how you see yourself. And in the case of sudden loss, like a cancer diagnosis, all your beliefs about the way things are "supposed to be" go out the window. You feel you've lost all control—of your health, of your body's processes, of your future—and it's a deeply disorienting feeling. Your body, mind, and spirit all react. And for healing to happen, you must acknowledge the impact cancer has had on all of those aspects of yourself.

Don't live in denial that this is not a huge loss, or fear that acknowledging it is "negative thinking." There's a *big* difference between accepting reality and indulging in "doomsday" thinking.

Remember, in order to move forward, you must first make peace with where you are.

New Losses Bring Older Losses to the Surface.

When they first begin to work with me, many of my patients assume that grief is a one-time process. Once you work through the pain you're feeling, they believe, you can and should move on with life. Revisiting past losses, as well as the unpleasant feelings that accompany them, isn't advisable.

These patients (and possibly you, too) are surprised to learn that you may need to grieve the same loss multiple times in your life. What's more, new loss—such as a cancer diagnosis—can bring older, long-suppressed loss to the surface of your mind, body, and spirit.

If you'll allow me to simplify some complex scientific concepts, everything is energy and vibrates at different levels (which we've already discussed). The pain of loss is stored in your cells as a low vibrational experience. When you grieve a loss in the present moment, the vibration of this experience will bring up similar vibrational experiences from your past, often making you feel overwhelmed with grief. It is as if you have an invisible thread attached to your present loss that is also attached to those of equivalent vibrations buried in your cells.

That's why, if you never gave yourself permission to grieve when your father passed away ten years ago, you may fall apart when your beloved dog dies. You're grieving your pet, but you're also grieving your father. Likewise, your cancer diagnosis and subsequent treatment may evoke emotional responses that surprise you. You may actually be grieving multiple losses. When you start to feel sad, it may be helpful to ask yourself, *What does this remind me of? When have I felt this way in the past? What am I learning from this?"*

Whatever you may be grieving in addition to your cancer, it's important to consciously let go of that pain. Not doing so can have further negative consequences for your health. In fact, I have worked with many patients whose cancer returned partially due to (I believe) a failure to let go of pain, resentment, guilt, and anger. Remember the ill effects that low energetic vibrations can have on your body!

In Chapter Eight, I'll share several tools, including Face/Embrace/Replace and tapping, that can help you to notice your pain, experience it, and send it on its way so that its low energy doesn't unnecessarily weigh you down and hinder your travels through life.

It's "Normal" to Feel the Way You Feel. So Honor Grief When It Comes.

That's right. How ever you're feeling in the face of this significant loss, it's normal. Grief wears many faces. Independent of your cancer's symptoms and your treatment's side effects, you may feel fatigue, stomach upset, headaches, or tightness in the chest. You may experience an inability to stay focused and remember things. You may lose weight (or gain it). You may have insomnia, intrusive dreams, or flashbacks. You may be numb or weepy or anxious or even panic-stricken. Just remember that all of this is normal. And if you think your loss—an easily treatable cancer or successfully removed tumor, for example—doesn't account for such powerful symptoms, you're wrong.

We all grieve differently. Your way is valid no matter what anyone says—and believe me, there are many people who will try to shut you down or hurry you up. Others may be uncomfortable with your grief and prefer not to witness it. Or they may, with the very best of intentions, want you to move forward so that you feel less pain.

Remember, it's okay to have the symptoms you're having, it's okay to cry, and it's okay to work with a professional if you need some extra help. Taking the time and the steps to process your grief, whenever it occurs, is the greatest gift you can give yourself.

And, please, do not allow others to rush you in your grieving experience. (And afford others the same courtesy!) We all grieve at our own pace. Here's another way to think about it: Each of us allows in the reality of our experience when we are ready to confront the truth of the loss. So if you recommend a book that helped you in your grief to a friend or family member who is grieving the loss of their health or a loved one, understand that they may not be ready to read it at the time you give it to them.

Remember, the body and the mind are so wise. They know what you can handle and what you can allow in. They will let you know when you are ready to read about your loss. You will pick up that book only when your inner wisdom recognizes that it can help you. If you do it too early, you will probably not finish the book. The same is true for seeking help, be it a group experience or one-on-one therapy. Listen to your inner wisdom and to your body for the guidance you need.

Don't Run from Your Grief Triggers.

If you know something is going to make you feel melancholy or will trigger tears, your first impulse may be to avoid it. If at all possible, *don't*. Sooner or later, no matter how you try to avoid it, your Higher Self will demand that you do the work of grief. Trying to escape the pain does not serve you. Healing is expedited when you do the best you can to express your pain, feel it, and let it go.

For instance, if you're watching a movie or eating dinner with your family and you suddenly feel an overwhelming sense of sadness, give yourself permission to cry. If you're in a doctor's waiting room or at a worship service, excuse yourself to a more private location where you can have a good cry and regroup (or even leave if you have to). And if you're feeling blue, you don't have to go to the dinner you had planned with your friends and feign merriment—but neither should you opt out of all social events and traditions because they make you feel sad.

Sometimes, it may even be good to face your grief triggers head on in order to work through your feelings. For example, just looking in the mirror and becoming aware of your loss of hair, eyebrows, or breast might be a powerful trigger, reminding you of what you have lost, as well as of the changes in how you view yourself and your identity. Rather than avoiding the mirror, choose to pair what you are seeing with the reminder that these changes are temporary. Say to yourself, *This, too, shall pass*, and remind yourself that you are looking at indications that the treatment of your choice is doing its best to help you heal.

Furthermore, listening to the music that makes you cry, or setting aside some time to look through your photo albums, writing a poem or two, or writing in your journal about how you're feeling, can be cathartic. These activities may bring on tears, but they're healing tears—and they are a good thing.

Linda Wrazen, a wise woman with whom I was honored to work, enjoyed life and found great joy in her writing and journaling. She also found peace and comfort in reading what others who are dealing with the challenge of cancer have written. She graciously offered to share with you a piece that her sister, Sharon, (who was challenged by ovarian cancer) wrote to her. It's a piece that dearly touched Linda's heart—and mine—and it helped Linda tremendously as a "trigger" in facing and working through her grief.

What makes this even more special is that it was written while Linda was meditating on a picture of her sister, shortly after her death. Linda felt enormously compelled to pick up her pen and write the words that began flowing through her—directly from her sister Sharon. This experience is known as automatic writing. Perhaps this piece will touch your heart as well, and trigger your own healing tears.

Sister,
I love you. Anytime you are afraid or weak, I am with you. We are human allies.
We are bound together by an energy that passes through space, time, and emotion. Know it, believe it, feel it.
Find me in the space between the clouds.
Find me in the corners of your mouth that lift your smile.
Find me in your breath.
Find me in your heartbeat.
Find me in the tingle of your tummy.
Find me in the eyes of
all children, yours and mine,
and in the eyes of strangers.
Find me in every touch that
you give or that you receive.
Find me in Reiki.
Find me in exercise.
Find me in dance.
Find me in music.
Find me in a glass of water, a glass of wine, in a margarita,
in a beer, and in a cup of coffee.
Find me in smiles, hugs and even tears.
Find me in rain, in sunsets,
in the warmth of sun.
Find me in crystals and in candles.
Find me in laughter, in silliness.
Find me in gifts, in stories
and in dreams.
You will never find me in fear,
in sorrow, in hate, in anger,

in depression.
I cannot feel these anymore-
their paths are blocked.
Turn around. I am here.
I am with you now and always.
I love you.

After the recent loss of one of my dear friends, Linda also sent me the following poem; one that she had written many years ago for a friend who had lost a new grandchild. She sent this with an exquisite cluster of crystals, along with the instruction to place the crystals in the window next to where I sit in my office. Linda wrote that her intention was for the crystals to represent the spirit and guidance of my good friend (who was a gifted healer) so that she might now be able to assist me in my work. I share this with you because it is something that may help you, too, as you grieve.

A tear shed is a crystal
With so many facets.
It carries joy;
It carries grief
To inspire a tear is an honor.

Grieve to Heal—but Don't Live in a Constant State of Grief.

I hope you're beginning to see that the grief that's associated with your cancer can be a gift. It can be the catalyst that pushes you to finally face and let go of long-held pain. It can push you to dig deep and figure out what's blocking the peace and joy you deserve to experience. It can force you to find inner resources you didn't know you had. It makes you stronger and more resilient. It opens you up to love.

But none of that can happen if you don't face your grief head on and consciously work through it. Once you do, you'll generally find that life has a richness and a color to it that you may have never imagined—yes, even in the midst of your cancer journey.

In the next chapter, I will share powerful methods to help you process your grief, and even use it to your benefit. For now, though, I want to leave you with an important caveat: Process your grief, certainly—but don't allow yourself to live in it.

You'll probably find that intense grief isn't constant. For most people, it tends to come in waves. Don't fight these waves—allow yourself to be "swept away" by each one so that you can experience and process the emotions you need to, when you need to. But once each wave abates, don't continue to wallow in feelings of sadness and negativity, which will cause you to vibrate at a lower, less healthy level.

Make Sure to Balance Your Energy as You Grieve.

As you know, grief and trauma are energetic emotional forces that have the ability to block the flow of your healthy energy so that it is unable to maintain your body's immune system. For the sake of supporting your health as you grieve, it's important to engage in methods of unblocking such energy. These may include activities such as tai chi, qigong, acupuncture, acupressure, working with an energy medicine practitioner, or maintaining a daily exercise routine. Keep in mind that talking with a professional who has expertise in grief, trauma, and illness is also therapeutically helpful for releasing blockages. In each of these activities, you are opening up blockages, bringing locked-in energy up to the surface so that it can be released, and rebalancing the energy within your body—all of which contribute to greater well-being.

Additionally, I encourage you to identify several go-to activities that consistently make you feel good. After you've dried your tears and begun to regroup emotionally after a wave of grief hits, it's a good idea to watch a funny sitcom, treat yourself to a bowl of ice cream, watch a sunset with your spouse, throw a ball for your dog, or do something else that will lift your mood. The idea isn't to negate your grief or to act as though it never existed; it's simply to balance out your sadness with happiness and pleasure. Remember, as often as possible, it's important to *choose* to participate in activities and thoughts that enhance your well-being and raise your vibrational energy.

Remember that your journey with both cancer and grief is greatly influenced by the perspective you choose. As the months go by, following your awareness of your loss, take a moment or two here and there to stop and ask yourself these questions: *How is this changing me? What is this teaching or showing me that I was not aware of before? Are there lessons I can take from this journey so far?* I assure you that with the passage of time your answers to these questions will evolve. It is my hope that you will feel a bit more conscious, more in control, and more empowered. If nothing else, asking these questions will help you to become more conscious of your own resources for handling a situation you did not see coming or were not sure you could face on your own.

To conclude this chapter, I'd like to share the stories of two of my patients. Both detail how these individuals were affected by grief, and how they were finally able to face and release it.

Daniel's Story

Daniel, a loving father, grandfather and husband, had retired from his very stressful job of many years in order to spend time with his grandchildren. Unfortunately, just a few years after his retirement, Daniel's son Robert died. Daniel reaffirmed his commitment to being there for his grandchildren.

Of course, Daniel never stopped missing, thinking about, and talking (nonverbally) with Robert. He dearly missed the loving relationship he had with his son—including the times they had spent doing Boy Scout projects, going to and watching Phillies' games, and playing basketball at home. With his mind so focused on his loss, every cell of Daniel's being felt the pain of his grief, making it difficult for his body to produce the cells needed to destroy any lurking viruses within the body. And as we know, cancer is a cell that does not waste time growing in size if it is not kept in check by our inherent physical resources.

Within two years of his son's death, Daniel was diagnosed with non-Hodgkin lymphoma. (This is far from unusual—studies show that after the death of a loved one, people tend to experience greater incidence of physical illness, and even higher death rates!)

After receiving his diagnosis, Daniel knew that he needed to do whatever was necessary for his healing so that he could return to caring for his family, especially his grandchildren, Jake and Josey. That determination led him to me. Only months before Daniel's diagnosis, his wife Maria had begun seeing me to better manage her own pain and her life. Daniel began coming in with Maria, and then chose to see me on his own.

While he had a positive attitude, it did not take long for me to see that Daniel was still grieving his beloved son. Each time he interacted with his grandkids, he experienced joy, but was simultaneously reminded of his son's death. The best word for such experiences, I feel, is *bittersweet*. Furthermore, Daniel was grieving the loss of his identity as a healthy man, capable of caring for his family.

As I've said, the important thing when grieving someone or something, as well as grieving your health, is to intentionally release the pain. Not doing so can have further negative consequences for your health. (In fact, I have worked with many patients whose cancer returned partially due to, I believe, a failure to let go of their pain, resentment, guilt, anger, and grief.)

So, in addition to Daniel's chemotherapy protocol, he and I worked on expressing his sense of loss. I explained to him that since the vibration of one loss pulls up all of the similar vibrations of loss that are stored in the cells, each loss he had experienced needed to be acknowledged and processed. One processing tool that that proved to be especially effective for Daniel was visualization.

Initially, visualization didn't come easily to Daniel—but it was a challenge that he took seriously. He chose to use the imagery of power washing, envisioning himself using a sprayer and brush. This imagery served two purposes: Not only was Daniel envisioning cleaning the cancer cells out of his body; he also envisioned washing away the low energetic vibrations caused by his grief that were blocking the flow of healthy energy within his body.

After feeling and acknowledging each portion of his grief, I encouraged Daniel to begin the process of balancing his energy by filling himself up with higher-energy vibrations. He did this by listening to meditation tapes and music, going on walks, swimming, reconnecting with old friends, spending time with his wife, resuming his carpentry hobby, and more.

Today, Daniel has experienced major healing. His scans are perfect, and his doctors have told him he is doing beautifully. Daniel and his family have also received a plethora of signs from their son, which has helped tremendously with Daniel's healing and his grieving. For instance, Daniel has found that when he is deeply missing Robert, a monarch butterfly will suddenly appear out of nowhere and either land on his shoulder, or circle him and those around him, as if to say, "I am here and I love you."

Daniel has also told me that when thinking about his son, he'll turn on the radio, only to hear one of Robert's favorite songs playing. And Robert has found a way to use hearts as a sign of his being present at family gatherings. Hearts simply appear on everything: menus, signs, napkins, in the sky, on airplanes, etc. And hearts are synonymous with love. What more can I say?

Amanda's Story

When Amanda came to me, she was deeply grieving the death of her beloved husband. (This was her second marriage; her first love had died many years before.) She was also preparing to retire from her position as a school principal, a transition that seemed especially difficult because she wouldn't be able to share the next chapter in her life with her loving partner. As much as Amanda was looking forward to having time to pursue activities such as traveling and going to the theater, she was also experiencing discomfort and anxiety when she thought about the future.

Essentially, with the relinquishing of her role as principal and the death of her husband, Amanda's sense of control, self-confidence, and security had disappeared. She slept poorly, she worried constantly, and her emotions were all over the place. Everything became relatively stressful for her: holidays, family connections, friendships, meeting new people, and being in unfamiliar situations. Life was being lived without her safety net, and it did not feel good.

Unfortunately, Amanda would face yet another significant loss. During the time between her husband's death and her retirement, Amanda's mother had begun to deteriorate. Amanda, a loving and caring daughter, would go to see her several times a week. But as the months and years passed, her mom became less responsive. Amanda felt that she was virtually alone, and her sense of loss and sadness increased.

Not surprisingly, Amanda's more recent losses caused the energetic vibrations of old losses, such as the death of her first partner, to reoccur. This further complicated her grieving journey. The good news is that Amanda responded to these challenges by doing what she needed to do to get through a day, a week, a month, and even a year—and more.

She had previously engaged in yoga and meditation, and these now became tools to help her restore her sense of well-being. She worked with a physician who prescribed medications to help manage her insomnia and her anxiety. She actively learned and practiced several cognitive–behavioral strategies for managing her state of mind, including Face/Embrace/Replace. And she eagerly learned and practiced Eden Energy Medicine and utilized the tapping techniques associated with Energy Psychology. (I'll discuss these techniques in more detail in the next chapter.)

In particular, Amanda strove to be conscious of when she was feeling down and of what she was saying to herself that contributed to these feelings. She learned to "tweak" her thoughts and remind herself that she had the ability to handle stressful situations. One of Amanda's go-to tactics was to envision herself on the stage in a theater, identifying with her own pain. As she walked to the back of the theater (in her mind's eye), she realized that in distancing herself from the situation she could diminish her pain and see things differently.

Amanda also intuitively knew that to survive, she needed community. She worked diligently to build a community of women with whom she had a sense of connection, and with whom she could go to the theater, call at the last minute to get together for dinner, or play a hand or two of cards. Over time, Amanda came to recognize that she was never alone, even when she was not with her friends and loved ones. Not only did her husband demonstrate that he was present through various signs; other angels and guides assisted her when she asked. This awareness brought Amanda, who was normally very left-brained and rational, great comfort.

Of course, Amanda continued to grieve while engaged in these healing activities. For some time, she had difficulty sleeping and felt anxious. Like so many people with whom I work who are grieving, she wondered if she would ever feel better and whether or not she would ever get a good night's sleep and not feel lonely. However, little by little, she realized she was healing.

I am pleased to say that in the years since her husband's death, Amada has built a fulfilling, positive life outside of her grief. She has re-entered the work world, and now holds a supervisory position at a major university in Philadelphia. She moved to the center of the city and loves being able to walk to the theater, the market, the gym, etc. She has indulged her love of travel by planning several successful trips. And recently, Amanda told me that she has found love once again and will be remarrying. I wasn't surprised. As Amanda has healed she has shifted energetically, and she is attracting and manifesting a high vibratory lifestyle.

While Amanda was not faced with cancer, her story is still one with which you may be able to identify. It is one of hope and serves to inspire us. Loss does not feel good. It is one of the hardest and most challenging of all life experiences, but it is also a powerful teacher. We learn that the choices we make about how we think, feel, and act have a significant impact on our life's trajectory after a loss. We learn that we have the ability and the resources to be resilient and to move through the pain to a place of peace. You can do this, just as Amanda did. The choice is always yours!

"Grieving is a journey that teaches us how to love in a new way now that our loved one is no longer with us. Consciously remembering those who have died is the key that opens the hearts, that allows us to love them in new ways."

THOMAS ATTIG, IN *THE HEART OF GRIEF*

CHAPTER 8

Utilize Crucial Tools for Healing

"Suppressed emotions may be felt … A part of the body may cease to vibrate at its normal frequency becoming numb or freeze and a hard lump may form. The lump may represent many different things energetically; an abrasive relationship, an unhealthy work situation, fear of change or anything that prevents nourishing of the soul. If the mass is physically removed, but the fear or issue remains, then the healing process will be incomplete. These areas may require specific energy work with a healer trained in body healing energy."

BETH DuPREE, MD, IN *THE HEALING CONSCIOUSNESS*

When you are fighting cancer, you're facing a significant loss. And as you navigate the grieving process, it's normal for you to experience a myriad of intense feelings. As we discussed in the previous chapter, it's important to allow yourself to feel these emotions as they come. Instead of bottling up the unpleasantness, you need to let yourself be angry, sad, cry, and scream. But once you've processed these emotions, it's very important for you to let go of them and move forward.

For example, Alycia was originally diagnosed with cervical cancer. As she was going into remission, she was diagnosed with brain cancer. Now, her cervical cancer has returned, along with extensive pain. This woman is feeling discouraged, fearful, and upset—and rightfully so. She *needs* to express her feelings if she is to survive, and to find acceptance and peace if this isn't the case. Expressing her feelings, along with talking to her family, her support group, and me (her psychologist) allows her to release her lower vibrational thoughts so that she can focus on what feels life-enhancing: humor, her grandchildren, and other loved ones.

In addition to talking about what she is feeling, I have shared several tools with Alycia to further aid her in raising her vibrational energy. (In fact, I share these tools with all of my patients.) In this chapter, I'll share them with you, too. Specifically, we'll learn about:

- Face/Embrace/Replace
- ABCs
- Energy Medicine
- Tapping (which is a specific tactic that falls under the Energy Medicine umbrella)
- Mindfulness

Any one of these tools can help you to deal with your pain at any given moment, whenever it arises. Many of my patients use the tool(s) that feels best to them when sitting in their doctors' offices, while waiting for test results, or when preparing for their surgeries and/or treatments—as well as when they become emotional contemplating their situations and their futures. First, let's look at Face/Embrace/Replace.

The Big Question: How Do You Feel?

To help you understand how the Face/Embrace/Replace process works, I'd like to review a few key points that we've already covered. First, you are an energetic, vibrational being, consisting of particles and waves of energy that vibrate at different frequencies. The higher your energy vibrates, the better you feel.

The problem is, all too often, we're not conscious of what we are thinking, and our negative thoughts cause us pain. And especially when a wave of grief strikes full force—which tends to happen often for cancer patients—we can feel totally helpless.

Personally, I have always approached healing with the understanding that you need to consciously be in touch with whether you feel good (peaceful) or not. Once you've made this basic determination, you can further examine your thoughts and decide how to tweak them.

That's where the Face/Embrace/Replace process comes in. I created this technique to help myself learn to feel better when I was stressed, and because it has helped me, I have been teaching it to my patients for many years. It helps you to be more mindful of how you're feeling so that you can do some repair work. Think of this tool as "conscious grieving": a way to direct your mind and spirit down a productive path instead of dwelling on your hurt and anger.

First, FACE your feelings and thoughts.

As soon as you feel disconnected from a sense of peace and well-being, place your dominant hand on your heart and ask yourself, "How am I feeling? Good or not good?" Of course, you already know that the answer is "not good"—but ask anyway. It's important to consciously face this feeling.

As soon as you are conscious of feeling "not good," take your dominant hand and place it on your forehead. Now ask yourself, "What's the thought that is creating the pain at my heart?" As you consider the answer, visualize an arc that connects the thoughts in your mind with the not-good feelings in your heart.

The thought you are facing may start with another being, such as, *She is such a difficult, even brutal, teacher/person/parent/etc.*, but ultimately, your thought should shift to beginning with "I." Often, not-good feelings can be boiled down to a few basic issues that all human beings focus on, including: *I (fear) I am messing up; I am failing or will fail; I can't do this; I have no value.* When you are facing cancer, your not-good feelings will probably include: *I am afraid of pain; I am afraid of dying; I don't know what's going to happen to me.*

Second, EMBRACE your feelings and thoughts.

Now that you've identified what you're feeling, you need to truly acknowledge it. In other words, you need to really feel and own your emotions—whatever they may be—rather than trying to avoid or discount them. As I explained in Chapter Seven, suppressing a feeling causes its low vibrational energy to stay within in your cells—and eventually, that emotion will bubble up to the surface, demanding to be acknowledged.

The more you repress your feelings, the greater their intensity becomes as they attempt to find a release. That's why I recommend embracing your feelings in a time and space that offers privacy. If you're at home, you might want to go into your bathroom or bedroom and close the door. If you're at work or at a doctor's office, take a walk or go to your car. Scream, curse, cry, and truly allow every one of your cells to acknowledge and release whatever it is that you feel. Embracing your feelings in this way may wipe you out physically, but I promise, it will ultimately enable you to feel better.

Believe it or not, you can use your breath to enhance the impact of this emotional release by cleaning out the residue created by your negative thoughts. Here's how to do it:

As you inhale deeply, imagine and see in your mind's eye the breath coming in from your Source (we'll talk more about your Source later in this book). Give that breath a color such as blue (for peace), green (for healing), or pink (for compassion). See and feel it traveling down to your heart, lungs, and stomach, concentrating on the peace it creates.

Now, as you exhale, imagine that your breath is a vacuum cleaner sucking up the particles of energy that your worries and fears have attached to your body. Part your lips slightly and allow those particles to escape. Simultaneously, be aware of how warm, heavy, and relaxed you feel as you exhale. In fact, with each breath in and out, be aware of a sense of warmth and peace flowing through you, and of a state of calm suffusing your being.

Whether you use this breath exercise or not (I hope you do), understand that the "embrace" step is critical because it enables you to release the negative thoughts and energy that are causing your suffering. You are releasing, letting go, and detaching from all that you have held within you, and that is not serving you.

As your intense emotions dissipate, notice how much lighter you feel. And give thanks to your Higher Self for taking from you all that you no longer desire. You have cleaned house, and you are now ready to bring in fresh, powerful healing energy.

Third, REPLACE your feelings and thoughts.

Now that you have faced and embraced your original thoughts and breathed out the pain, you are in a position to replace those thoughts with a feel-better thought that makes your heart sing. You'll enjoy this last step because you get to create a movie within you that has the power to raise your vibrations. You'll feel greater peace and well-being, and you'll attract to you equivalent vibrational experiences. Here's how to "replace":

While continuing to relax by breathing deep, healing breaths, close your eyes and see yourself going to your heart. Envision a treasure chest there. It's filled with meaningful photos, images, or memories collected at special moments during your lifetime. (I suggest that you spend some time consciously filling this treasure chest so that you'll be able to easily pull out a positive image or memory at will. Examples include making love with your partner, holding your baby for the first time, experiencing a sunrise or sunset with a loved one, or being surprised by friends and loved ones at a special celebration given in your honor.)

After you open your heart's treasure chest, select a precious image and, still breathing deeply in and out, in and out, allow yourself to create your own personal movie. Experience the image with every one of your senses. If, for example, you are at the beach, hear the lapping of the waves as they roll onto the beach. Smell the divine scent of ocean water, feel the hot sand beneath your feet, taste the salt air, and enjoy the breeze as it gently kisses your face. Fully imagine yourself stretched out on your warm towel, your body completely relaxed and at peace in this heavenly place of your choice.

By engaging in your own feel-good movie for 30 to 60 seconds, you will energetically raise your vibrations and shift to a feel-better place. You can, of course, extend your movie a bit, but that's not strictly necessary.

When you've completed the Face/Embrace/Replace process, immediately place your attention on another task, errand, or item on your to-do list, such as cleaning a closet, calling a friend or relative, or writing in a journal. The idea is to distance yourself from whatever triggered your initial stressful thought or feeling. When the trigger reappears, go through the same steps. You are teaching your mind that you have the ability to overcome habitually disturbing images and thoughts.

I love Face/Embrace/Replace because it is an easy process to learn, and it can be used on a frequent basis to help you process anxiety, worry, distress, or any other imbalance of your energy. And especially as you face cancer, it can be a valuable tool for healing.

ABCs: An Alternate Method

ABCs is a method of releasing your pain that is very similar to Face/Embrace/Replace, and also helps you rebalance your body's energy flow so that you return to well-being.

Over the years, I've noticed that there are some who feel more comfortable with the ABCs process than with Face/Embrace/Replace. If that's you, please feel free to use this tool instead.

- **A is for AWARENESS and ACKNOWLEDGMENT.** Become aware of your thoughts and images at the "head" level that do not feel good at the heart or belly level. Here, you're actually facing the feelings and thoughts that are causing you to feel bad.

  Put your hand on your heart or belly and ask yourself, *Am I feeling good (or okay) or not good at this moment?* If your answer is "not good," put the same hand on your forehead. Be aware of and acknowledge the thought that created this feeling by asking yourself, *What is my thought, picture, or image that makes me not feel good?*

Now, if you wish, Acknowledge or "Embrace" the feeling by giving yourself permission to really feel the pain associated with your thought or image. Kick, scream, or cry it out—for a few moments, or more, if needed.

- **B is for BREATH and BREATHING OUT YOUR PAIN.** Learn to use the Gift of Breath and then use your ability to shift yourself energetically to a higher level of well-being. Take three deep breaths. As you breathe in, visualize yourself breathing in the colorful and magnificent energy of the Universe or God. (Yes, actually give it a color so you can "see" it more readily.)

  See and feel this powerful healing energy entering and filling every part of your body with amazing warm, relaxing energy. You may feel so relaxed, warm, and heavy and, at the same time, so light that you are aware of your body energetically shifting to a higher level of vibration.

- **C is for CHOICE and CHOOSING THOUGHTS and IMAGES THAT FEEL GOOD or BETTER.** Here's where you "Replace" your negative energetic thoughts with those that are positive. You choose thoughts and images that lighten your vibrations and enable you to allow in those experiences you have viewed as your intentions, hopes, and dreams. Every moment is about choice. Be conscious of how you are feeling, moment by moment, and choose to focus on anything and everything that brings you relief and feels better or good, including your kids, pets, loved ones, or your favorite funny video.

Use Energy Medicine to Rebalance and Heal Your Life.

As we stated in Chapter One, everything is energy. That includes our bodies, thoughts, and feelings. Most of us are not aware of this—unless we read a book like this one! However, we *do* learn about energy in biology class, where we conduct experiments that establish that energy never dies. Instead, it undergoes a nifty transformation act when necessary (Where did that boiling water go?). Well, guess what? That principle can apply to your body, thoughts, and feelings, too. Here's how.

When your energy is flowing as it needs to flow, you feel good! (Remember, healing is all about establishing balance, harmony, and peace.) But when your energy is unable to flow as it needs to flow, it becomes unbalanced, and you do not feel well. The normal pathways through which your energy needs to flow to care for your organs, etc., are blocked, meaning that excess energy is trapped in the "wrong" places. (Remember, energy never dies!) Your body is counting on you to be conscious of how you feel so that you can take the necessary steps to balance the flow of energy throughout your body and maintain wellness.

Stress (which is a normal reaction to fighting cancer) is one of these factors that tends to throw our bodies out of balance. Your brain notifies your organs, tissues, and cells that you are struggling to maintain control and balance. And before you know it, you are out of balance. The energy that *should* be flowing elsewhere in your body is being used to handle stress, and other areas of the body (like your immune system) suffer as a result.

That's where Energy Medicine comes in. Energy Medicine is not medicine in the traditional sense; rather, it is an energetic, therapeutic way of helping you to heal by balancing the flow of energy through your body. (One of these tactics is tapping, which I'll talk about in the next section of this chapter.) Ultimately, Energy Medicine gives you the power to shift your own low energetic vibrations to higher levels that produce endorphins, new vitality, mental clarity, increased calm, and well-being.

If you'd like to delve more deeply into the "whys" and "hows" of Energy Medicine, I encourage you to read *The Little Book of Energy Medicine: The Essential Guide to Balancing Your Body's Energies* by Donna Eden, as well as the award winning *Energy Medicine* by Donna Eden and her husband, renowned psychologist David Feinstein.

In the meantime, you can immediately put Eden Energy Medicine (so called because it was pioneered and developed by Donna Eden) to work for you by watching Donna Eden's *Five Minute Energy Routine,* which is available from many online sources, including YouTube at www.youtube.com/watch?v=gffKhttrRw4. In the video, Donna demonstrates each step of the routine, which includes tapping, full-body motions, breathing, and postures. The routine is designed to balance you energetically and counteract stress hormones.

I do Donna's *Five Minute Energy Routine* every morning and throughout the day when I am feeling tired, stressed, and in need of replenishing my energy. It balances me, calms me, and enables me to think, concentrate, and focus better. I used this routine many times during a recent emergency hospitalization once I felt strong enough. (Yes, I am just like you and become unbalanced and ill on occasion!) I believe that this routine enabled me to more quickly leave the hospital. And it felt so good to be doing something that helped me feel better!

It probably won't surprise you that I also teach this routine to my patients who are anxious, depressed, grieving, or ill. My patients who have taken the time and energy to practice this routine have successfully shifted to feeling more self-confident, less anxious, and healthier. If you are deeply grieving (which is likely to be the case if you're facing cancer), this routine restores much of your energy, revitalizes you, promotes peace, and enables you to feel emotionally stronger.

Also, remember that you have the choice to integrate Energy Medicine into your cancer treatment plan, along with your traditional treatments. Today there are more opportunities than ever for helping your body engage its natural healing forces. Hospitals throughout the country are integrating energetic types of medicine like tai chi, Reiki, Therapeutic Touch, and others.

If you wish to work with a certified and trained energy medicine practitioner, go online and Google *Energy Medicine with Donna Eden – Directory – Innersource*, or call Innersource directly at (541) 482-1800.

Your body is waiting for you to take charge in a good way— one that benefits the work of your cells. Before moving on to the next healing tool, I'd like to share how Energy Medicine helped several individuals do just that.

Bea's Experience with Energy Medicine: "I Always Feel Better."

A piece of Bea's legacy is the following account she chose to share with me a year and a half before her passing about how Eden Energy Medicine enabled her to have a better quality of life while dealing with her cancer challenge.

Bea had been happily working with Diana, her Eden Energy Medicine (EEM) practitioner, since receiving her third chemotherapy treatment for ovarian cancer. "The sessions are so gentle," Bea explained. "I look forward to my time with Diana because I always feel better."

Bea was diagnosed in June of 2013. At the end of July 2013, she had a hysterectomy and began her chemotherapy a few months later in October. Bea, who was 63 at the time of our interview, lived by herself and co-managed a family-owned store in Princeton, New Jersey for close to 20 years. When she was diagnosed, this family graciously and lovingly purchased a gift certificate so that Bea could have a number of EEM healing sessions with Diana. This gift proved to be invaluable to Bea.

Bea's chemotherapy protocol required five months of three-week treatments, and a double dose of chemo during one of every three weeks. Chemotherapy can be a challenging experience for many reasons, one being that it depletes you of your energy. But Bea was a fighter who persevered through challenges like this. "You do it and keep going," she said. Bea continued to go to work, even on the more difficult days. In fact, she noted that she had only taken a few days off during the entire span of treatment. She would have done this differently and taken more time off to heal, she said, if she had to do it again.

What helped her to manage the effects of the chemotherapy? It was the Eden Energy Medicine. She told me, "My biggest regret is that I did not start sooner with Diana, because I know it would have helped me better handle my surgery and chemotherapy. But Diana's schedule was full and I could not get into see her regularly until after my third chemotherapy session."

When I questioned Bea as to how EEM helped her, she replied, "My sessions made a huge difference in how I was feeling. The symptoms were the same, but after my sessions, they were much less. My headaches, including migraines, were fewer in number. In fact, I could gauge the difference between when I was seeing her and when I was not. The chemo really hits you. I always felt worse when I was unable to see Diana for a session. I just wish I could have begun sooner."

When I asked Bea if she planned to continue EEM, she vehemently said, "Absolutely, I plan to continue! This is a lifelong thing … It is noninvasive, it is natural, and I don't have to take any pills—which could be a problem."

When I questioned her as to what she would want other cancer patients to know Bea said, "I wish people could just be open-minded about this. It truly works—and you have nothing to lose. I would strongly encourage people to start it on a regular basis as soon as they are diagnosed because it can help diminish the effects of your treatments ... and you will feel better!"

Julia's Experience with Eden Energy Medicine: A Family Affair

After working in the corporate world for twenty years, Julia was beginning to feel unhappy and unfulfilled. She often found herself wondering, *What do I want to do with the rest of my life?* She knew that she was not where she was supposed to be—but had no idea where she needed to go! This nagging feeling, in conjunction with an overwhelming sense of unending fatigue, the stress of her work responsibilities, and worsening allergies was becoming too much. Yet when Julia was evaluated by her family doctor, he told her that he could find nothing wrong with her.

During this time, Julia recalled reading an article in which an oncologist had discussed Eden Energy Medicine. She found the article again, reread it, and thought to herself, *Since nothing seems to be available to help me, why not give it a shot?* So she made an appointment with Eden Energy Medicine Practitioner Diana Warren.

Julia admitted to me that in that first session, she did not understand the energetic concepts that Diana explained to her. However, she felt very comfortable with Diana. Julia says, "Though I had no clue about what it was all about, I decided that I would place myself in the hands of this warm, caring healer."

After seeing Diana for weekly Eden Energy Medicine (EEM) treatments for four months, Julia noticed that she was feeling better. She was off both of her allergy medications and her inhaler. She was no longer experiencing chronic sinusitis and bronchitis, as she had for the previous two years. "I felt whole and complete," she says. "I knew I was functioning differently. My body was in sync with itself."

During this time, Julia also experienced an "epiphany" regarding her career. She described it as a gentle knowing, yet simultaneously a powerful insight. She knew that she wanted to move in the direction of professional coaching. This made total sense to her, given her personal and professional strengths. Within ten days Julia had researched leadership coaching programs, contacted, applied to, and was accepted by Columbia University. She began her program in April of 2012 and has since graduated. All of this felt perfect and completely right to her. This, she knew, was what she was here on Earth for.

Regarding the value of Eden Energy Medicine, Julia told me, "Without this energy medicine, I would never have chosen the work I am now doing. EEM helped me to reprioritize what was important in my life. It helped me to distance myself from what was sucking my life energy and it opened up my heart so that I could align myself with what is good. It was because I was open that I could experience all of this. Thanks to EEM my body is now in balance and I am at peace with things that used to drive me bonkers—but which I now recognize as being out of my control."

The benefits of Eden Energy Medicine didn't stop with Julia, though—EEM also helped her son. Julia's son had been dealing with moderate to severe anxiety, exacerbated by his ADHD. The specialists he had been seeing and the medications he had been taking had not helped him. However, Julia's son *had* noticed that his mom was improving as she worked with Diana.

And so, at the age of 12, Julia's son started Eden Energy Medicine sessions with Diana. Though he initially did not know what to make of them, he, like his mom, allowed himself to be open to the experience and to trust Diana's ability to help him. He found each session fascinating, and spent much of his time asking Diana what she was doing and why. In fact, he became Diana's student, absorbing as much as he could about the art of energy medicine. He would say to his mom and dad, "I can't put it in words and I can't describe what is happening but I feel better; I feel I am where

I should be. I feel an alignment with myself!" Julia noted that after many months of Eden Energy Medicine sessions, her son was able to cut back to a very low dose of anxiety medication.

Julia and her son view their EEM sessions with Diana as a gift. In Julia's words, "As you get your energy in sync with yourself, you heal. And as you heal, your heart opens and you are able to see your place in the world from a different perspective. This opening of your heart allows you to grow and evolve and your soul opens to greater possibilities."

Use Energy Medicine to Tap Away Your Fears, Worries, and Stress.

It's likely that you have never heard of tapping, but it's a gift that all energetic beings have, and it's routinely used in Energy Medicine. Believe it or not, if you tap certain spots on your face, torso, and hands while thinking or talking about an upsetting image, you can unblock energies and send a new, better signal to the brain. (Unblocking negative energy is enormously helpful when facing the challenge of cancer, since your mind and body desperately need healthy, healing energy to flow unimpeded.) Tapping helps you to manage your stress and negative emotions in the short term, and in the long term, it enables you to reprogram a healthier response to the original disturbing thought, memory or image. Best of all, tapping is incredibly easy to do.

In this chapter, I'll share a simple tapping exercise with you. But know that this is just the tip of the iceberg—as I've mentioned, there are multiple places on the body where you can tap, as well as multiple tapping methods. If you'd like to learn more, I recommend reading *The Tapping Cure* by psychologist Roberta Temes. You can also seek out the work of Roger Callahan (Thought Field Therapy), Gary Craig (the Emotional Freedom Technique), and David Feinstein (Energy Psychology). There's a wealth of information about these tapping variations online, as well as videos that demonstrate where and how to tap.

I share the following tapping tool with many of my patients because it can be unobtrusively performed anytime, anywhere. Its purpose is to assist you in reducing or dissolving your fears, worries, and overall anxiety.

To start, you need to find a place on your hand called the "gamut." The gamut is located on the outside of your hand, approximately halfway between your wrist and the point where your pinkie and ring finger meet.

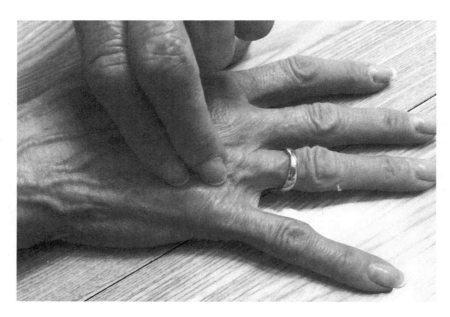

Begin by closing your eyes and scanning your body to assess your level of distress, using a scale of 1-10 (with 10 the highest and 1 the lowest level). Tap this spot with the middle three fingers of your other hand to the count of 10. Stop tapping and count to 10 again. Then resume tapping for about a minute and a half. Be sure to take deep, cleansing breaths in and out while tapping. Now, repeat the process while tapping on your other hand in the same place. (This represents one set.) Do two more sets of tapping. Then, rescan your body and rate the extent of your distress (10 being the highest level and 1 the lowest). If your sense of discomfort remains, repeat the process with three more sets and a rescanning of your body to assess your new level. Continue the process until you feel completely comfortable. You will notice that with each three sets, your numbers begin dropping and you feel more at ease.

Especially if you're new to tapping, I understand that this tool might seem strange to you. *How can tapping my hand, or any other part of my body, influence my emotions?* Here's the short answer: In the exercise I just shared, you are manipulating an energy channel called "triple warmer." This meridian is considered to be the commander in chief of the body because it "decides" when you are in danger (even if you are really not), and tells the body to prepare for war. Tapping is a way for you to "talk" to and calm your triple warmer meridian, letting it know that you are going to be okay, that you are safe, and that there is no need to worry. (If you want to know more about meridians in general and triple warmer in particular, the resources I've shared above can help, as can a quick Internet search.)

There are many variations of the triple warmer tapping exercise I've just shared. One is to simply tap on the gamut for about a minute, while deeply breathing in peace and breathing out your stressful thoughts and feelings. Another is, while continuing to tap on the gamut, to silently or verbally repeat on your in-breath, what is bothering you (e.g., *Even though I feel sad, angry, etc.*) and, on your out-breath, finish it with, *I deeply love and accept myself, love and accept myself, love and accept myself.* This programs a new, more positive wisdom into your body. After a few taps, you can shorten this phrase to, *Sad, Love myself* while continuing to tap, breathe and talk.

I encourage you to try these tapping methods and see which works best for you. My patients love tapping on the gamut because it helps them to quickly shift from a place of angst and fear to one that is more comfortable. It is especially helpful while waiting for test results or when traveling. Please believe me when I say that your body finds comfort in gentle tapping—which, if you think about it, mirrors the comforting rhythm of your heart's constant beating.

Immerse Yourself in the Present by Being Mindful.

When you experience any type of concern, grief, worry, fear, agitation, frustration, or similar emotion, you are not living in the moment, but rather in the past or future. (For example, you might be regretting past choices or worrying about what might be in store for you down the road.) And let's face it—you tend to feel a *lot* of these low-vibrational emotions when you're facing cancer. That's why mindfulness is such a crucial tool for healing—it keeps you in the present moment, where you are happiest and at your best.

Specifically, mindfulness is the practice of staying in the "now" and focusing on your thoughts, feelings, internal sensations, and external experiences with an open heart and a nonjudgmental attitude of acceptance. Research has demonstrated that mindfulness bolsters your immune system, enables you to balance your moods, improves your relationships, and creates positive changes in the parts of the brain's gray matter that influence learning, memory, empathy, and emotional regulation. Mindfulness also has the power to assist us with relaxation, and with reducing anxiety, anger, frustration and aggression.

(If you're curious about the scientific history of mindfulness, I encourage you to learn more about Jon Kabat-Zinn, who brought the many benefits of mindfulness to the public's attention when he conducted the Mindfulness-Based Stress Reduction Program at the University of Massachusetts Medical School in 1979. Kabat-Zinn's work has demonstrated how valuable and helpful mindfulness is, especially for parents, teachers, prisoners, and veterans.)

Here, I'll share a mindfulness strategy that I learned from several mindfulness teachers many years ago. I love to use it because it is simple, takes little effort to use, and best of all, it works!

To start, sit and quiet yourself with deep breathing. Focus on the in-breath entering through your nostrils and traveling to your heart, lungs and stomach. Then, watch as your out-breath carries stagnant energy up and out from your heart, lungs, and stomach and travels up through your esophagus, throat, mouth, and lips. Do this for several minutes until you begin to feel more and more relaxed and peaceful.

Now, while breathing in and out, in and out, consciously focus on the sounds that come to your attention. Attend to them, and without thought or judgment of any kind, label them *Sound*. Release your awareness of these sounds with your out-breath. So, for example, if you hear cars going by on the highway, you can label your awareness of the cars driving by as *Sound*, then detach from and release this awareness as you breathe out.

Next, focus on your thoughts while continuing to breathe deeply. When a thought rolls in (such as, *I wish I felt better*), observe it, label it *Thought*, and then release or detach from it via your out-breath. With subsequent breaths, continue to notice what comes in at the level of your mind, observe it, label it *Thought*, and release it or detach from it before you make a connection to it—all via your breath.

Now, focus on your bodily sensations. While breathing deeply and consciously, scan your body and observe or notice any sensations that capture your attention. Perhaps you notice a pain in your right arm. Observe it and label it *Sensation*, and then release it or detach from it by breathing it out.

Finally, while breathing comfortably in and out, choose to notice any scents or movements that come into your awareness. Do the same routine: Notice and observe the experience, label it *Movement* or *Scent,* and breathe it out in order to detach from your awareness of it.

As you've no doubt noticed, the pattern here is to notice, observe, label, and release or detach via the out-breath. The key to this mindfulness exercise "working" is that there is absolutely no attachment to what you observe or notice. Things come in and leave *without* you becoming emotionally or mentally attached to them, which often creates stress or worry. This helps you achieve a relaxed, peaceful state of being.

Mindfulness can be practiced anywhere, bringing you a wonderful sense of calm—and it can be done with or without labels like *Thought, Sound,* and *Movement.* Since mindfulness is an "in the moment" strategy that naturally fills you with peace, it is wonderful to use when you are feeling anxious about test results, treatment, diagnosis, and prognosis.

It is my sincere hope that some or all of these healing methods will be a huge help as you navigate some of the incredibly challenging moments that come with cancer. Just knowing that you have these tools at your disposal anytime you need them can be a source of tremendous reassurance. This is especially true once you've tried them out and found that they truly do work.

It's kind of like having a tire-changing kit and a spare in the trunk of your car, along with the knowledge of how to use them. It's no fun to break down on the side of the road, but there's so much peace in the certainty that you can "fix" the situation and find your way home again!

CHAPTER 9

Face Your Fear of Death (Synchronicities and Stories Can Help!)

~⦿⦿~

"It's only when we truly know and understand that we have a limited time on earth—and that we have no way of knowing when our time is up—that we will begin to live each day to the fullest, as if it was the only one we had."

ELISABETH KÜBLER-ROSS, MD

I know from personal experience that if you have been diagnosed with cancer, a frightening thought has almost certainly crossed your mind: "What if I die?" A huge amount of the fear associated with cancer relates to our fear of death. And while greater numbers of those people diagnosed with cancer are surviving, this disease is firmly associated with mortality in our culture's consciousness. Thus, it's perfectly normal for you to worry that cancer will lead to your death, even if your prognosis is hopeful.

Specifically, you might be grappling with one or both of these particular fears:

- What happens after death? Is there an afterlife? If so, will I suffer? Or does everything just end?
- It's not *death* I'm afraid of so much, but the *process* of dying. I dread the pain, treatment, and decline that might be ahead of me.

In this chapter, I'd like to address each of those fears.

Death is a Transition.

You may believe—or fear—that "you" will cease to exist after death, or worse, that you will be painfully punished for the transgressions you committed on earth. My intention is not to belittle any religious beliefs you may hold, but right here, up-front, I want to emphasize that death is not "the end," nor is it a punishment. It's merely a transition. Energy does not die; it changes from one form to another. In this case, the physical energy of the body is transformed into nonphysical, spiritual energy.

I'm not saying that only to reassure you, but because I firmly believe it's true. In both my research and my work with grieving patients over the past several decades, I have gathered a wealth of evidence that an afterlife is real. There is much evidence that suggests that this afterlife is certainly not an isolated realm of eternal suffering, but rather a wonderful spiritual realm that is intertwined with the waking world.

The experiences of my patients, as well as my own experiences, have convinced me that after the body dies, the spirit transitions into pure loving energy that retains awareness and continues to exist within the fabric of the universe. Following death (whether cancer is the direct cause or not), you can continue to observe and touch the lives of the people you love, just as your own deceased loved ones are able to touch yours.

Yes, your deceased loved ones are still with you, aware of what you're doing, thinking, and praying. And often, they reach out to let you know that you have grieved enough, that they are safe, that they still care, and even—sometimes—to influence your decisions and actions. I find this an amazingly comforting and even joyful perspective. I believe that if you can accept and internalize this truth, it can completely eradicate your fear of death.

Think back on your own experiences. Have you ever felt close to a loved one who has passed away? Perhaps you occasionally catch a whiff of your grandmother's perfume in an empty house or hear the clicking paw-steps of a beloved pet that has passed on. Or you consistently see the type of bird your friend loved to watch, even in unexpected places. Or maybe you've simply *known* something you were never explicitly told, or have been vividly visited by a loved one in a dream.

It's easy to write these incidents off as coincidences, but I truly don't believe they are. Instead, they are *synchronicities*, and they can be a valuable tool in helping you face your fear of death.

Synchronicities Bring Beauty, Comfort, and Lessons.

Synchronicities are events that *appear* to be coincidental, but actually, they're far too meaningful to be called coincidences. The truth is, miracles are happening every moment of every day. We often do not realize we have just experienced a miracle or synchronicity because our perspective may be just a bit too narrow to include such a possibility. But as we journey through life, we develop maturity and the willingness to consider thoughts, ideas, and perspectives we could not and would not entertain in our earlier years. Recognizing that there is more to life than what we can see, touch, or feel is a significant part of this experience called life.

A willingness to open yourself to synchronicities can bring comfort to those who are experiencing the pain of anticipatory fear and grief. Think about it: Especially as you face your challenge with cancer, if you were given indications that once out of the body you might continue to be present for your loved ones who are alive, wouldn't this bring you some comfort and, on some level, reassure you that life and your relationships do not necessarily end with physical death?

Each time you listen to an inspirational story, read of a synchronicity, or learn of signs and miracles others have experienced, you open the door of your heart a bit more to the possibility of possibilities. These possibilities gradually chip away at your long-standing beliefs and rational ways of approaching life and death. You get to choose whether to fear or not fear what follows this lifetime. I've found that the more stories you hear, the more you realize you can either live stuck in your fears and your grief, or you can adapt to a new way of looking at your situation—one that will be more soothing and peaceful for you.

Personally, the stunning stories shared with me by my patients and the research I have conducted have enabled me to be at peace with what comes next … though, at this time, I am far from ready to leave those I love.

Joni James Aldrich, author of numerous books including *The Saving of Gordon: Lifelines to W-I-N Against Cancer* and *Connecting through Compassion: Guidance for Family and Friends of a Brain Cancer Patient*, had a similar experience. In the years following the death of her husband Gordon from multiple myeloma (a rare blood cancer), she began considering the possibility that loved ones and angels may very well be a part of our reality.

This topic came up when Joni interviewed me on the *Ladies Who Inspire*, a radio show she hosts for The Cancer Support Network. At the beginning of the interview, Joni and I discussed a recent event in which a teen who was trapped in her crushed car after being hit by a drunk driver asked rescue workers to pray for her. As they began praying, a man dressed like a Catholic priest appeared—seemingly out of thin air. His presence brought a gentle, warm calmness that touched everyone, and he promised that more help would soon arrive. Once it did, he vanished. Everyone who experienced the event—the teen, the rescue workers, and even a news reporter who covered the story—felt that the man had been an angel and that Katie's rescue and survival were a miracle.

After discussing this story with me, Joni asked her listeners to send her their extraordinary stories of signs from loved ones, the divine, and angels. And they kept coming and coming. Joni says that stories like these have opened her heart to the ongoing connection our loved ones maintain with us, and have provided her with great comfort. She acknowledges that our fear of death diminishes with each and every story we process and integrate.

Others' Stories Can Help You Come to Terms with Your Fears.

Whenever you are preparing to face anything new and different (death, and what happens after, certainly qualify!), or even if you "only" fear that a dreaded event *might* happen, you will experience fear and anxiety. The more you know about the situation you are going into, the more control you'll feel that you have, and the more comfortable you will be. Remember, low-vibrational emotions, no matter their origins, will impede your healing journey.

This is why I strongly recommend reading stories from those who have had experiences with the afterlife, with dying and returning to life (near-death experiences, or NDEs), and with what we view as spiritual (Heaven, God, Angels, and all that is Divine—often, these stories involve synchronicities). Great examples of these books include the recent bestsellers *Proof of Heaven* by Eben Alexander, MD, and *Dying to Be Me* by Anita Moorjani.

Other excellent books dealing with NDEs I highly recommend include:

- *Embraced by the Light* by Betty J. Eadie
- *Death Is of Vital Importance: On Life, Death, and Life After Death* by Elisabeth Kübler-Ross, MD
- *On Life after Death* by Elisabeth Kübler-Ross, MD
- *Life After Life* by Raymond A. Moody Jr., MD
- *Reflections on Life After Life* by Raymond A. Moody Jr., MD
- *Life After Loss: Conquering Grief and Finding Hope*, by Raymond A. Moody Jr., MD and Dianne Arcangel
- *The Light Beyond* by Raymond A. Moody Jr., MD
- *Closer to the Light: Learning from the Near-Death Experiences of Children* by Melvin Morse, MD with Paul Perry

- *Transformed by the Light: The Powerful Effect of Near-Death Experiences on People's Lives* by Melvin Morse, MD and Paul Perry
- *Parting Visions: Uses and Meanings of Pre-Death, Psychic and Spiritual Experiences* by Melvin Morse, MD with Paul Perry

I also suggest that you read stories from professionals who work in a hospice situation because the repetition of patterns they write about will be sure to challenge your thoughts about death and dying process, as well as the afterlife. In particular, I recommend *Final Gifts* by hospice nurses Maggie Callanan and Patricia Kelley.

All of these stories will serve as inspiration for you and will help you to heal, relax, and vibrate at a higher level during your journey and at the time of your transition—whenever and for whatever reason that takes place.

Finally, I myself have written two books, *Touched by the Extraordinary* and *Touched by the Extraordinary: Healing Stories of Love, Loss and Hope*, that describe how numerous people—many of whom are my patients—were visited and reassured by departed loved ones. In particular, Book Two of *Touched by the Extraordinary: Healing Stories of Love, Loss and Hope* is filled with stories that my patients and friends shared with me. All demonstrate how the power of love makes it possible for our deceased loved ones to continue their loving role in our lives.

Here, I would like to share a few of the stories I have collected. They demonstrate that our essence—or spirit—lives on in a meaningful way after death.

Allie's Signs

Allie, the daughter of Elena, lost her life in a freak horseback riding accident in 2004 at the age of nine. During our many sessions, Allie's mom shared numerous stories with me of how Allie would creatively come to say *Hi* and give *I love you* messages to her family.

Allie, a true animal lover, often chose a Northern Mocking Bird, which the family came to call the Allie Bird, as well a particular squirrel. The Allie Bird even traveled from Georgia, where Allie died, to the family's new home in Pennsylvania. There it would come and sit by the house, follow Elena when she drove into and out of their driveway, and even into and through their home. The squirrel would come and sit for hours by their front door.

Here's my favorite Allie story: Within days of her death and funeral, Allie chose to express her presence through her favorite stuffed animals—and Allie had many, many stuffed animals. The family had gathered in Allie's playroom for the purpose of each choosing one of Allie's special stuffed animals to take home. Almost immediately, the family heard a bark coming from the pile of animals in the room. Elena went over, picked up a white poodle, and turned it off. No sooner had she done this than they heard barking coming from another toy, a little brown dog. However, *this* dog was voice-activated—and no one in the room had the microphone into which you spoke to activate the toy. This toy also walked, sat, and stood.

Allie's beloved Uncle Bill was seated in the room watching this. You can imagine his surprise when the toy dog walked right over to him while barking. Elena pulled the toy back, but to the delight and amazement of everyone gathered there, the little dog walked right back to him. All of this was too much for Uncle Bill. He got up and moved to the other side of the room. And what do you think the toy dog did? Well, of course it walked right over to him.

When it was time to leave for home, Elena explained to Uncle Bill, who hadn't planned to take the little brown dog home, that he needed to do this because Allie had made it clear that this was the toy she wanted him to have. Elena also explained that if Uncle Bill wished for Allie to communicate with him, as she had done with the dog, he needed to ask Allie for a sign.

As for Elena, she chose the small white toy poodle, which she keeps on her dresser. She has told me that often, while she is reading a book, the toy dog has unexpectedly barked at her. Elena knows this is her Allie saying *Hi, Mom. I'm here and I love you.*

A 93rd Call for Malika

This is another favorite story of mine because it has the power to diminish our fears of dying while simultaneously demonstrating that our loved ones find ways to offer us their guidance, love, and assistance. Essentially, they find ways to continue taking care of us … because this is the power of love.

Malika, a high school senior whose mom had died several years before, was in need of $800.00 to pay for repairs on the old car her dad had purchased for her. Malika's dad had been working to pay off the medical bills that had accumulated during her mom's illness, and therefore could not financially help his daughter.

Malika explained to me that she had been home doing her homework when she felt an intuitive nudge to turn on her radio. She heard the message, *Dial this number, and if you are 93rd caller, you will win the prize.* Malika called in, but the line was busy. A few minutes later, she felt nudged once again to call back. This time, Malika made it through and, much to her amazement and delight, learned that she was the 93rd caller and would be receiving a prize of one thousand dollars!

Malika later told her dad, *It was Mommy who told me to call again.* Malika now had the money she needed—and then some—

to pay for her car repairs. And even more important, she had received loving validation that her mother was aware of her circumstances and was always with her.

Signs of Forever Love from Alicia's Parents

Alicia's parents died too early in her adulthood. Her dad died several years after an accident had left him with significant brain damage, and her mom died a little more than a decade later. Alicia had grieved deeply for her parents, knowing that they had left her far too early in her life's journey. However, Alicia found comfort in their creative ways of letting her know they were with her—ways that have brought her gentle comfort and that have lessened her fear of death.

Alicia's father will say hello to her on the highway by means of large trucks that bear his name (Werner) in huge letters. Alicia also described to me how both her mother and her father let her know they were present by gently touching her on the back while she was sleeping, or by becoming an invisible force field she bumped into when moving through her hallway.

Recently, Alicia shared with me that when she is experiencing significant stress, her mom will let her know she is right there with her and will comfort her in a very special way. While in the midst of feeling overwhelmed, Alicia will feel a warmth suddenly move over and through her. She intuitively knows that this is her mom, and the experience has always brought great peace. In particular, Alicia recalls feeling this warmth while preparing for her daughter's sweet sixteen, graduation, and more recently, while preparing for her daughter's wedding shower and wedding.

It is moments like these that enable Alicia and many others to feel a genuine awareness that death does not end either who we are or our ability to lovingly connect with our loved ones. In fact, there is not a day that passes in which a patient, friend, neighbor, family member, or even stranger shares with me a story that has helped to diminish their own fear of death, as well as provided them with needed comfort.

If you allow yourself to become open to them, the vibration of these stories has the ability to help you perceive life and death differently—and more comfortably. The choice is yours.

You Have the Power to Manage Your Treatment.

As I noted at the beginning of this chapter, perhaps you are at peace with death, but desperately fear your illness's treatment and/ or the process of dying. This is more than understandable. Cancer can be a painful disease, and its treatments, while meant to heal you, can also be very unpleasant. I know this firsthand. And over the years, many of my patients have shared with me that they do not fear death as much as the dying process—and more bluntly, the pain that may be associated with it.

In fact, as I write this book, my friend Shana has just been diagnosed with non-Hodgkin lymphoma. Shana is an outstanding intuitive healer and is not afraid of death. However, she knows the power of the chemotherapy her doctors want to use to restore her body, and she *does* have concerns and fears about that—though I know her well enough to believe she will overcome all that she has to endure. And Elliot, a gentleman in my practice, has recently made the significant decision to move to Hospice care after being on a ventilator for an extended period of time. Justifiably, he is also afraid.

In the second half of this chapter, I'll discuss several options that may soothe your fears and help you manage the process of dying.

Energy Medicine Can Provide Peace.

In Chapter Eight, I talked about Energy Medicine: what it is and how it works. I have watched specific forms of Energy Medicine (like Reiki, Therapeutic Touch and Eden Energy Medicine) transform patients', friends', and loved ones' agitation, discomfort, and concerns to a more peaceful and comfortable state.

I recall being in the hospital room of a dear friend of mine who was dying. I placed my hands across her head, stroked her arms, and gently ran my hands through her hair. (Not having received my training in Eden Energy Medicine at the time, I was using my own form of energy medicine, combined with Reiki.) When the hospital hospice nurse entered the room and began caring for my friend, she commented that she was aware that the energy in the room had changed, and asked if I had been using Reiki with her patient. In other words, this nurse validated for me that my loving intentions had helped to shift the energy, providing her patient (my friend) with greater peace and comfort. I was touched, and more than a bit comforted myself.

Hospice Can Diminish Discomfort.

Hospice is intended to provide those who are extremely ill and/ or dying with access to the circumstances, people, medications, and environment that make living as comfortable as possible, and the dying process both peaceful and one not to fear. It focuses more on quality of life rather than the illness. And while there are occasional exceptions, this is usually what occurs. Fortunately, we live in a time in which we have the medication and technology to make dying "better" by making it more tranquil and pain-free.

Sometimes, families choose a hospice program that allows their loved ones to be cared for and/or to die at home, providing the patient with a sense of soothing stability and familiarity.

Others choose a hospice program in a nursing home, assisted living facility, or in a hospital. So many hospice facilities are designed to look like a home setting in order to provide family, visitors, friends, and the patient with what is emotionally, physically, and spiritually needed for support and saying goodbye.

Caregivers Can Assist the Process of Dying.

Here, I want to speak directly to readers who are caregivers for a dying loved one. (If you yourself are facing cancer, you may want to ask your caregiver to read this section.) Wherever your loved one is, be sure to be his or her advocate. Being the advocate for your loved one (or having your own!) is an excellent way to provide or restore a sense of some control in a situation where control often feels out of your hands.

First, do what you can to ensure that your loved one is comfortable. Too often, without an advocate, the patient's need for pain medication is not met. He or she may be over-medicated or under-medicated. Trust your intuition if you sense that your loved one is having too much discomfort, and get help! Call the hospice agency or even your own doctor if you are not hearing back or feeling dissatisfied with what is occurring.

Secondly, if your loved one is preparing to die, know that he or she may fervently wish to have family and close friends present. He or she may also explicitly wish to say goodbye. I have been with many patients over the years who appear not to be conscious and alert in the days leading up to their departure. But often, just before they die, they become alert enough to say their goodbyes to family members who have come to be by their bedside. In fact, many often have a deceptive burst of energy just before their departure. Keep in mind, though, that goodbyes need to be done with gentleness and peacefulness while honoring your loved one, rather than creating a circus-type atmosphere.

On the other hand, some people would prefer to make their departure with no one present—often because they know their family members can't handle their death, or simply do not wish them to leave just yet. Psychiatrist Elisabeth Kübler-Ross wrote of this numerous times throughout her many works dealing with death and dying. She described stories of her patients, especially children, waiting until their loved ones had left the room (perhaps to get something to eat or to go to a restroom) after sitting for hours by their bedside. That is when the patient would choose to die.

Please know that the departures I have described are applicable for the majority of people. Yet, in my years of working with those dealing with cancer, death, and dying, I have had less than a handful of individuals who made it clear they did not wish to go peacefully. They wished to fight their cancer to their final dying moments—and they did. I am saddened by this, but it was their choice. My sadness comes because I know that it is in our soul's best interest to leave the body in a higher vibratory state. Our departure and transformation from the physical to the nonphysical state is less painful when we choose peace.

Again, Others' Stories Can Enlighten and Comfort.

Already in this chapter I've pointed out that others' stories can be a tremendously valuable tool in facing your fear of death. Here, I'd like to look at near-death experiences (or NDEs), which can help you face your fear of the *process of dying*, specifically.

My research dealing with consciousness and my work with the dying have convinced me that in the days leading up to our physical departure, our consciousness (the part of us that is separate from our brain and body, and that allows us to communicate with others, mind to mind) travels between the physicality of the body to a nonphysical realm. Those who have had near-death experiences have written stunning and amazing accounts that reinforce this truth. Their stories of moving up to ceilings and out of the buildings, and of observing events in the rooms next to where their body rests, are impressive and powerfully convincing.

Additionally, the research concerning those who have had near-death experiences and the observations of those who work with individuals nearing their final transitions each provide numerous stories of patients being visited by deceased family members and friends. In *Touched by the Extraordinary*, there are several stories from my patients and friends whose dying parents spoke to them of their family members coming to see them during the night. Transitions usually occurred within hours or a few days of these visits.

I share this information with you because hearing about the experiences of others has the power to open your heart and mind to new perspectives and possibilities. Reading about near-death experiences may reassure you that throughout the process of dying you will not be alone.

Spend the Time You Have Left Living Fully.

Ultimately, of course, all of us—cancer patient or not—will face death. And we must come to terms with that reality in order to live a rich, joyful life. One of cancer's "gifts" is that it pushes people to confront the fear of death *now*, rather than avoiding and suppressing the topic indefinitely. Again, to reiterate an important point here: Giving yourself permission to hear, read, and discuss stories and research that highlight the real possibility that life does not end with death can and does contribute to a change in your perceptions. Making peace with death—and even welcoming its spiritual aspects—will allow you to spend the time you do have left (whether it's measured in months, years, or decades) living fully and without fear.

CHAPTER 10

Connect with Your Higher Power and Grow Your Spirit

"There's nothing you can do with love. All you can do is experience it. That's as intimate as you can ever be with another human being. You can hug him, you can kiss him, you can pick him up, take him home, cuddle him, feed him, give him your money, give him your life—and that's not it. Love is nothing you can demonstrate or prove. It's what you are. It's not a doing. It can't be 'done,' it's too vast to do anything with. As you open to the experience of love, it will kill who you think you are. It will have no other. It will kill anything in its way."

BYRON KATIE

"The truth is that we are always moving toward mystery and so we are far closer to what is real when we do not see our destination clearly …"

RACHEL NAOMI REMEN, MD

Let me start out by saying I know that words like "Higher Power" and "Spirituality" are loaded. While some readers will feel quite comfortable with them, others may not. In fact, for some readers, these references may evoke feelings of scorn, betrayal, disappointment, and confusion. Others might be uninterested in spirituality, or at best, apathetic. Still others might consider themselves outright nonbelievers: atheistic or agnostic. (I can't tell you how often I've heard people say wistfully "I wish I could believe in a Higher Power but I just can't.")

That's why, before you read any further, I want to clear some things up:

This chapter, and this book, are not affiliated with any particular religious tradition. You don't have to be affiliated with a particular tradition, either (or indeed, "religious" at all) to benefit from them.

When I use words like "Higher Power," "Source," and "God," I am not referring to any particular being. Instead, I hope you will read them through the lens of your own beliefs. To you, a Higher Power might mean Jesus, Buddha, the Virgin Mary, Allah, Nature, or the Universe.

Especially if you're atheist, agnostic, or simply unsure of how you feel about spirituality, it may help you to know that my research and conversations with those who have had NDEs (near-death experiences) points to the truth that *we* are our Higher Power. What I mean is, we are not separate from our Source; it is not a vengeful or judgmental being looking "down" on us. Rather, we are one with, or connected to, our Source. Additionally, this means that we are Love—unconditional Love—something we tend to not see or accept, but which we are here to learn.

However you choose to perceive your Higher Power, your Higher Power can help you to grow spiritually, connect you to the universe's divine love, and raise your vibrational energy.

Cancer Is a Catalyst for Growing Your Spirit.

In the introduction to this book, I mentioned that cancer can be a catalyst for growing your spirit. What I'm saying is that even if you've never considered yourself a "spiritual" person, the journey you are on can help you access a part of yourself that has previously been unawakened. I've seen nonbelievers become fervent believers, or at least find that the solid rock wall of their doubt is worn away, leaving a dawning sense of hopefulness that perhaps there *is* a loving God out there after all! Here are a few reasons why:

- **Cancer slows you down.** Because cancer drains you of the energy to support a fast-paced life, for the first time in a long time (and in some cases, for the first time ever), you may have time to connect with God, your Source, or your Higher Power, and focus your energy on your spirit. Connection often takes place when you are "forced" to be still; when you are unable to run around completing errands or taking care of your personal or professional obligations.

- **Cancer shifts your priorities.** A cancer diagnosis prompts you to re-evaluate your life through a new lens: "What is *really* important to me? What legacy do I want to leave? Am I living for myself or for others?" If religion and/or spirituality were once part of your life but have been pushed to the back burner, the answers to these questions might cause your priorities to shift, bringing nourishing your spirit back to the forefront. What you are doing is letting go of the past and shifting to what you need in the present moment. This is a good thing, because you're choosing to love yourself first, rather than feeling responsible for the rest of the world. After you learn to love yourself first, then you can begin to re-evaluate your need to be responsible for others.

- **Cancer makes you realize you may need help.** Because cancer also strips you of your feelings of safety, stability, and power, it may prompt you to ask for help from a Being higher than yourself. (I have noticed that this is true not only for religious cancer patients, but also for individuals who have not previously believed in a Higher Power, or who may have distanced themselves from a Higher Power in the past.)

  Several patients in my practice have demonstrated that even clergy who are challenged by cancer become more aware of the nature of their relationship with their Source. They, too, ask for help, and find that cancer has the power to shift their perspectives of what is sacred and holy in their lives. Cancer has this effect on all of us, sometimes causing us to scream out in fury to our Source that this could be happening (especially if we feel we have been good souls trying to do the right thing), and other times, causing us to ask for assistance in navigating our path to wellness from a place of deep humility.

Here's how cancer can help you grow your spirit ... and help you heal.

- **Cancer prompts you to look for hope.** After a cancer diagnosis, you are physically and emotionally vulnerable. And being vulnerable forces you to open your heart to the possibility that possibilities *other* than decline and death exist. Hope comes to you from books (like this one) that share stories and tools to help you learn the art of surviving and thriving. Hope can come from support groups, from choosing to connect with other cancer patients on the Internet, and from simply making the decision to adopt a more positive attitude. Wherever hope comes from, it allows in higher energetic forces—angels, guides, masters, or your Source—that can step in and assist you.

- **Cancer shows you that miracles do exist.** Difficult times are gifts because they enable you to discover that you are not alone, that your prayers are answered (though not always immediately or in quite the way you requested), that miracles do happen, and that love is what you are here for. As you experience these positive energetic forces, you grow your spirit.

Those who are challenged by cancer and other illnesses have frequently shared stories with me of their experiences they call synchronicities (not coincidences, because they involve a meaningful connection that feels miraculous ... and perhaps *is* miraculous!). As you navigate your way through the journey of healing, you'll begin to notice these strange but wonderful moments in which your needs are being met, such as an appointment or hospital room suddenly showing up when needed. Patients have frequently told me that just when they had the thought or need to see me, my assistant would call them to arrange the appointment they desired. These moments and synchronicities have led them to feel that they are being watched over and protected.

When synchronicities happen in your own life, you'll begin to wonder *why*—how it is that your desires are being addressed. Just by considering other possibilities, you'll begin to shift to a higher vibration that feels better and enables you to experience more hope and inspiration: just what the doctor ordered! And as you consider the meaning of synchronicities, why you are here, the reasons for your illness, and the lessons you are learning, you'll gradually recognize that there is so much more to reality and to *you* than what you have been taught! Your head and mind might grapple with this experience, but your heart will find comfort in finally sensing an alignment with your intuitive knowing of who you really are. It is in this manner that you connect with your Higher Wisdom or Power and grow your spirit.

- **Cancer can help you feel empowered.** My patients come to me initially feeling frightened, unsure, and wondering what steps they need to take to become the victor in their new life challenge. Yet, when they leave my practice, they almost all feel a sense of increased self-worth, greater empowerment, and more connected with their inherent gift of intuition.

    I listen to my patients as they share extraordinary experiences that include a heightened awareness of forces working in their lives—forces of which they'd previously had little awareness. I notice that their perspectives about life and death are slowly changing the nature of reality, and are inviting miracles into their lives. My patients become more willing to accept the possibility that they may not be alone and that love continues even after death. As a result, they feel more at peace, more confident, and more joyful. They have learned to listen to their inner wisdom, which results in the expansion, growth, and healing of their spirits.

Before sharing tools that you can use to grow your own spirit, I'd like to tell you about three individuals I know, and how being connected to their Higher Powers helped them to heal.

Linda's Story: Angels Bring Healing!

Linda had been extremely vigilant regarding the medicines her oncologist prescribed to prevent further growth of her tumor. The problem was that she was experiencing so much discomfort throughout her joints that she felt like "an old woman", to use her words. Linda felt that her quality of life had been significantly impaired by these medications, and she wished she did not need to be taking them so often and in such high doses. These were her thoughts as she and her husband traveled to Florida for a few days of vacation.

Being an exceptionally organized woman, Linda kept her medication in the same pocket of her handbag at all times. Shortly after arriving in Florida, she went to her bag when she knew it was time to take the medicine. To her amazement and distress, she found only an empty pocket where her bottle of medicine should have been. Naturally, she thought that she had probably placed the bottle in another section of her bag. But, after emptying the contents of her handbag, retracing her steps, checking her car, and having her husband, Bob, help her in the search, Linda knew the bottle was missing.

The couple's problem seemed to increase in severity when they tried to order another bottle from the drugstore—and were told that their insurance company was not permitting a duplication of the medication. Bob spent hours trying to find a way for Linda to be able to have what she needed while they were away.

As with everything in life, though, another side of this situation was evolving—a side that seemed to be a gift! Linda began noticing within a day that she had fewer aches and pains, and that she was feeling years younger. Her vitality was returning, and she felt better.

Within a few days, Bob was finally able to get permission from the insurance firm to have a local drugstore provide Linda with medication. What was especially interesting and fascinating was that when Linda went to put the new bottle in her handbag, in the same place she always kept it, her old bottle was right there in its usual place.

Linda broke into smiles and laughter. She knew her angels had been lovingly caring for her and just wanted her to have a break.

You see, Linda talks to and works with her angels on a moment to moment basis. As she began to experience an improved quality of life, Linda repeatedly thanked her angels for creating circumstances that prevented her from taking the medication that caused her discomfort. She was grateful for her respite. Additionally, she was becoming aware of the possibility that perhaps she did not need to be taking as high a dose of this particular medication, and she knew that she would be addressing this possibility with her doctors.

For Linda, this certainly wasn't an isolated incident. When Linda was diagnosed with breast cancer, she knew she would have to make choices that would contribute to the direction her healing journey would take. She and her husband moved forward with as much spiritual guidance they could enlist. An integral part of Linda's journey has been her awareness of her angels and the connection she has with her Source. She is receptive to her higher wisdom, and regularly asks for its guidance. Linda is aware of how much her cancer journey has enabled her and her husband to grow spiritually, and she is grateful for the peace and power they have garnered along the way.

Barry's Story: The Healing Power of Prayer

Barry is an old, dear friend of mine. And while he has not been faced with cancer, his experiences still strongly demonstrate how powerful prayer and a spiritual connection can be.

Barry, a very religious and highly spiritual soul, prays daily upon awakening and in the evening before retiring. He feels exceptionally close to his angels, to God, and to friends and family who are no longer here physically. In fact, he has experienced an extraordinary number of experiences that I view as miracles. (Many of his stories have appeared in both of my *Touched by the Extraordinary* books.)

For close to seven years, Barry has been experiencing increasingly intense pain in his feet. This is a significant problem because his work requires that he be on his feet for as many as eight hours a day! Barry recently told me that about six months ago he added some additional requests to his morning prayer ritual. Specifically, he began asking God to bless his heart with even more love, to bless his hands so that he could continue doing his work effectively and productively, and to bless his feet and ankles so that he would have a reduction of pain and an increase in his comfort and ability to work.

Sure enough, Barry's pain levels have receded. In fact, as of this writing he can stand on his feet for hours without discomfort. In other words, his prayers were answered. Barry smiled as he told me this story, fully aware that when he puts out requests to his Source, he is heard.

Hanna's Story: Prayer and Intention Invite a Miracle.

This story was shared with me by the mother of a young child, Hanna, who was taken to the hospital and diagnosed with possible leukemia. Her parents were, of course devastated, and were told that if there was no change in their daughter's platelet count by the early part of the following week, they would need to immediately begin treatment for her. Hanna's parents brought their daughter home and called their friends, neighbors, and family members, requesting that prayers be immediately offered for their daughter.

Hanna's mom and dad were also familiar with the research regarding the power of energetic intention and the power of touch. Throughout the weekend, they made a point of sending their daughter healing and loving energy. They visualized this energy coursing through her each time they walked by her, held her, and hugged or kissed her.

When the family returned to the hospital on Monday morning, they were delighted with the change in Hanna's platelet numbers, which had dramatically shifted. Over the next week, the numbers continued to improve, though not as dramatically as during the first few days. The family was, of course, relieved and delighted. They had experienced the amazing power of prayer and intention.

How Can You Nourish Your Spiritual Foundation?

According to David R. Hawkins, MD, PhD, spiritual development is not an accomplishment but a way of life. It is an orientation that bring its own rewards, and what is important is the direction of one's motives.

I agree with that assessment. To grow spiritually and connect with your Higher Power, you can't use the tools I'm about to share once or twice—they have to become habit. As you engage in any or all of them, I encourage you to request the help you need from the Universe, God, your angels, or your Source. And remember, as we discussed in Chapter Six, the healing you need may be spiritual as well as physical. All of us, cancer patients or not, are spiritual beings (which refers to our awareness that we are so much more than a physical body and mind), and the part of us that is Divine love and energy needs to seek growth and balance.

Here are a few tools you can use to grow spiritually during your cancer journey:

- **Pray.** Set aside time to pray for others, for the planet and, of course, for yourself. Prayer is as simple as saying the words, "Please help me (or a loved one)." It can be more—much more—if you wish. But what matters is that you ask. You need to ask, affirm, and to be open, in order to receive. Direct your requests to your personal Higher Power—again, that might be God, Nature, Divine Love, or any other divinity, deity, or force that resonates with you. What's important are the thoughts, intentions, and vibrations that you are releasing into the universe, and those that you, in turn, are receiving.

In *The Lost Mode of Prayer*, Gregg Braden suggests that you need to pray with your heart full of gratitude and appreciation, and affirm that your prayers have already been answered. I have been praying in this manner for many years, because it feels right for me. Rather than focusing on what you are lacking and do not have, focus on what you wish to have as though you already have it. A simple, powerful prayer can be "Thank you, God, for helping me with this," or, "I am so grateful to you for making this possible for me." It is all about that feeling of acknowledgement—that what you're praying for is a "done deal."

Remember, everything is vibration. Approaching prayer from a place of lack puts low energy vibrations out into the universe. However, praying with gratitude—affirming that what you want is already yours, or at least is on its way to you—is a higher, more positive, more hopeful energy. Praying from lack leaves you feeling without power; praying as if you already have your heart's desires empowers you. Honestly, we need to feel in every cell of our being that our prayers have already been answered ... and express our heartfelt thanks for this as well.

When I pray, I have a prayer list that I use to guide me as I offer several of my favorite prayers on behalf of my patients, loved ones, friends, family, and pets. I would like to share one of my favorite prayers with you. It's from Lorna Byrne, author of *Angels in My Hair*. It was created by God, given to the Archangel Michael, and passed on to

Lorna who works as a healer in Ireland. I have memorized it and offer it for everyone I care about—myself included. It is nondenominational and serves everyone!

A Healing Prayer from God to Michael

Pour out Thy healing angels,
Thy Heavenly Host upon me (or, upon any name you would like to insert)
And upon those that I love. (or, upon those that another person loves)
Let me feel the beam of Thy (or, Let her or him)
Healing Angels upon me, (or, upon him or her)
The light of Your Healing Hands.
I will let Thy healing begin,
Whatever way God grants it.
Amen

- **Connect with the Divine in Nature.** After an unexpected major surgery related to my cancer I found myself sidelined from many of the activities that had previously filled my days. I needed to give my body plenty of rest so that it would be able to heal. And so I found myself sitting for long periods of time in my garden room or on my back porch, observing rabbits, squirrels, deer, and an array of fascinating birds as they went about their business.

  This turned out to be a profound gift. Surrounded by Mother Nature, I felt the rhythm of my thoughts change, and I knew that my spirit was healing along with my body. Tuning into nature allowed me to reconnect with God and feel a oneness with my Source, everyone, and everything. The bottom line is, nature was and is an integral part of my healing—and can be for you if you allow it to be.

I'll discuss the healing properties of Nature, as well as how you can tap into them, in Chapter Twenty. For now, know that distancing yourself from the busy, chaotic, stressful, and often-artificial rhythm of everyday life and immersing yourself in Divinely-inspired nature can help you to find calmness, balance, and spiritual peace.

- **Tune into your inner guidance system via meditation (It's as easy as focusing on your breath!).** This may be the first time you've ever realized you have an inner guidance system. You do, and you need to learn to use it! In fact, I always explain to my patients that healing is an inside job, driven by your intuition (or inner wisdom). It is through your intuition that you receive guidance from your own Higher Wisdom, as well as from the people who are working to assist you in your healing endeavors.

Your inner wisdom is available for the asking, but first, you need to relax your entire being so that you can shift to a higher vibration. This will allow you to more easily receive the guidance you desire. A simple meditative exercise enables you make this shift. Here's how to tune in:

First, set the mental intention, such as "I wish to receive guidance from (or connect with) my Higher Power and those who work with me, regarding my concern." Then state your concern, such as "What are the best treatments or doctors to consider, meet with, or engage in?"

Now, use meditative breath to shift your energy to a higher, more receptive energetic vibration. Here's how: Focus on your inhalation breath entering your nostrils and then traveling to your heart, lungs, and belly. See and feel this taking place. Next, focus on your exhalation breath traveling up from your belly, heart, and lungs and out through your throat and mouth, carrying away the negative energy attached to your thoughts of stress and discomfort. Notice how your body increasingly relaxes with each breath.

And now, once again, ask to receive, and then observe what pictures, images, and videos come pouring in. Note them as you continue breathing in and out in a relaxed fashion—while simultaneously remaining aware of how your body is feeling heavier, warmer, and more relaxed. Record your observations when finished.

"To become more conscious is the greatest gift to give the world; more-over, in a ripple effect, the gift comes back to its source ..."
RACHEL NAOMI REMEN, MD

Once you have learned to tap into your inner guidance system, you can also use it to live consciously. Let your inner voice tell you how you're feeling at each moment, and if necessary, do the work of shifting away from what causes you distress so that you can focus on what makes you feel better. Yes, this does take practice, but by practicing the techniques I've shared in this book (Face/ Embrace/ Replace, the ABC's, Mindfulness, Tapping, etc.) you can learn the art of living consciously. You will know you are succeeding because you will begin to catch yourself shifting toward higher vibrational experiences, and you will feel so much more joy—an important component of healing and growing your spirit!

• **Feed your mind spiritual food.** Seeking out and reading inspirational materials can answer questions you may have about spirituality, help you to better understand the Divine, and provide tools and tactics to help your spirit heal and grow—all at your own pace. These materials can be religious in nature, or not. That said, feeding your mind is also a highly personal activity. Don't force yourself to do, read, or participate in anything that doesn't feel intuitively good to you.

In the appendix at the back of this book, you'll find a list of recommended resources, many of which may help to nurture your spirit.

• **Connect with a supportive community. All of us need to feel we belong to someone or something. Belonging expedites healing!** Knowing there is a niche in which you can and do feel safe and comfortable contributes to a healing of mind, body, and soul. Spirituality isn't something that you have to pursue alone. If you're comfortable doing so, it's wise to allow the words, wisdom, and experience of other people—and even entire communities—to guide, teach, support, and nourish you. You might choose to attend worship services, pray or meditate with others, or even seek out a cancer support group with a religious or spiritual aspect. Don't underestimate the power of being connected to a group or movement bigger than yourself. As with reading spiritual materials, interacting with other like-minded seekers can provide you with insights, explanations, and stories that nourish your spirit and broaden your view of the Universe—as well as how you fit into it.

In Chapter Five, I wrote of the extraordinary women in my cancer support group, the GyniGirls. The women in this group are courageous, strong, wise, and loyal (to one another and to their families). Additionally, they have repeatedly shared with one another their extraordinary stories of synchronicities, the awareness that they are not alone, that they feel guided and protected, that they are more powerful than they ever thought themselves, and that their cancer has been a gift which has blessed them with lessons that have elevated them to a higher place in their spiritual evolution. Together, this group has learned the power of love in ways that have heightened their ability to enjoy each and every moment of life. This is the power of a community of like-minded souls.

I love this quote from Pierre Teilhard de Chardin: "We are not human beings having a spiritual experience. We are spiritual beings having a human experience." I believe this. We are wired to connect with our Higher Power, which is why the words of another famous spiritual figure, "Seek, and ye shall find," resonate so powerfully. This "seeking" is one of the most life-changing endeavors anyone can undertake … and now is the perfect time to start!

Whatever personal beliefs you may hold, I hope that you will consider making spiritual nourishment part of the fabric of your daily life. My personal experience, as well as my work with patients over a 25-year period, has convinced me that spirituality is a crucial part of healing.

CHAPTER 11

Use the Law of Attraction to Affirm Better Health

~⟨∞⟩~

"People deal too much with the negative, with what is wrong ... Why not try and see positive things, to just touch those things and make them bloom?"

THÍCH NHAT HANH

As you've probably gathered by now, I believe vibrational energy (specifically, the Law of Attraction) is one of the most valuable and effective tools at your disposal for cancer—and indeed, for building a healthy, joyful, and fulfilling life in general. If you'd like, you can look back at Chapters One and Two for my initial explanation of how the Law of Attraction works. Here, I'll share a brief recap before giving you a tool you can use to attract higher-energy experiences into your life.

The Law of Attraction Can Create Negative or Positive Experiences.

Every morning when you wake up, the ball is in your court regarding how you want to spend your day. In other words, your thoughts—and the vibrational energy they transmit—are under *your* control. If you choose to dwell in anger, bitterness, and grief, not only will you feel bad emotionally; the low vibrations you're emitting will also weaken your immune system, slow healing, and lower the tone of any interpersonal interactions you may have.

The good news is, you *can* shift your thoughts to content that uplifts, inspires, and gives you hope. (This is especially important when you're facing a life-challenging illness, which makes it more likely that your dominant vibrations are quite low.) Since like energy attracts—or allows in—like energy, your feel-good thoughts will begin to attract—or allow—more uplifting, joyful, and healing experiences into your life. As I explained in Chapter One, this is exactly what happens when you strike a tuning fork and the corresponding strings on musical instruments begin to resonate.

Specifically, when you make the choice to consciously shift your thoughts to a higher level, you will promote healing. Your brain will ramp up its production of healing chemicals, including feel-good endorphins and immune system-boosting hormones like DHEA. You'll also transform the tone of your relationships and the opportunities that materialize in your life. And on a very basic level, you'll feel less stressed, and more at peace.

To illustrate the power of the Law of the Attraction, I would like to share the story of an extraordinary woman named Jennifer.

Jennifer's Story: Transforming Life from the Inside Out

How do you go on with your life when you learn that your spouse has been diagnosed with brain cancer? This is a question Jennifer often found herself asking—and then answering, nonverbally, with the obvious: *You just do, that's all.* But, of course, that's easier said than done.

Jennifer's husband, Gary, avoided talking about his diagnosis and chose to continue living his life as though he were healthy as long as he possibly could. But denial wasn't a coping strategy that worked for Jennifer. She felt the need to talk about what was going on and to express her feelings. To complicate the matter, Jennifer, who was the more organized and structured partner, found herself making Gary's appointments and keeping track of the many details that had to be addressed—all while working full time. She also knew that eventually, she would be assuming caretaking responsibilities once her husband's cancer progressed. So, for support during this difficult life challenge, Jennifer began working with me.

When she came to me, Jennifer was experiencing low vibrational thoughts such as *I am so tired, I do not know how much more I can handle,* and *I wish this situation would end,* followed by intense feelings of guilt. (This is very common for those who become caretakers of family members who are ill.)

Jennifer used our sessions to gain clarity and a perspective that enabled her to view her situation with greater comfort, ease, and wisdom. She has always understood the basic principles of energy, and she knew that if she allowed herself to be aware of her thoughts and feelings, she could then modify them or choose different thoughts that could enable her to feel uplifted, content, and peaceful.

Sometimes she practiced the Face, Embrace, and Replace technique in which she acknowledged her feelings and thoughts, breathed out her pain, and replaced it by focusing on something delicious or pleasant. Other times, she allowed herself to express her anger, and then would breathe in peacefully and shift to a feel-better thought. She often tapped to alleviate her pain. Going on a walk with her beloved dog, Wendy, would always help her to shift from stress to joy. Humor and support groups also helped lift Jennifer's mindset to a higher vibrational place. The bottom line was, Jennifer knew she had tools and resources to see her through her journey—and she made full use of them.

In the years since I met Jennifer, her beloved husband Gary has died. Looking back, we can both see how caring for her husband and healing her grief have enabled Jennifer to claim her power, better listen to her intuitive wisdom, and live with clear intentions. Jennifer now lives her life adhering to the principle often quoted by the teacher Abraham: *The path of least resistance is the path of greatest allowing.* In other words, because she seeks to live in a genuine state of peace and joy (without resistance), Jennifer can and does manifest whatever she needs. I have often marveled at her ability to state her wishes and needs and then see how quickly they are satisfied by the Universe.

For example, in the year and a half following the death of her husband, a friend had introduced her to a new man, and love entered her life once again. Feeling ambivalent and unsure of whether or not this was good for her to pursue, Jennifer often asked Gary for signs—and received them in the form of feathers appearing on her pillow, furniture, or the path from her front door.

As Jennifer and I know, and as you know too, life can be bitter at times. Always remember that we live by the choices we make.

How we choose to think about and respond to the things that come across our path determines the quality of our journey. My hope is that, like Jennifer, you will learn the art of happiness by allowing yourself to live fully in the Now—yes, *especially* in the midst of your cancer journey. You need not live your life in state of unhappiness and fear. Claim your extraordinary power and choose to attract and accept trust, faith, and love.

Now, let's look at a simple, and very direct, tool you can use to raise your vibrational energy and attract the experiences you want into your life.

The Words You Say to Yourself Matter.

As we've established, the words you say to yourself are *much* more than mere sounds and syllables. They actively determine your vibrational energy levels, which in turn have an impact on your spirit, your cells, your relationships, and much more.

Unfortunately, most of us live our lives without being aware of the power of the words we choose. Thus, without awareness or consciousness, our mental commentaries are full of negative thoughts. How often do you tell yourself things like: *I can't do this; I am no good at this; I am hurting and in so much pain; I can't find a way out of this; I am in a hopeless situation* etc. You get the idea! Please, never make the mistake of believing that thoughts like these are harmless.

From this point forward, your job is to learn to live consciously, fully aware of your thoughts and their implications concerning your well-being. First, I want you to recognize that in the vast majority of situations, there is an opposite for your thoughts. If you're thinking (and therefore feeling) something negative, you can choose to flip that thought into a positive.

For example, let's say that you're having a particularly bad day. Since you woke up, you've been plagued by nausea, body aches, and dizziness. You might instinctively say to yourself, *I hate feeling this way. And the worst part is, things are only going to go downhill as the day wears on. There's nothing I can do to feel like my old self.*

When you catch yourself thinking this way, stop and consider the impact your chosen words will have on your cells. Then, turn your previous thoughts around. Reshape them into words that your cells will consider to be kind, gentle, loving, comforting, and healing. For instance: *I love and value my body, and am giving it what is necessary for its healing.* Or, *I have all that I require to get through this. This is my wake-up call to give myself the rest and care I need.*

Note that you're not denying that you feel bad or pretending that your reality isn't what it is. (That never works!) But you are shifting your thoughts away from negativity and toward loving self-talk. In other words, you've used positive affirmations to energetically empower your body, mind, and spirit.

By intentionally using the strength of specific words to create your own well-being, you can encourage your cells to produce what you require to fight cancer and heal your body. I promise, when you think before you speak and decide to express and affirm what you want rather than what you do not have, you will feel better!

My Experience with Healing Affirmations

In my work with those who are challenged by cancer and other illnesses (including diabetes, cardiac situations, chronic fatigue, and autoimmune disorders), I encourage the repetition of positive healing affirmations because I know from personal experience that they work.

For instance, after my own recent major surgery (the removal of a—thankfully—benign tumor, as well as both ovaries), I was having a hard time managing my pain, especially after taking myself off prescribed pain medications. When I caught myself using adjectives like *struggle, hard time, hurting,* etc. to describe my pain, I made a conscious decision to feel better and to expedite my healing by affirming how I wanted to feel.

After I began to monitor what I was thinking and saying to myself, I would often catch myself expressing thoughts like, *Oh, this is really painful.* I would then quickly shift my thoughts to an affirmation similar to one of the following: *I can handle this, I can see myself feeling stronger and better with each passing hour (and day), I am healing little by little, the universe is giving me everything I need for my body to heal, I feel better when I think of what makes me happy,* etc. Then, I would consciously focus on something that would make me laugh or smile, such as an activity I was looking forward to doing or person I was looking forward to seeing.

The more I did this, the more I realized that the process of thinking and speaking in the most positive and affirmative manner truly did contribute to my shift in feeling more comfortable. I engaged in affirmations repeatedly for a number of days, always aware that the uplifting message of managing the pain was getting to my cells (my team), and that they were supporting me and enabling my body to heal more quickly. I could actually feel this taking place.

You have the power to do the same thing. Each morning, evening, and throughout the day, use affirmations to shift you into a state in which your immune system is operating full force and at top speed.

Harness the Healing Power of Positive Affirmations.

So, how can you begin to incorporate affirmations into your own healing? First let me share a list of affirmations you can use. To start, simply fill your mind with those that resonate most with you (or compose your own!). Repeat them upon awakening, through-out the day, and before going to sleep. And keep in mind that healing isn't *just* physical—you might also need to heal your emotions, your attitude, your outlook, or your spirit. The following affirmations can serve you on many levels:

- I am healing, little by little.
- I am peace.
- I am feeling peaceful and fulfilled.
- I am aligned with my heart.
- I am Love and I am loved.
- I am being given what I need for my own healing.
- I am attracting everything and everyone I need.
- I am healing moment by moment.
- I am at peace and I am joy.
- I am getting stronger with each day, hour, and moment.
- I am one with my Source.
- I Am that I Am.
- I love life and life loves me.
- I am attracting people I love to me.
- I am feeling better and better.
- I am joyful.
- I am happy.
- I am blessed.
- I am living in alignment with my soul's purpose.
- I am living in integrity with my heart.
- I am smiling because I feel loved.
- I intend to be in peace today.
- I am receiving everything I need for the fulfillment of my hopes and dreams.
- My body's cells are taking such good care of me.
- My chemo and medications are helping me to eliminate cancer.
- I am free from discomfort.

- I am held lovingly by the Universe.
- I am well.
- I choose to focus on what makes me smile.

Next, I'll share a few strategies you can use to "supercharge" these affirmations:

- *See* **them while you** *say* **them.** As you know, affirmations are vibrations you are offering your cells to enhance their ability to care for you. You can further empower your affirmations by allowing yourself to see in your mind's eye (your imagination) what you are affirming and, as you say them, feeling your body responding to them.
- **Make affirmations a constant habit.** Saying each affirmation once or twice a day is certainly helpful. But the more frequently you repeat your affirmations, the more of an impression they will make on your cells (your healing team). Get into the habit of repeating your affirmations whenever your mind isn't actively engaged elsewhere. For instance, you can affirm while you're folding laundry, walking your dog, or receiving a treatment. Cumulatively, all of these positive healing vibrations will result in the brain's production of chemicals such as neuropeptides, endorphins, and hormones that are needed by your immune system to heal you and to keep you healthy.
- **Write them out.** I have found that it helps to write out your affirmations and post them in places you are sure to notice them, such as your bathroom mirror, your nightstand, the refrigerator door, your kitchen counter, your desk, and the dashboard of your car. Read the affirmations and repeat them several times each time you see them.
- **Combine affirmations with breath.** Breath reinforces all good things: prayers, meditations, intentions, tools for reducing worries and anxiety, and simply relaxing.

Try this exercise the next time you repeat your affirmations: Breathe a warm, deep, healing breath in through your nostrils. See it travel down to your heart, lungs, and belly. As you breathe out through your mouth, with your lips slightly parted, repeat your affirmation a few times. Your body's 60 trillion cells respond well to the guiding wisdom of your words when you are relaxed by your breath.

As often as needed, remind yourself that you have what you need, that you are healing, that all is well, etc. And finally, remind yourself that Divine energy is a part of every cell of your being, and that you are never, ever alone.

"Change your thoughts and you change your world."

Norman Vincent Peale

CHAPTER 12

Forgive Those Who Need to Be Forgiven

"The weak can never forgive. Forgiveness is the attribute of the strong ..."

GANDHI

Life is about finding, healing, and maintaining the balance of energy between your body, mind, and soul. Your words, thoughts, and deeds are all expressions of your own personal energy—and that energy has the ability to impact the functioning of your body's immune system. But you are more than "just" your biology and your mind. You are also love.

The highly respected NDE (near-death experience) body of research includes numerous descriptions of those who have physically died and returned to write of it. These individuals report becoming aware of a state of being that is infinite, eternal, expansive, and most of all, unconditionally accepting and loving. They learned that we are love, and a part of everyone and everything. (It is their work, along with that of the quantum physicists, that has forever changed my perspective on life and death, as well as my approach to healing.)

The energy of being unconditionally loving has the power to help you heal—period! That's why it's important to consistently choose to *be* love. And when you choose to *be* love, forgiveness comes with the territory. In fact, love and forgiveness may be thought of as two sides of the same coin.

In this chapter, we'll look at two types of forgiveness—forgiving yourself and forgiving others—as well as why each is a crucial part of your healing journey.

First, Love and Forgive Yourself Unconditionally.

Why is loving yourself relevant to your cancer journey? It's simple: Most of us tend to be very hard on ourselves. And unless you can let go of low vibrational damaging thoughts and feelings that are directed at yourself (like fear, guilt, resentment, anger, disappointment, etc.), you will impede your physical and spiritual healing. In other words, by carrying around thoughts, feelings and issues that fill your being with fear and anger, you are making it difficult for your body to do the work of keeping you healthy.

Also, before you can forgive others, you need to first make peace with *yourself.* Usually, the anger we feel towards others is a projection of what is going on within our own being—but about which we are in denial because it is too painful to face. For example, fear is so often behind the thoughts and emotions that we call anger. We might fear revealing our sense of inadequacy, worry about losing our control over a situation, or be concerned about failure—so we lash out at others. However, by denying that we feel fear, we are not being true to who we are and are not allowing ourselves to experience what comes our way. Consequently, we are not experiencing well-being.

Many of my patients who are facing cancer have come to recognize that the person they are angriest at is themselves. For instance, some are angry that they did not take steps to repair a damaged or dysfunctional relationship before the other person died. They are frustrated with themselves for not saying, *I am sorry* and/or *I love you* while there was still time.

Others are angry because of decisions their young adult children have made. Eventually, these parents recognize their anger as self-anger, with the fear being that they somehow "messed up" in their parenting role. Let's look at this scenario—and how it can result in self-forgiveness—in a little more detail.

My goal is to help upset parents understand that they did their best, bringing to each decision all the love and wisdom they had at that time. Yes, these parents might have made a very different choice a month or year later, but they *did their best* at that time, with loving intentions—and that is all any of us can do! Additionally, I remind parents that they need to let their children learn to fend for themselves, and that their children are here to learn to take responsibility for their own lives.

Finally, I point out to parents that if we can choose to remember that we are love and that we love unconditionally, we can *allow in* what takes place with our children, make the choice to feel our pain (for it is real and it is part of who we genuinely are), and forgive ourselves for whatever thoughts we are experiencing that have to do with self-blame. Our task is to forgive ourselves and learn from the lessons provided to us by the experience.

Before moving on, I'd like to share one more common scenario that involves self-forgiveness. Many of us have long held, but never spoken of, the anger and fears that result from trading our lives (including our dreams and desires) to make others happy. Over time, we become angry that we did not love ourselves enough to have the courage to speak up for what was important for us. Remember, your cells are aware of the vibration of this fear and anger, and over time, these negative emotions impact the release of the chemicals that are needed to keep you healthy. Again, for the sake of your current peace and health, it is essential that you forgive yourself for doing what you thought was right at the time.

Please think about whether you have been beating yourself up and blaming yourself for your past actions and decisions. If you *are* harboring resentment and anger toward yourself, I encourage you to do the work of forgiveness, which is what we'll talk about next.

What Is Self-Forgiveness, Exactly?

Essentially, forgiving yourself means that you accept the fact that right now, you are exactly where you are supposed to be on your spiritual journey. That doesn't mean you should stop striving to improve the aspects of yourself you know need work. It *does* mean realizing that your past mistakes and regrets do not make you in any way unworthy. You can say to yourself, *I messed up, but I am still okay. I accept my faults and mistakes. In fact, they enabled me to learn the lessons I needed to learn. Today and always, I love myself wholeheartedly.*

You may find it helpful to familiarize yourself with the findings of those who have had near-death experiences. Their realization that we are love and that we can choose to live in a state of *being* love is powerful and valuable for you and me—and all humanity. Actually, an attitude of unconditional love mirrors Divine (Infinite or Source) Energy—the energy that created the universe—which is the energy of Love. Infinite energy loves and accepts you unconditionally, warts and all. (Near-death experience research validates that this is the message received from our Source—whomever you believe that Source to be—when we die: that we are loved along with all our faults and errors.) It makes sense, then, that self-love moves you to a much higher vibrational plane.

Having written this, I must emphasize that your willingness to forgive yourself and love unconditionally occurs only when you are ready—when it feels right for you. Self-forgiveness should not occur "just" because your therapist or someone else says so (though he or she can recommend or suggest it), but when *you* intuitively feel that it is time.

Move Forward with a Tool for Self-Forgiveness.

Of course, forgiving yourself can be easier said than done! Here is an exercise that I've found helpful. (As a side note, this strategy will also help you to forgive others—but be sure to focus on self-forgiveness first.)

First, you need to have the clear intention of choosing forgiveness for yourself. Next, quiet yourself and become conscious of how you are feeling. Focus in on how awful, guilty, bitter, angry, etc. you feel toward yourself. Allow yourself to really *feel* that feeling, and give yourself permission to stay with it. (As was the case with the Face/Embrace/Replace and ABC tools, this process can include crying or shouting, so find a place where you can have some privacy, such as your car, your bedroom, or the shower.)

When you are ready, take several deep breaths, and with each, intentionally release—or, if you prefer another term—let go of or detach from the energy associated with your terrible feelings. Affirm to yourself: *I am a normal being who has come to learn lessons—lessons of love and forgiveness. I choose to love myself enough to affirm that I did my best.* (Even the masters and the saints erred as they were trying to do their best!) *By choosing to love and forgive myself first, before others, I will no longer carry this unhealthy burden around with me.*

Continue with, *I choose to surrender all of this to my Higher Power.* If you believe in a forgiving Source and Universe, you can add, *If my Higher Power* (God or Jesus or Buddha or Allah) *accepts and unconditionally loves and forgives me, then I must be able to do this for myself. I choose to see and feel myself releasing these feelings, surrendering them to God, and then feeling myself to be so much lighter.*

Now, Choose to Forgive Others.

Aside from withholding forgiveness from yourself, refusing to forgive other people for their wrongs (or for what you perceive as their wrongs) is one of the most toxic acts you can commit against yourself. Remember, illness occurs within our bodies when we are not physically, emotionally, mentally, and spiritually balanced. Maintaining unresolved fears and anger creates imbalance and makes it difficult for the wisdom of our biology to care for us. By choosing love and forgiveness, we are physiologically better off.

Here's my point: One of the strongest choices you could possibly make as you seek healing is to let go of any unresolved anger you have toward others, as well as the fears that may contribute to your anger. When you don't forgive, you deny yourself a higher energetic payoff—as well as potential healing.

Who, exactly, should you forgive? If bad or uncomfortable feelings arise whenever you think of a certain person—even if you can't put your finger on why—that's a sign that you have some unresolved issues with him or her. Extending forgiveness will dissolve the tension between the two of you and will make your relationship far more pleasant.

Keep in mind that forgiveness does *not* mean that you're condoning another person's bad behavior; simply that you're choosing not to let that offense *continue* to harm you by consuming your thoughts and emotions. You're not offering forgiveness to benefit the other person—though this may, in fact, occur—you're doing it for *you*.

The forgiveness exercise I just shared can help you to forgive others as well as yourself. Simply replace your negative feelings toward yourself with your negative feelings toward others as you work through the exercise. And know that it's okay to keep your forgiveness to yourself. You can practice it in your imagination or even in a letter. In other words, you do not need to forgive other people in person. What matters is *not* the other person knowing you have forgiven him or her, but that you have released your negative feelings from your own being. Again, forgiveness is for your own healing.

Yes, I acknowledge that choosing forgiveness often feels unbelievably difficult, if not impossible, whether you're forgiving yourself or another. But I can promise you that time is a beautiful healer, magically softening your thoughts, heart, and being. What you can't imagine doing initially will become easier to consider over time ... and even more so when you choose to perceive yourself as you really are: a being of unconditional love who is connected to other beings of unconditional love.

Knowing that *you* are love, and that you are loved—by yourself, by the Universe, and by other people—with all of your faults and errors, may enable you (as it has me) to choose to love those with whom you have issues. The more you affirm, "I Am Love," the more you will come to remember your true identity, and the easier it will be to let go of low-vibrational emotions.

Forgiving the Tough-to-Forgive

But what if there's someone in your life you are simply not ready to forgive? The reality is, many of us will be confronted with powerful and extreme challenges to our forgiveness. Whether you are struggling to forgive a person like Hitler who has robbed your family of loved ones, someone who has taken the life of a family member or friend, or your own loved one who has taken his or her life, extending forgiveness may feel impossible right now. That's okay. You cannot *force* spiritual growth and healing. Forgiveness needs to come from your heart and on your time schedule for it to be genuine. Do not allow yourself to be forced into forgiveness because someone else feels it is the right time or place.

For now, until you *do* feel ready to forgive, continue loving yourself unconditionally, and remember that everyone on earth is walking their own path and is trying to do the best they can. Also, you'll need to accept that there is a price to be paid in terms of your own peace of mind and vibrational energy as long as you withhold forgiveness. But because life is about constant growth, know that one day you may be better equipped to let go of old grievances. When that day comes, here is a tactic that may help you move forward:

First, engage in stopping the unforgiving thoughts by simply saying "Stop! Stop! Stop these thoughts!" Then remind yourself of who you are. Return to seeing yourself in a state of unconditional love, feeling this love in every one of your cells. Now, if you can, intentionally focus on loving qualities the other person displays— qualities that have touched you and/or for which you feel grateful.

For example, let's say that someone you love or care about has said mean, harsh words to you. Go within, and while intending to release your need to be angry with this person, recall times when he or she was especially kind, thoughtful, loving, and caring. Replay these memories while affirming unconditional love. By focusing on the other person in a feel-good way, you will vibrate at a higher level and will experience greater compassion—which may make forgiveness easier.

You may also find it helpful to read *Remarkable Recovery: What Extraordinary Healings Tell Us About Getting Well and Staying Well* by Caryle Hirshberg and Marc Ian Barasch. In it, you'll find the story of Edith Eva Eger, a psychologist who survived the concentration camp of Auschwitz. Edith had many reasons to withhold forgiveness, yet here are her words: "If you create an 'us' and 'them' mentality, you create another Auschwitz. It is important now we create peace and love in the world."[1]

Edith's entire story is truly remarkable, but it's especially noteworthy that she had the wisdom to understand that only by forgiving those who had taken her family and nearly her own life as well, could she live a life in which she was free. Freedom is the gift of forgiveness.

A Mother Heals: A Case Study in Forgiveness

I would like to end this chapter by sharing two powerful stories of forgiveness. The first involves a psychiatrist named Sue Chance.

When Sue's son Jim took his life unexpectedly at the age of 25, she used journaling to help herself heal by processing her intense feelings of guilt, anguish, and anger. In *Stronger Than Death: When Suicide Touches Your Life*, by Sue Chance, MD, you learn how this gifted psychiatrist, loving mother, and suicide survivor navigated her way back from a personal, hellish abyss to a place of peace and recovery. Ultimately, she came to forgive both herself as well as her son.

As I stated earlier in this chapter, parents feel an enormous sense of responsibility for their children—especially when they choose to end their lives—and often have trouble accepting that their child has come to be responsible for his or her own journey. So how did Sue come to grips with this realization?

It was the expression *"You did your best."* These words came at the right moments from a good friend and from her brother. They reminded Sue that Jim was an adult, that she could no longer control his life, and that she had done the best she could with all that she had at that time. Yes, those four deceptively simple words were powerful enough to shift Sue out of her overwhelming sense of responsibility for her child's death.

In her book, Sue writes of owning responsibility for her part in this tragic event, but she also writes of her recognition that her son was not able to bear his personal suffering and, therefore, made the decision to take his own life. Now, Sue knows that she could not control her son's life. She strongly feels that death was his choice, and his alone—and that this was not a condemnation of her as his mother. As the months and years passed, she was slowly able to forgive herself for her responsibility in Jim's death, and in the love she felt for her son, she allowed him the right to choose to die as he wished.

While Sue did not have a near-death experience, she *did* experience a life-altering event when her son took his life. And as I've mentioned, such experiences send us into the next energetic plateau of our lives. It's not surprising that within a few years of Jim's death, Sue found herself living in a state of Buddhist consciousness and being guided by Buddhist principles.

Sue had come to a place in which she recognized that she was a part of the Whole or Source, that she was whole and perfect just as she was, that to live in joy and peace she needed to embrace and allow in whatever came to her ... and most importantly, that she is love and is here to unconditionally love everyone and everything. (If you're interested, Sue's realizations mirror those of cancer survivor Anita Moorjani after her near death experience. I highly recommend Anita's book, *Dying to Be Me*.)

Tom's Story: Quenching the Fire and Connecting with Love

Before Tom first came to my practice, his loved ones (who referred him to me) warned me that his anger defined him. They described in detail his low level of tolerance and his high levels of frustration and impatience. Yet when I finally met Tom himself, the reality I uncovered was very different from the description I had been given. I met a gentle soul who had an awareness of his spiritual roots but who had also experienced a great deal of pain. Not knowing what to do with this pain, Tom released it at the wrong times and in the wrong situations.

It did not take long for Tom to explore why he had so much pent-up frustration and pain. In our first sessions, Tom shared long-held feelings of disappointment related to growing up without support, approval, and validation. He also admitted to feeling resentment for having to put some of his dreams on the back burner in order to support his family. As a short-term coping mechanism, he had learned to suppress his thoughts, feelings, desires, hopes, and dreams. This, in conjunction with engaging in relationships that were not healthy and fulfilling, contributed to Tom inappropriately releasing his feelings in explosive outbursts of anger when tested by stress and difficult circumstances.

What therapeutically helped Tom was seeing his situation from a Higher Perspective. By looking at his life with greater objectivity, he was able to better understand that his outbursts were sudden releases of pent-up feelings he had held onto since

his childhood. He also began to see that he had carried this unhealthy dynamic into relationships with his wife and others.

This understanding enabled Tom to experience greater love
for himself and his family, and to begin the process of forgiving
first himself, then others. Gradually, Tom was able to let go of the
old hurts, resentments, and frustrations that had been defining
him since childhood. With the increased expression of his feelings, his anger diminished and he became much more empathic,
understanding, and compassionate regarding the feelings of other
family members. Essentially, forgiveness helped Tom to remember, reclaim, and honor his true self.

Tom also recognized that his challenges were providing him
with life lessons. He gradually came to realize that each event that
could possibly trigger his anger was also a teaching moment in
which he could lovingly choose compassion for himself and the
other person. He took the time to learn and use tools such as Face/
Embrace/Replace to help him in this endeavor. In small but significant baby steps, he was learning to make choices that reflected
forgiveness, love, healing, and balance.

Life has not always been easy for Tom, but he is finally at
peace. While his marriage has since dissolved, his relationships
with his children have strengthened a great deal, and he has their
loving support. He now lives in the country where he pursues his
passions, often aided by meditation and journaling. Tom is an
extraordinary role model for all of us when it comes to healing the
mind and soul through the power of forgiveness!

Forgive Constantly.

You too can use forgiveness to aid your healing journey. And that
brings me to one last piece of wisdom I'd like to share with you:
Like Sue Chance, Tom, and so many others, you may find yourself needing to forgive the same person (which might be yourself!)

more than once for the same hurtful behavior. Work through the forgiveness exercise I've shared as often as you need.

"Re-forgiving" doesn't mean that you failed to forgive the first time; simply that you need to continue processing whatever is bothering you. Remember, past traumas are stored vibrationally within our cells, so it's possible that over the course of your life you may find yourself dealing with the same past hurt multiple times. Don't be discouraged if this happens. Instead, proactively choose to experience your anger or grief, then replace it with a higher-vibrational emotion.

Forgiveness, like healing, is a journey. You rarely reach your destination overnight, but once you do, you're always glad you kept putting one foot in front of the other.

CHAPTER **13**

Live in Alignment with What Is in Your Heart

"Living more in harmony with who we truly are isn't just forcing our-selves to repeat positive thoughts. It means being and doing things that make us happy, things that arouse our passion and bring out the best in us, things that make us feel good—
and it also means loving ourselves unconditionally ..."

ANITA MOORJANI, IN *DYING TO BE ME*

In theory, living in alignment is simple. It means that you are honoring and living your own truth—not another's truth. In other words, when you are living in alignment, you are clear on what your values are, what feels right to you, what's important to you, what makes you feel comfortable and safe, and what fills you with happiness and joy—and you are consciously making sure those things are present in your life.

Like I said—alignment *sounds* simple. But in reality, many of us ignore what we intuitively know is best for us in favor of making other people happy, fitting in, or living a certain lifestyle. We try to live our lives for others, ignoring what we need to feel fulfilled and at peace.

You know how it goes: You stay in a career you dislike because it's lucrative, and anyway, how are you supposed to switch gears at this point in your life? Or you continue to invest in a stale friendship because "I've known her for 20 years—I can't just cut her out of my life!" Or you allow yourself to become burdened with tasks (from your spouse, from your child's school, from your church, etc.) that you don't really want to take on, simply because you don't want to disappoint others. Or you eat foods you know are bad for you because they're convenient. Or you go into debt because you think you "need" that car, those clothes, or that house.

At this point, I advise you to take a look back at Chapter Three (A Life That Isn't Working). It describes many of the symptoms of an out-of-alignment life in detail, ranging from a lack of quiet time to unhappy relationships to financial problems and more. As I pointed out there, many people's lives have spiraled so far out of alignment that they feel utterly trapped: by money, by social obligations, by career expectations, by bad relationships, etc. What often keeps us in these situations—and out of alignment—is the fear of choosing to leave them for the unknown.

If that describes you, you probably *want* to get back on track but have no idea where to start; no idea which string to pull to begin loosening the tangle. So you do nothing. It feels easier to stick with the dissatisfying status quo than to do the work of bringing your life into alignment, *especially* with the challenge of cancer looming.

Now, it's time for some tough love: If you want to experience healing and better health, you can't afford *not* to bring your life into alignment, no matter how daunting the task may be. Just think of the low vibrational energy that a life of stress, dissatisfaction, fear, and inauthenticity creates. Then, consider the detrimental effect that those vibrations are having on your health.

For the vast majority of my patients, cancer has been the universe's way of screaming that they are not living in balance, harmony, or peace! That's why you need to begin making changes now. Yes, even in the middle of your cancer journey. In a very real way, your cancer can be seen as a wake-up call.

Cancer Makes the Path Forward Clearer.

The good news is, cancer may clarify what steps you need to take in order to bring your life into better alignment. For many people, a life-challenging illness shines a light that enables you to finally see what you need to release, and what you need to keep.

Specifically, cancer forces you to make choices concerning your lifestyle from a *survival* standpoint, not from a social one. Many of my patients tell me that just about everything on their former to-do lists takes a backseat to dealing with their new visitor. They realize that they no longer care about pleasing that demanding, draining friend, for instance, or that they're no longer willing to prioritize time spent at the office over time spent with family.

I have watched my patients clear out amazing amounts of unnecessary "debris" from their lives, including activities, objects, relationships, obligations, and routines. By choosing to focus on what feels good and detach from what doesn't, these patients have helped to restore balance to their lives and enable greater healing.

The same thing has happened to me, too. Each time I have been diagnosed with a life-threatening illness, that illness's gift to me has been the opportunity to reflect on what contributed to my being so out of balance. What also came to mind were several age-old and universal questions: "Who am I—really? Am I a psychologist, wife, author, healer, mother, friend, etc.? What are my priorities? And how can I balance those priorities with my joys and passions, which include my family and friends? Finally, what do I need to change to live a more healthy, peaceful, and balanced lifestyle?"

These questions forced me to reflect not only on my identity, but also on what I could release from my life in order to be healthy and live joyfully. As I focused on treatments, healing, and recovery, I formulated the steps I would need to take when I returned to work: reducing my work hours, increasing my time to exercise, spending more time with loved ones and friends, and getting more sleep, for example.

These were my personal choices. They may or may not mirror yours. Remember, each of us is a being with the ability to decide for ourselves the direction in which we wish to move.

"But I Can't Quit My Job!": A Common Concern

For many of my patients (and perhaps for you, too) an unfulfilling or demanding job is at the center of their pain, stress, and unbalanced lifestyle. These patients understandably feel trapped by practical and financial concerns. While they may *want* to hand in their notice or reduce the number of hours they work, they fear doing so because they need their current paychecks and insurance. Since this is such a common—and very weighty—concern for so many cancer patients, I'd like to address it directly.

If you feel that you're locked in to your current job whether you want to be or not, there are other strategies you can adopt to regain the sense of running your own show—a feeling that cancer has most likely taken from you. I recommend working within the system until you can disconnect and create a life that does enable you to feel genuinely better, happier and more balanced. Here are some ways to do that:

- **Find small but significant ways to bring greater peace into your life.** You may not be able to change much of the stress that comes your way at work. That's why it's so important to take control of what you can in your personal life, and infuse as much peace into your non-working hours as possible. For instance, you can choose to meditate for 20 minutes instead of watching the (depressing) evening news. You can choose to let go of your rigid need to maintain a spotless house in order to spend more time working on art projects with your kids. You can place a calendar on your desk and fill it in with events you're looking forward to sharing with family and friends. Sometimes these small changes—taking control of what you can rather than fretting over what you can't change—have the power to transform your outlook and greatly enhance your well-being.
- **De-stress with relaxing breaths.** In Chapter Eight I discussed breath, as well as several healing techniques, in detail (and we'll look more at breath in Chapter Fourteen). Here, I'll share a quick exercise you can do whenever you're feeling stressed or anxious. If you're at work, close your office door—or even go into the bathroom to get some privacy! Close your eyes and count to ten while breathing in. Hold your breath to the count of ten, then exhale to the count of ten (or higher). As you exhale, *see* the breath leaving your body. Feel your body become warmer, more

relaxed, and heavier with each breath in and out. This works. It is your time-out, and enables you to release and replenish.

- **Build breaks into your workday.** Whenever you can, take time during the workday to disconnect from your job's demands and recharge a bit, both physically and mentally. For instance, whether you're eating lunch in the break room or off-site, do not talk work! If you can go outside for a short walk, take advantage of the opportunity. If you like to knit, keep a ball of yarn and knitting needles in your desk drawer so that you can pull them out during lulls. Maybe you can even form a yoga group with colleagues and practice before or after the workday. Essentially, do anything that feels good, relaxes you, and raises your vibrational energy.
- **Balance your energy with the Donna Eden Five Minute Energy Routine.** I mentioned this extremely helpful technique in Chapter Eight, and I'm bringing it to your attention again here because it's so easy to do before starting work, during your lunch break, and any time in the day when you feel stressed, tired and unable to concentrate. This routine will both balance and boost your energy, which will make it easier for you to make decisions that support living in alignment. You can watch Donna teach and demonstrate her 5 Minute Energy Routine on YouTube at www.youtube.com/watch?v=gffKhttrRw4.

As you incorporate these tools, I also encourage you to use any "forced" downtime you have in the course of your treatments to begin exploring other positions, jobs, or opportunities that might eventually enable you to live in a greater state of alignment. I have worked with many patients over the years who have succeeded in shifting to a more fulfilling career, either during or after cancer. I want to assure you that you can do this too—and you will reap the benefits of living a life that feels better than what you've previously experienced!

Tools for Building Greater Alignment

In the remainder of this chapter, I will share several tools you can use to pursue alignment in your own life. No matter what your circumstances are, they will help you to identify what you need to let go of and gravitate toward, and to make meaningful changes that will promote health and happiness.

TOOL 1: Use the ABCs to Identify What Needs to Go.

Like my patients and me, you may already have a good idea of what is keeping you from living in alignment. Still, it's a good idea to look at each area of your life (I recommend using the topics presented Chapter Three as a guide) to clarify what is and isn't in alignment with your higher self.

You may remember the ABCs and Face/Embrace/Replace tools from Chapter Eight. Here, we'll use a modified version to help you focus on each area of your life, determine how you feel about it, and—if alignment isn't present—begin to move toward balance.

- **A is for AWARENESS and ACKNOWLEDGMENT.** First, "Face" each area of your life and determine whether it's in alignment with your higher self, or not. Find a place you can be alone for a few minutes and sit quietly in a chair or on the floor. Think about the area in question (whether it's your diet, the way you spend your free time, your marriage, or something else). Picture it in your mind.

Now, put your hand on your heart (this is the center of truth) and ask yourself, *Am I feeling good (or okay) or not good at this moment?* If your answer is "not good," put the same hand on your forehead and ask yourself, *What is my thought, picture, or image that makes me not feel good?*

Now, take time to Acknowledge or "Embrace" the picture or thought. If you feel pain, fear, or anxiety, give yourself permission to really feel it. Don't be surprised if you have a strong emotional reaction. Kick, scream, or cry it out—for a few moments, or more, if needed, but not too much more, if possible.

- **B is for BREATH and BREATHING OUT YOUR PAIN.** Take three deep breaths. As you breathe in, visualize yourself breathing in the colorful and magnificent energy of the Universe or God. (Yes, actually give it a color so you can "see" it more readily.)

  Watch and feel this powerful healing energy coming in and filling your body with amazing warm, relaxing energy. Be aware that you are breathing in peace and breathing out the pain and anxiety that this unhealthy area of your life causes you. As you breathe, you experience heaviness, warmth, and deep relaxation, as well as a feeling of lightness, enabling you to shift to a higher energetic level. Be sure to visualize yourself breathing up the energy of pain and suffering in your heart and belly and releasing it through your mouth, lips slightly parted.

- **C is for CHOICES THAT FEEL GOOD or BETTER.** Here's where you "Replace" your negative energy with positive energy. Be conscious of how you are feeling, moment by moment. It's time to make a conscious choice: Do I want to continue approaching this area of my life as I currently do, or should I change my habits, attitude, relationships, etc.? Make your decision. Then feel the healing energy of your choice flow through your body.

Once you have assessed each major area of your life, you might choose to use your newfound clarity to create an "alignment visualization" that will help you to stay focused on your goals and/or mission as you continue on your cancer journey.

To do so, draw an umbrella and write your goal or mission above it. Along each of your umbrella's multiple spokes, write an action you can take to expedite your healing. Look at this drawing often, and continue to add spokes to the umbrella as other impediments to alignment become clear.

TOOL 2: Create Moment-by-Moment Alignment with Intention.

Learning to live in alignment with what is in your heart is often as simple as noticing that you are not at peace in the moment. It does not feel good to always be harried, rushed, stressed, and not peaceful. I advise starting your day with the intention of doing your best to be mindful of how you are feeling in each moment.

Since it's all too easy to get caught up in the momentum of everyday life and forget these intentions (*especially* when you are battling cancer), leave reminders for yourself. You might place a Post-it note that reads "Mindful and Aligned" on your bathroom mirror, for instance, or on your refrigerator, car's dashboard, or desk.

I also recommend keeping a 3×5 "My Alignment" card in your wallet or pocket. Each hour, take it out, perform an alignment self-check, and note that you have assessed your state of peace. For example, your card might say:

- Play – Aligned?
- Work – Aligned?
- Home – Aligned?
- Gratitude – Aligned?

You might also want to include a reminder to yourself to perform the ABCs or Donna Eden's Five-Minute Energy Routine if you need help in assessing a particular area.

If you aren't at peace, you can make an immediate difference in your state of mind by saying simple affirmations such as, *I am so thankful for my blessings; I am at peace; I choose peace; I choose joy; I choose to be grateful; I love life and life loves me; I am attracting everything I need right this moment as I breathe in peace; I release resistance; I allow and I feel; I choose to detach;* etc. While affirming, visualize your intentions and feel their energy vibrating through every one of your cells.

TOOL 3: Learn to Say No (Finally!).

As I've pointed out, cancer teaches us that our time is finite. It stops us in our tracks and forces us to love ourselves first and foremost—or else. It might surprise you to hear that for many of us, the biggest obstacle to loving ourselves and living in alignment is a two-letter word: "No." Specifically, we have trouble saying it to others, and meaning it.

Believe me, I understand. Saying no, even when you intuitively know it's the right thing to do, takes courage. After my own recent surgery, I knew that I needed to focus my energy on wellness and healing, not hosting visitors. Still, I actually had to picture myself gathering my courage in order to thank my friends for offering to visit, while lovingly saying "no, thank you" at the same time. And, of course, they all understood!

Another example involves my friend Sandy, whose wife's father was diagnosed with a terminal disease. Having been a caretaker for his own ill parents, Sandy knew that he did not have the emotional or physical energy to go down that particular road once again. He also recognized that he wanted to be free to enjoy this particular time in his life, and that his wife would benefit spiritually from caring for her father herself.

Yet, Sandy still had trouble telling his wife, "No, I cannot be your father's primary caretaker. However, I will have your back in loving support." After I helped him understand that a refusal was a form of self-love, not selfishness, Sandy was able to tell his wife how he felt. She accepted his decision with grace.

My point is, learning to say *no* is challenging, but it is also an essential part of taking your power back and reclaiming the life you were meant to live. Whether it's something "small" like choosing not to go out to dinner after receiving a request from a relative, or something "large" like declining to lead an activity you've spearheaded for years out of a sense of obligation, saying no will lead to higher-vibrational experiences.

As was the case with Sandy, it may help to remind yourself that declining what's not in your best interests is an expression of self-love; one that is necessary for healing as you face cancer. And I'm giving you permission to play the "cancer card" if you have to—no one can argue with that!

TOOL 4: Rate Your Long-Term Alignment Levels.

It probably won't surprise you to learn that achieving lasting alignment isn't as simple as flipping a one-time switch; it takes time and commitment. This exercise is designed to help you increase your alignment by regularly infusing healing, high-vibrational experiences into your life. It will give you a simple, tangible way to see and feel that you *do* have control over your life.

- **First, write down five or more people, places, and/or activities that bring you pleasure.** They might include spending time with friends and family, interacting with a pet, listening to your favorite music or comedian, getting a massage or a manicure, spending time outdoors, cooking, volunteering, doing yoga or tai chi (or any physical activity, playing a musical instrument, etc. The possibilities are endless, as long as they make you happy and raise your vibrational energy.

- **Second, reflect upon the ways you can integrate each of these items into your life.** To name just a few possibilities, you might offer your services as a volunteer for a phone hotline, sit outside in nature where you can focus on your connection to something greater than yourself, listen to a favorite CD or comedy tape whenever you're receiving treatment, or take a class in meditation or nutrition. You get the idea. And don't forget: Building time into your schedule for a short nap also has the power to raise your vibrations and bring you a sense of peace.

- **Third, do a quick assessment each day to determine if you are feeling more at peace.** Across the top of a 3×5 notecard, list the pleasant activities in which you've begun to engage. List the days of the week down the left side. At the end of each day, rate each activity on a scale of 1 to 10 (10 being the highest). If your numbers are in the upper range (7 to 10), you'll know that you are living in greater alignment with your heart's truth. I also encourage you to write in any additional activities that brought you pleasure and contentment. Maybe you said "no" to someone, stood up to your boss or supervisor, or read an inspirational article that touched you, for instance.

  If your numbers are lower, replace your activities with others that may bring you more joy and restore a greater sense of control. For too long, you have engaged in life events and activities that have not fostered a sense of inner peace and joy. It is your turn, your right, and your privilege to begin building into your life what you love.

Remember, alignment is a moment-to-moment endeavor. Working toward it will take dedication, perseverance, courage and work (which, in some cases, may be play!). Yes, try to honor your responsibilities as an employee, parent, spouse, etc., but begin integrating things that make you feel good, happy, and satisfied into your life. In other words, as you face cancer, carve out time to live your joy and your passion. Self-love and healing begin with you making time in your schedule to do what fulfills you, be it sitting by a lake, going to the library for an hour in the middle of the day, or taking guitar, acting, tennis, or singing lessons. You are not being selfish; you are showing yourself the love and care that you need to be healthy.

It is also important to remember that opportunities for re-alignment come when you are feeling fearful and anxious, and when you are aware that others' expectations of you do not match what you feel to be authentic and genuine within your heart. Keep in mind that love is the energetic opposite of fear. When you love yourself enough to gather your courage and say "no" or "I forgive you," or to detach and let go, you gain the physical, mental and spiritual energy to realign, feel more at peace, and focus on health-affirming activities.

Elena's Story: Finding Alignment through Forgiveness and Reclaiming Power

I would like to close this chapter by sharing the story of a dear soul and patient, Elena, who reclaimed her power by aligning with her soul. She grew spiritually by consciously making loving choices that enabled her to experience greater peace. Some of these choices centered on choosing to forgive those with whom she had experienced personal pain and suffering. Other choices contributed to her experiencing a sense of quiet joy and inner peace. Her ultimate goal was to re-align with the wisdom of her heart and achieve a sense of balance, wholeness, and well-being.

When Elena first came to me, she had been re-diagnosed with breast cancer. Her first occurrence was in 2003, at which point she'd had a lumpectomy. And while she had agreed to undergo breast surgery for the re-occurrence, she made it clear to me and to her doctors that she did not wish to partake in the recommended course of chemotherapy because of the impact it would have on her body and her quality of life. Instead, she wished to pursue a variety of integrative treatments that included working with an oncologist for hormonal treatment, a physiatrist, a naturopath, a chiropractor, an energy medicine practitioner, and Reiki practitioners.

I am not sure I would have or could have had the courage to make similar choices. However, as I have previously written, healing is the restoration of balance in order to return to a state of being at peace—which occurs when we are aligned with our heart's bliss. Thus, as Elena's psychologist, I worked to help her achieve balance between her mind, body, and spirit.

As we talked, it became clear to me that the emotional struggles of Elena's childhood may have been a contributing factor to her cancer, in addition to her carrying the BRCA gene. (Elena had already lost her mother and sister to cancer.) The oldest of her siblings, Elena did not feel valued and tried to win approval by being a "good girl" at home and in school—but her efforts never met with success. The nuns at her school, she said, rejected the drawings she had colored with such pride because she colored outside the lines! And while she knew her mom loved her, Elena spent her childhood repressing her own thoughts, feelings, and wishes. She grew up doing whatever her mother, whom she described as being strict, told her to do.

As a result, Elena lacked the confidence and self-worth to confront those in authority, even when her own best interests were at stake. As she grew into adulthood, she held onto the hurt and anger that had arisen during her childhood, especially toward her mother (although their relationship did eventually improve), and she continued to avoid confronting authority figures. In other words, as Elena matured, she lacked her own voice and a sense of her own power.

For Elena, cancer's gift was that it enabled her to heal these wounds, work toward alignment, and reclaim her own power. Her disease was a wake-up call that gave her courage to meet with doctors locally and throughout the country, many of whom had written of their unique integrative approach to healing cancer. It took courage for her to travel with her husband to speak to these individuals who served as authority figures for her and with whom she knew she might disagree.

Gradually, Elena became more and more comfortable composing letters to her doctors and speaking with them in person. She was able to express her need to be listened to and have her thoughts respected, even if she did not follow the prescribed protocol. She was no longer afraid to say what was on her mind. Elena's courage helped her to achieve a sense of heartfelt satisfaction, self-perceived strength, value, and peace within her being. Each conversation with a medical authority figure provided her with an opportunity to love herself enough to align with her own sense of Truth—and to feel good!

Along with taking her power, Elena learned to practice the art of Unconditional Love. To do this, she had to forgive herself and others, as well as release the feelings of pain and suffering she had been carrying around since childhood. She made peace with her mom and dad, with the nuns in her childhood schools and other authority figures, including her physicians, and with her present family members.

Elena came to realize that she had been projecting her childhood pain onto present relationships with those she loved, and that it had been very destructive. For instance, Elena had experienced differences with her son-in-law due to his parenting style, which reminded her of her mother's. She feared that her grand-children, too, would repress their feelings if their father treated them as her mom had treated her. Elena wanted her grandchildren to grow up feeling special, loved, and valued—and aware of their own unique power.

She was determined that there would be healing—and there was! Elena was able to release the vibration of anger and expressed her feelings to her son-in-law, who understood and forgave her. He told her that he was aware of how much she had shifted.

Throughout the process of taking her power and learning to forgive, Elena found joy in researching spiritual matters. She and her husband enjoyed attending seminars and taking classes in matters of spirituality. She especially loved learning about Angels and their work. These events buoyed her spirit, enabling her to feel greater peace, joy, and a sense of living in alignment with her heart's desires. Elena was equally passionate about learning and understanding everything she could to assist in the healing impact of her energy medicine sessions. They, too, enabled her to feel a stunning sense of peace, improved well-being, and inexplicable wholeness, despite the pain that often accompanied her on a daily basis.

And Elena loved to write. In fact, she was a very gifted writer. Journaling and writing affirmations seemed to sustain her and to give her needed hope—all of which helped to achieve alignment. Daily, she wrote and verbalized affirmations such as: *I love love; I love life; I am drawing to me what I need for my healing and well-being.* She had a repertoire of healing tools and she used what felt right at the time—all with the goal of re-aligning with her heart and using love to eradicate her fears.

I can honestly say that Elena became a rare being who actually lived in a state of love. Even with all that she was going through, Elena would become distressed when she learned that a friend, relative, or even one of her healers was not doing well. She would pray for that person and do whatever she could to help.

Many thought of Elena as an earth angel. I share all of this with you because every one of Elena's actions helped her to achieve alignment and healing.

But do not think that Elena was Miss Goody Two Shoes! Elena was quite human and struggled with the same things that most of us who are challenged by cancer do. She often spoke to me of how difficult the nights were because of the thoughts that would overtake her regarding her cancer. It was during those long nights that she would make the choice to breathe deeply; to allow herself to have a good cry; to pray; to practice her tapping, mindfulness, and face, embrace and replace techniques; and to focus on what brought her joy, especially her grandchildren.

As you may have guessed from my use of the past tense, Elena did not experience physical healing. However—and this is very important—she left feeling no resistance, only peace. For her, this was true healing. Finally, she was living in total alignment with her heart.

Know that I very much wanted Elena to live, survive and thrive, as did her family and all those who knew her. Elena's legacy is her courage and how she chose to live while on her cancer journey. She could have felt sorry for herself and not have used the time for anything except self-pity. However, realizing that the quality of her life had to do with her choices, Elena chose to use this time to grow spiritually, learning powerful lessons. These lessons enabled her to shift her perspective and realize that she had never, ever been alone—and that if the soul is eternal, then she, too, is.

"And while his mother's lecture had gone over his seven-year-old head, Pasquale saw now what she meant—how much easier life would be if our intentions and our desires could always be aligned."

JESS WALTER, IN *BEAUTIFUL RUINS*

CHAPTER **14**

Breathe Mindfully

―cho᠆oᠯᡅꝋ᠆

"Feelings come and go like clouds in a windy sky. Conscious breathing is my anchor."

THÍCH NHAT HANH

If you've read every chapter up to this point, you know that many of the exercises I've shared to help you find healing, balance, and clarity involve breath work. That's no coincidence. Breath is one of the major gifts with which we were all born.

Of course, your breaths keep you alive. But beyond that, I prefer to view breath as loving energy that is drawn into the body every few seconds—energy that can provide you with all you need to achieve well-being and peace. When approached mindfully, breath is the basis of relaxation, meditation, prayer, and healing, and it can be a powerful tool in helping you achieve a higher vibrational state. It can also help you to connect to the intuitive wisdom you'll need to survive and thrive during your cancer journey.

If you've always thought of breath as a natural and necessary bodily function—but nothing more—I encourage you to expand your understanding of it and begin using it as a tool to aid your healing by relaxing your body and spirit.

The Science of Breath

I have been teaching variations of breath exercises to patients for close to thirty years, and I have witnessed firsthand the dramatic power breath has to help restore balance and inner harmony. The breath that I teach is a variation of the breath originally taught by Dr. Herbert Benson, also called The Relaxation Response.

Dr. Benson, a cardiologist at Harvard, developed his technique as a way to help patients in need of healing. He conducted major research, delving into Transcendental Meditation, Biofeedback, and even traveling to study with Tibetan monks. Dr. Benson discovered that breath is a common element that can enable every one of us to experience increased feelings of warmth and well-being. In 1975, he published a very small, but very significant book, *The Relaxation Response*, to share his discovery with the world.

Specifically, Dr. Benson's research shows that when you choose to rhythmically breathe in and out for a few minutes, you set in motion a physiological response in the brain which reduces the stress hormone (cortisol) while releasing feel-good chemicals (such as endorphins) and hormones (such as DHEA) that guide your body to a deep state of relaxation. Rhythmic breathing also facilitates greater mental clarity and increases physical and emotional energy.

My version of Dr. Benson's healing technique combines the physiological mechanics of breath with imagery (just another word for the pictures you play in your head), which supports and sustains the impact of each breath on your cells. Both rhythmic breathing *and* imagery are needed to maximize this exercise's relaxing, calming impact on your physiological, psychological, and spiritual being.

My 15-Minute Peace Plan

As you'll see, my breath-driven "peace plan" only takes 15 minutes to complete, so I suggest you practice it daily. You can also adapt this exercise into a shorter "mini version," which you can practice as needed throughout the day. Doing this work regularly will help you conquer fear, sharpen your intuition, speed healing, and live your life with a sense of love and gratitude. Here's how:

- **Set the stage.** Choose a room that feels good and that has a chair or a comfortable place to sit: peaceful, safe, and inviting. If possible, use the same location and sitting position every time. You want to create a sense of strong association. This scene will become a trigger in your mind's eye. With enough practice, you will be able to immediately quiet and center yourself just by thinking of the space.

- **Play quiet, gentle music.** Of course, whether or not to listen to music is up to you—but I find (as do many of those with whom I work) that certain types of music help you to feel at peace. Personally, I enjoy listening to music by Johann Pachelbel (especially his "Canon in D") or Native American flute music during my breathing exercises. However, anything that helps you relax and get centered is fine.

- **Assume the "meditative or intuition posture."** Sit comfortably with spine relatively straight, feet flat on the floor, palms up. With your feet on the ground, you can visualize that you are connected to the earth. With palms up, you will feel more inviting and that the universe is open to your energy—and that you, in turn, are open to receiving the energy and wisdom of the universe.

- **Count slowly to ten as you begin to quiet and center yourself.** Then, hold your breath to a fast count to ten; then very slowly release your breath to a count of ten or higher. (If you find it helpful, bend the tips of your fingers in to touch your palms as you recite each number.) While you are exhaling, visualize your breath moving through the body, traveling through each cell. (The next two tips provide more details on how to do this. Understand that these tips are not necessarily sequential; some of them will happen simultaneously.)

- **Give your breath color and shape.** See *and* feel the warmth of your breath as you breathe in. Visualize that your breath has a shape and color. You might find it helpful to choose a color that symbolizes your intent. For instance:

    Green = Healing
    Blue = Peace
    White = Divine energy
    Pink = Compassion

Research with imagery has validated the importance of visualizing your breath. As you consciously breathe deep relaxing breaths, chemicals in the brain are released to help you feel greater warmth and relaxation.

- **Follow your breath on its travels.** *See* the breath enter through your nose and mouth, and watch it start the journey through your body. You want to *see it* and to *feel it* in your mind's eye and in your body. Visualize each breath going through every organ, limb, vertebra, muscle, and tissue. Picture it flowing through your bloodstream. Envision every cell delighting in the breath. Notice yourself feeling the increased warmth and *see* yourself feeling well. This facilitates progressive relaxation.

  While doing the breathing, you will experience an increased sense of heaviness. The paradox is that you may also notice a feeling of lightness!

- **Find your mantra.** *I am experiencing healing. I'm feeling more relaxed. I'm feeling more peaceful. I'm becoming pure love. I am in alignment with my higher self.* These are just a few suggestions. Your mantra can be a favorite expression, the first line of your favorite prayer (e.g., "The Lord is my Shepherd"), or something that just helps you relax like "Shalom." Whatever you choose, associate the tone of your mantra with finding peace and healing. Then say it over and over in your mind. This creates your "mind's ear" connection.

- **Make a connection with something greater than yourself.** As we discussed in Chapter Ten, it doesn't matter whether your "something greater" is God, Jesus, Mary, Buddha, Universal Energy, or Mind. Just imagine breathing in Its divine energy. Ask your Higher Power for help, guidance, and healing.

- **Begin with gratitude.** Be certain to give thanks. The vibrations of "thank you" and/or the vibrations of "blessings" are very powerful. They draw to us what we secretly desire and what we need for healing and alignment. Gratitude is a higher state of consciousness.

- **Love is the key. Fill your body with love.** Imagine your whole body being filled up with love. Not romantic love, but pure, unconditional love—the kind you would feel for a baby, a puppy, or a kitten. Make it your intention. Give it a color and a shape. Visualize and feel yourself becoming loving energy.

- **After you've made the shift, state your intention.** After about ten or fifteen minutes of breathing, you will feel an inner shift of consciousness. The shift may be very subtle and the time required to reach it will shorten with practice. You will know this subtle shift when it happens; it means you have established a connection with your higher wisdom. This is the time to state your intention. (You may also state your intention at the beginning of the process, before you begin your breathing.) For example, *I wish to receive healing energy* or *I will focus my attention on living in alignment and feeling calm and at peace.*

  You might also use this time to make a request, knowing that rhythmic breathing enhances your intuition. For instance: *I wish to tune into* _____ (fill in whatever questions for which you're seeking answers). *I would like to receive information for either myself, or a particular person or situation. Please enable me to receive this information.*

- **Listen for your answer.** It may come in flashes of insight, which can easily be overlooked if you're not paying attention. Or it may take the form of a feeling in the gut or the head. Stay focused. Ask "What do I need to know?" It is important to realize that the answer you're seeking may not come right away. Often you may need to "sleep on it" or lose yourself in another activity for the answer to come to you.

Remember, this exercise is meant to help you learn to shift your consciousness more quickly, to sharpen your intuitive sense, and to promote healing, peace, and well-being. (All of which are especially needed during your cancer journey!) With daily practice, you will find yourself making better, healthier, self-honoring decisions, and you'll just *feel* better in general. Safer. More grounded. More in control. Your self-esteem and confidence will increase while your fear decreases.

Over time, and with continued practice, you will learn to notice if you aren't feeling well and to shift so that you can connect with this higher energy. More and more, you'll come from a place of love and gratitude instead of from a place of fear. And that's a change that can transform your whole life, regardless of cancer's role in it.

"Breath is the bridge which connects life to consciousness, which unites your body to your thoughts."

Thích Nhat Hanh

CHAPTER **15**

Open Yourself to Miracles and Extraordinary Experiences

"I no longer feel that life is ordinary. Everyday life is filled with mystery. The things we know are only a small part of the things we cannot know but can only glimpse. Yet even the smallest of glimpses can sustain us

...

Mystery seems to have the power to comfort, to offer hope, and to lend meaning in times of loss and pain. In surprising ways, it is the mysterious that strengthens us at such times."

RACHEL NAOMI REMEN, MD

Gabriela was referred to me by her physician following the un-expected death of her son. She wanted to heal. Yet Gabriela was not one to accept easily what she could not see, touch, or feel. (Perhaps you can relate!) However, over the years we have worked together, she has become more open to extraordinary, miraculous experiences. Now, Gabriela will often share a story with me that can't be explained by normal means. We'll both smile in awe of the situation, and I'll take comfort in the fact that my patient is feeling peace. (The most recent synchronicity was the fact that her grandson was born on the date of her son's death!)

Over the years, other patients and friends have shared sight-ings, signs, and events that they know are outside the ordinary, and that have an immediate healing impact on their well-being. You, too, have the capacity to experience the extraordinary—and to let these experiences contribute to your healing as you proceed on your healing journey.

Like so many of the healing tools I share in this book, becom-ing open to the extraordinary is an inside job. When you choose to view the world, or even a specific situation, with a different viewpoint or perspective, you will find that your world changes. In this chapter, I hope to help you cultivate an open, accepting mindset, and give you the tools to invite miracles large and small into your life.

Miracles Are Part of the Human Experience.

Overall, I've noticed that humans—regardless of spiritual be-liefs—seem to intuitively know that miracles occur. Many of us have experienced them firsthand, and from what I've observed, most of us would welcome them into our own lives. A survey released by Pew Forum on Religion a few years back supports my observations. It shows that nearly 80 percent of Americans believe in miracles. This group of believers included many people who described themselves as being unaffiliated with any particular religious tradition.[1]

Having spent more than two decades studying the nature of miracles and the conditions under which they occur, I firmly believe that *everyone* (yes, including you!) can receive these natural gifts because we are all spiritually connected to God, Source, Allah, or whatever you choose to call this wellspring of goodness. I think that we're all hungry for more hope, joy, and spiritual growth—even diehard skeptics. *Especially* diehard skeptics!

Why is that? Well, we'd all like to experience a connection with loved ones who have passed away, which miracles often provide. Beyond that, when people experience a miracle firsthand, they tend to see it as a blessing that makes them feel safe, holy, divine, not alone, protected, and taken care of—and frequently, just makes them smile. All of those are good, high-vibrational feelings, which are good for your spiritual, emotional, and physical health.

Miracles and Cancer

I encourage my patients with cancer to remain open to miracles and to read stories about them, because stories provide inspiration, comfort, and hope. All of these things help to restore internal balance, enabling the immune system to take better care of you. I do *not* choose to focus on miracles in the sense of radical healings and cures, but rather encourage awareness that when balance is restored, the body is better able to heal itself. This can (and usually does) take time and patience.

Of course, if you are dealing with an illness such as cancer, you would like to be free of this burden. But remember, this journey is about finding the ability to be at peace with where you are, and choosing to love yourself first—unconditionally. Unconditional love is at the heart of making miracles because unconditional love allows you to release anything and everything that keeps you disconnected from you remembering your true essence (which is love).

With the release of your fears, doubts, judgments, self-criticism, regrets, and anger, your immune system can begin to produce what is needed to lovingly care for you ... and you can begin to experience various types of healing, including physical, emotional, mental, and spiritual healing.

Invite Miracles into Your Life.

In order to live a life rich in miracles, from the small to the momentous, you simply have to foster your ability to invite them in. Here are a few suggestions and insights that will prepare you to receive your own miracles:

- **Give yourself permission to be open to extraordinary experiences.** After working with patients who have shared countless stories of miraculous events in their lives, I have come to recognize that the ability to experience miracles is often dependent on whether or not you allow for the possibility of miracles in your life in the first place. To put it more simply, the odds of experiencing a miracle dramatically increase when you choose to believe that they are a part of our world. Accept that you will allow the Universe to do its good, and it will respond accordingly.
- **Rediscover your spirituality.** Take time to connect with your own soul and with the Source by returning to—or visiting for the first time—prayer, ritual, and faith. Learn to meditate while breathing deeply, or do yoga. Most of all, try to reach a point at which you feel your connection to the Universe and everything in it. (Look back at Chapter Ten for more specific tactics.)

- **Commit to making significant changes in negative thoughts, feelings, and beliefs.** This is especially important for a person suffering an illness because, as we've discussed, anxiety and desperation have a strong tendency to block your ability to heal. To review, in order to change this stone-set pattern, you must always be aware of what you are feeling and then consciously replace negative or disturbing thoughts with positive and empowering ones.

  Here's the "miracle connection": If you think uplifting, feel-good thoughts the majority of the time (so that they are your dominant thoughts), you will attract and allow positive things, people, and events into your life. Above all, keep your heart brimming full of love and compassion. Filling yourself with this type of high-level energy is the most important factor in inviting miracles into your life.

- **Keep a synchronicity journal.** Synchronicity is the flow of "meaningful coincidences" that indicate that life, *all* life, is connected in a complex web of psychic moments, signs, symbols, and shivers of spiritual connectedness. The sheer volume of these subtle miracles that happen in so many different lives adds up to powerful evidence of "something greater." That's why I recommend keeping a list of "meaningful coincidences" that happen in your own life. For instance, make a note if:

  - You think of an old acquaintance you haven't seen for a while, only to receive a phone call from her that evening.
  - You can't shake the feeling that you should call your mother, and when you do you find her sick in bed.
  - You have been thinking of your father who passed away years ago, and while alone in your home, catch a whiff of the cologne he always wore.

- Your dentist recently moved, and you need to find a new practice. Later that day, a coworker begins raving about the new dentist he just saw.

When you begin to identify the meaning behind synchronous occurrences in your own life and realize that they *aren't* random, you will find yourself attracting more and more miracles ... and being conscious and appreciative of them as they occur.

- **Write down your intentions.** In detail, record on paper with joyful enthusiasm and gratitude exactly what you desire from the Universe—daily. That might be reconciliation with a loved one, clarity regarding an upcoming decision, or even physical healing. Expect good things to be placed in your path and they will come—be it a spiritual visit from a passed loved one, a new chance in a waning relationship, or the return to living a joyful, meaningful life.

As you clarify and record your intentions, remember, miracles are determined by your perspective, as well as by the meaning you assign an experience. Let's use physical healing as an example. It helps to realize that healing takes many forms, any of which may be perceived as a miracle by you. For some, physical healing may be seen as the ability to regain energy and return to a relatively full life, though it may include continuing treatments of different sorts. For others, physical healing may mean going into remission, and for still others, it may mean the sudden and complete disappearance of the illness.

Thus, you might write out one of the following intentions: *I intend to live a meaningful, joyful life again. I intend to experience greater balance, energy, and well-being in my life. I intend to heal on as many levels as is possible ... emotionally, mentally, physically, and spiritually.* As you write your intentions, visualize yourself becoming them, and feel the reality of the experience moving through all your cells.

- **Immerse yourself in stories of the miraculous.** Many, many people have had miraculous experiences. When you read about or listen to the amazing things they've experienced, you mentally, emotionally, and spiritually "set the stage" to notice the small miracles you might be overlooking in your own life. You also open yourself up to receiving new ones.

Think about it this way: Someone can tell you all day long that the soul survives death, that your loved one is in a better place, that God loves you, that there's more to life than science can explain, and that against-the-odds healing can occur. But until you hear these pieces of information in the context of a story, they don't resonate, and they might even be easy to disbelieve or dismiss. Essentially, stories speak to us in such a way that bypasses the thinking brain and connects to visceral truths.

That's one reason why I decided to write *Touched by the Extraordinary, Book Two*. It's a collection of real-life occurrences—including messages sent from loved ones who've passed on, angel visitations, and signs—that can be defined only as the stuff of miracles. My hope is that this collection of stories will enable readers to experience comfort, healing, and peace—and to become more open to experiencing miracles in their own lives!

Accordingly, to conclude this chapter, I will share a few stories that might help you incorporate the extraordinary into your cancer journey.

A Mom's Healing Presence

Linda, who was dealing with breast cancer, lymphedema, and lung issues, told me about one of the most powerful, meaningful, and miraculous Reiki sessions she has ever had. She deeply felt that it impacted her cancer healing journey.

Linda received a call from a friend who was also a Reiki Master. At the time, this friend was helping her students learn and participate in a distant healing session. She asked for permission to share with Linda what she was receiving during the healing session, and to describe to Linda what she and her students were doing to expedite Linda's healing. She also indicated that they were working with Archangel Raphael, the Archangel of Healing.

Linda's Reiki Master friend indicated that she could perceive a river of green healing energy flowing through Linda's body. The Reiki Master then told Linda that she was aware of a white light presence in the room that was "mother-like," and that the presence—Linda's mom—was there to enable Linda to let go and release her pain from their relationship. Keep in mind that Linda's friend had no idea that Linda had been working with a therapist on childhood issues related to her mom!

Linda spoke of her struggle with talking about the emotional pain her mom had caused her as a child, while at the same time feeling she was dishonoring her mom by speaking about it. Linda's mom then used Linda's friend to channel this message to Linda:

My dear sweet one, I am so light and free here and I know such deep love here. I was not free in my earthly body and often felt trapped. My dear sweet baby, I love you. My dear sweet baby, I am sorry ... and my dear sweet baby, I do love you.

Linda was then told to continue to feel the green river of healing energy flowing through her body—which she did feel. Raphael gave her one more message: *"Your mother's presence in your life had the purpose of helping you to reach your highest self."* Linda shared with me that these messages both humbled and empowered her, and added to her healing.

After the Reiki sessions, Linda noticed her mother's necklace hanging on a jewelry hook on her bedroom closet door. While she especially loved to wear this piece, Linda had been unable to do so because pain from her lymphedema restricted her range of motion, making it impossible for Linda to place the necklace on herself. This time, though, Linda's arms lifted with ease. She was able to clasp the necklace in place around her neck without feeling guilt, pain, and ambivalence—only love. Linda knew that without a doubt, an extraordinary miracle had just taken place. For this, she was extremely grateful.

Wings of Hope

In *Touched by the Extraordinary, Book Two*, Mary Ellen, who had been challenged by non- Hodgkin lymphoma (and is now thriving), described her encounter with red cardinals as she was returning to her teaching position following her surgeries and chemotherapy treatments. She had prayed to a statue of the Virgin Mary that her friends had given her the day before. In her prayers, Mary Ellen requested signs of inspiration and hope for healing. When a red cardinal flew directly in front of her car window while on the way to work, several days in a row, Mary Ellen felt that these events were signs from Mary that she would heal. She was filled with hope and joy.

Angels Among Us

A number of my patients share with me that they enjoy ongoing communication with their angels and feel more at peace knowing that their angels are always there for them. When you are dealing with a life-threatening illness, it is exceptionally comforting to know that you are not alone and you are being watched over.

Recently, a breast cancer patient, Heather, told me that she had been asking her angels to help her with her sense of hope and purpose by lining up clients to build her pet sitting business. The following day she received two calls that dealt with referrals for her new business. Heather believed this was in response to her request, and she was delighted.

One way my patients know their angels are with them is through the use of Angel Cards (created by Doreen Virtue to communicate with your angels). So often, patients share with me that following our session, the cards they end up selecting (by chance) reflect the very subjects we discussed, be it forgiveness, patience, love, intuition, protection, etc. My patients are always amazed—and so am I! I especially love Marcy's experience with Angel Cards, which I'll share next.

The Gift of Asking and Receiving

Marcy, a wife, mom, and healer in her own right, who also worked with breast cancer patients, was experiencing her fourth challenge with breast cancer. By the time she and I met, Marcy was feeling that enough was enough. When cancer continues to reoccur, it begins to erode your sense of confidence in all being well, in your health, and in your sense of control. Normally a confident, strong, determined young woman, Marcy had begun to doubt her own intuitive wisdom.

In our work together, Marcy and I addressed, processed, resolved, and released many issues. However, she knew that what still remained was a major decision regarding a surgery she needed. As a researcher of intuition and consciousness, I encouraged Marcy to take the time to meditate and ask for guidance.

Over a period of several months, Marcy experienced a connection with her Higher Wisdom through her meditation and the use of her Angel Cards (created by Doreen Virtue). The guidance she was receiving about the best route to take (regarding which surgery to have and where to have it) countered what her doctors—with the exception of one—were telling her.

Having the courage to listen to the voice that spoke frequently to her during her quiet times contributed to Marcy's decision to travel to New Orleans for her surgery. This was a decision that was not supported by most of her doctors.

When Marcy returned from New Orleans and was seen by one of her physicians, he was kind enough to let her know that he felt the surgery was done beautifully and that, thanks to her, another option was available for his patients. This was the same physician who had initially recommended a different surgical option, believing there was no other way to go.

Marcy knows she does not travel the journey of this lifetime alone. She knows guidance is available to her at all times, if she only assumes responsibility for her life by asking and listening. Because she trusted in this wisdom, she chose to quiet herself, go within, and ask for what she needed.

All of this is miraculous and significant because Marcy now feels a greater sense of confidence and empowerment, enabling her to release her fears regarding her health and her future. She is thriving and deeply grateful for all that she receives from the universe.

When Cancer Gifts You with Life

I have written elsewhere in this book about how my breast cancer saved my life. But since I consider this to be miraculous, I'd like to share the story again here! Had it not been for my breast cancer treatments, I would never have received the body scan that revealed a tumor on my adrenal gland. This rare tumor, called a classic pheochromocytoma in the medical books, was life-threatening because it caused my blood pressure to skyrocket to dangerously high levels. I was told by one of the doctors who saw me that I had been a walking time-bomb.

This diagnosis explained why I had on two occasions during the six months leading up to my surgery felt like I was going to die, and why my blood pressure kept rising higher and higher with each of my surgeries. Had the tumor not been discovered and removed, I would not be here writing these words. Yes, this was a miracle, and as I perceive the experience, a gift from the universe so that I could continue enjoying a quality-filled life.

"There are only two ways to live your life. One is as though nothing is a miracle. The other is as though everything is a miracle. I choose the latter."

ALBERT EINSTEIN

CHAPTER **16**

Don't Be the Strong, Silent, Solitary Type

"Trouble is a part of life, and if you don't share it, you don't give the person who loves you a chance to love you enough."

DINAH SHORE

It's not unusual for people to withdraw from the world when they are sad, frightened, or anxious—which is often the case after a cancer diagnosis. There are many specific reasons why you may become withdrawn:

- You're depressed, and don't have the energy to interact with other people.
- You feel that you're somehow "responsible" for comforting others who are upset by your diagnosis, and you want to avoid dealing with *their* grief, fear, etc.
- You want to avoid talking about your cancer altogether. The less you think about it, the less real it seems.
- You've convinced yourself that you're strong enough to "handle this" on your own, and that you really don't need anyone else.
- You don't want to be a burden—emotional or physical—on your friends and family.
- Other's solicitousness feels cloying and suffocating.

... and so on and so forth. But no matter why you're withdrawn, please believe me when I state that it is *not* in your best interests to isolate yourself from others. As John Donne accurately and poetically stated, "No man is an island"—and scientific research bears this observation out. Many researchers have conducted studies that demonstrate the impact of social support on quality of life, longevity, and health.

For instance, in a lecture titled *Healing and Feeling: Stress, Support, and Breast Cancer,* David Spiegel, MD (who is Professor and Associate Chair of Psychiatry and Behavioral Sciences at Stanford University School of Medicine and Medical Director of the Center for Integrative Medicine at Stanford University School of Medicine) emphasized that it is imperative to meet the psychosocial needs of the patient. He spoke of his major study, which demonstrated that women with advanced metastatic breast cancer who participated in a breast cancer support group and received traditional medical care lived 18 months longer than women who did not participate in such a group. The women in support groups also experienced less anxiety, depression, and physical pain than those not in a support group. For more information on this talk, go to http://www.shlnews.org/?p=55.

The Amazing Story of Roseto, Pennsylvania

One of my favorite studies that substantiates the impact of social support, community, and love on our physical health focuses on the town of Roseto, Pennsylvania. (If you'd like to read a more detailed account of "The Roseto Effect," I suggest visiting http://www.uic.edu/classes/osci/osci590/14_2%20The%20Roseto%20Effect.htm.)

When researchers Stewart Wolf, MD and sociologist John Bruhn originally visited the town of Roseto in the early 1960s, they found the incidence of heart disease to be half of the national average for men ages over 65 and to be zero for men 54-64. This came as a surprise to the researchers, given the lifestyle factors of the men. They worked long days in the quarry, ate a high fat diet (fried foods and lard), smoked, and drank wine. Some were diabetic and obese. All of this was a stark contrast to the men in a neighboring town whose heart events and mortality met the national expectations.

What the researchers discovered was that Roseto was a tightly-knit town of Italian-Americans where people genuinely cared for one another. Relationships mattered. Several generations of families lived together, with the elderly being honored members of their society. Mealtimes were family time for nourishing the soul. In fact, all the town's people tended to eat a set menu depending on the day of the week. The rituals of the town, including celebrations, holidays, religious services, and social clubs contributed to everyone's well-being. The goal of the people was to work to create a better life for their children via hard work and education.

Roseto's residents took pride in their life of predictability and conformity. Wealth was not flaunted in homes, cars, or clothes. This was a community based on a strong work ethic in which women worked in the small blouse factories in the town and the men deep in the quarries. There was no competition because everyone shared values centered on family, rather than material possessions. Everyone knew their place, roles, and goals. Consequently, there was little stress, essentially due to not having much freedom to make different choices. Each person felt safe and comfortable. What mattered most were the relationships with family and friends. Amazingly, Roseto experienced no crime, nor were there any applications for public assistance.

The researchers believed that there would be significant changes in their findings when they returned 25 years later—and there were! When the researchers returned to Roseto, they found an increase in heart disease. The number of heart attacks and the mortality rate equaled that of the rest of the country. There were several reasons.

First, Roseto's children had grown up and chosen to move away to attend school and to follow the American dream (and make money). Additionally, the values of the members of the community had changed, with a stronger emphasis on material possessions rather than relationships and connectedness. They were experiencing the impact of stress on their health.

Think about this for a moment. Like the people of Roseto, most of us have shifted away from the values held by our grandparents, which were much more strongly centered around family and relationships. Now, many of us have less time for social relationships as we strive to make money. We are trading off what we need most—social support—in order to achieve less fulfilling goals. Stress abounds and impacts the body's immune system, resulting in an increase of cardiovascular disease, autoimmune disease, and cancer.

My point? It's important to stay mindful of the ways in which our stressful modern lives may be impacting your health, and consequently arrange your life so that you have time for friends, family, and fun. As the case of Roseto powerfully demonstrates, community and social support can be an incredibly powerful factor in achieving health and overall wellness. The bottom line is, if you are facing cancer and want to promote healing, you cannot afford to be the strong, silent type.

Plus, keeping in mind (once again!) that everything is energy, your immune system needs to vibrate at a high level in order to take good care of you. And I promise, your own energy will be enhanced when you surround yourself with people who care about you, and who are compassionate, caring, and loving.

That being the case, in this chapter, we'll delve into authentic relationships: what they look like, and how to find and cultivate them. Remember, other people can be one of your biggest assets in your fight against cancer!

Identify Relationships That Aren't Working.

Before you can fully focus on creating meaningful relationships, you need to weed out the ones that aren't working—those that are draining your time, energy, and emotional well-being. Here are several tactics you can use to identify toxic relationships:

- **Get clear on what your values are.** Really spend some time thinking about how you want to live your life and what you look for in others. Trustworthiness? Honesty? Mutual respect? Forgiveness? It might help to write out a list. When you have consciously identified what is important to you, what feels right, and what makes you feel comfortable and safe, you'll be able to determine whether those things are present in your relationships. (This exercise is all about living in alignment, which we discussed in Chapter Thirteen.)

Remember, your thoughts are energy, and energy vibrates. When you're interacting with another person, you intuitively sense his or her energy. When you're clear on your own values, you'll know whether the two of you are a good fit. You'll feel safe, and the relationship will feel authentic.

- **Start paying attention to how people make you feel.** Chances are, at some point in your life, you've met another person who just didn't feel "right," even though you might not have been able to put your finger on why. Maybe you called it a gut feeling, a premonition, or intuition, but you simply knew deep down that this relationship wouldn't go anywhere good. Trusting such feelings is usually a smart idea even if there is no "rational" reason to do so.

  When you're with someone and you start to feel uncomfortable—edgy or ill at ease—pay attention. *Especially* when you're fighting cancer, you don't want to regret becoming embroiled a toxic or draining relationship. It is so important that you listen to your own inner wisdom, especially if you are beginning to notice that something does not feel right deep within your core.

- **Listen with your heart, not your ears.** Whether you've just met someone or are spending time with a friend, coworker, or acquaintance you've known for years—or even when you're interacting with a member of your medical team—*really* listen during your conversation. That doesn't just mean using your ears—it also means using your heart. In other words, look for a lack of congruity between the words being said and the way those words make you feel.

When someone is trying to lie to you, mislead you, or fool you—whether they're malicious or "just" telling a white lie—you can usually tell. Try to get into the habit of assessing yourself physically and emotionally on a regular basis. How are you feeling? Are you off-balance, is your energy dropping, or do you not feel totally "there"? Remember, when your values are aligned with another's, you'll feel good. And also, keep in mind that a disagreement in this area doesn't necessarily mean that another person is *bad* ... just bad for *you*.

- **Let cancer sharpen your clarity.** As we've discussed several times before, cancer has a way of clarifying whether or not we're living our lives in alignment. On a very regular basis, my patients tell me that they've "suddenly" realized who their true friends are and aren't, as though blinders had been lifted from their eyes. They have a new understanding of which relationships are toxic, and which are healthy.

  The fact is, cancer throws into sharp relief the fact that you have limited time on this earth. So don't be surprised if you find yourself instinctively drawn to spending more time with certain people, and less with others. By the same token, don't be surprised if some individuals you expected to support you pull away, and if your staunchest allies come from unexpected places. Above all, trust your intuition in terms of who you choose to spend your time with. Now more than ever, it's important for you to nourish relationships that promote healing and well-being, and to stop enduring others out of obligation.

Don't Feel Bad About Letting Relationships That Don't Work Fall Away.

As you begin to get more comfortable with trusting what your intuition tells you, you'll inevitably identify relationships that are unhealthy. (Again, another person or group can be bad *for you* without being inherently bad itself!) Your first instinct might be to try to "make it work"—after all, no one wants to hurt another's feelings unnecessarily.

Realize, though, that it's okay to extract yourself from a negative relationship, or at least to back off and relate to the person on a more superficial level. If it helps, remind yourself that you're not betraying or dishonoring the other party—you're honoring yourself. This is something we all need to do more often, and it's especially important when it comes to cultivating high-level, healing vibrations.

Of course, you won't necessarily have to end relationships that aren't working for you. (And in fact, you usually shouldn't without first working to ease the dysfunction.) As demonstrated by the two stories I'm going to share next, your illness may prompt you to take back your power and proactively make changes that need to happen for the sake of your healing.

The Clarity That Comes with Cancer: Diane's Story

After meeting and marrying the love of her life, my patient Diane had a daughter, Liza. Liza was adored by her grandmother who, over time, became an integral part of the family. Liza and her grandmother became exceptionally close: a good thing for Liza, but problematic at times for Diane. Not wanting to hurt her mom's feelings, she often let situations with which she was uncomfortable pass without telling her mom how much they bothered her.

Life is sometimes filled with heartbreaking challenges, as was the case for Diane. Precious Liza died at the age of four, leaving her parents and her grandmother absolutely devastated. Diane chose to work on her grief and to put the pieces of her life together. She went on to eventually feel emotionally, mentally, and physically healed enough to have another daughter, Samantha (Sam). Again, Diane's mom returned and stayed with the family to be present for both Samantha and Diane.

Diane experienced two more challenges: The first was the occurrence of breast cancer, and the second was the reoccurrence of the cancer. With each bout, her mom lovingly stepped in to help the family. However, over time, Diane became aware that she often felt responsible for her mother and husband's feelings. Diane was carrying this responsibility deep within her, and it, along with her need to remain connected to Liza, was affecting her health. In other words, Diane was not able to live being fully present.

In our work, Diane came to realize that for her to be able to take back the reins of her life and to focus on what she needed for her own healing, she needed to evaluate the dynamics of her relationships with her mom, husband, deceased daughter, and even her dad.

Being an astute and intuitive woman, Diane gradually communicated her feelings to her mom and husband, and released the need to feel responsible for their happiness. She needed to let them figure out what they could do to find their own peace. She also took her power by letting them know what she did and did not need from them, in terms of responsibilities. Furthermore, Diane emotionally released her need to hold onto her Liza, allowing herself to be more present for her daughter Samantha.

Finally, Diane came to realize that she needed to consider releasing her longstanding anger toward her dad, and to forgive him. She knew this process was essential, and that her father did the best that he knew how to do.

Take Back Your Power in Order to Heal: Darlene's Story

Darlene came to me physically, emotionally, mentally, and spiritually depleted and on the verge of becoming extremely ill. Like so many women, Darlene intuitively knew that something was terribly wrong with her life. I soon discovered that she was depressed and that she lacked energy, confidence, and power in her relationships with family members.

Darlene grew up in a family in which it was difficult to balance being noticed, doing what made her happy, and not being rejected for saying or doing the "wrong thing." Darlene adored her parents, but felt a greater sense of being understood and loved by her mom, who was a nurse. Like so many women, Darlene loved her dad but felt somewhat disconnected from him for much of her early life.

Darlene is extraordinarily bright and intuitive. Yet, to learn her life lessons, she drew to her a partner and children (each a beautiful soul) who would test her in many ways (as did her parents) by creating challenges that prompted her to remember just how powerful she was and is. As human beings, this is what we do. We tend to energetically choose partners who will help us learn our life lessons. If we have not worked out our "issues" with a parent, for example, we tend to find a partner who will push us to do the same type of work. Our partners become the resistance against which we push to eventually remember how strong and resilient we are.

Darlene is like many women in that she relinquished her power early in life, believing that she was here to put the needs of others first. Many of her own desires were put on the back burner.

When this happens, the body recognizes that something is amiss and registers the vibration of not feeling content. And after a lifetime of these lower-level vibrations, women often develop illnesses (such as breast or gynecological cancers) in their forties and fifties that serve as a wake-up call. For Darlene, the wake-up call included asthmatic breathing problems and multiple sclerosis.

When Darlene first came to see me, her children were in elementary and middle school and she was actively involved in parenting. There were issues in her marriage and her family that she wanted to address. She knew that she was entitled to be treated with respect and to be valued, but she needed to learn how to express her needs and to fight for the right to have them met. The bottom line is, Darlene's journey was about reclaiming her power and using it to experience the peace and joy she realized she deserved.

Little by little, month by month, and year by year, Darlene began healing herself emotionally, mentally, and in her relationships. The lovely thing was that gradually, as we worked together, her asthma became less and less problematic. This was due, I believe, to the fact that she no longer felt smothered by grief and powerlessness.

While Darlene still deals with MS, she is grateful that due to her efforts her family is lovingly present for her, and will continue to be. Darlene is one of my heroes. I admire her constancy of vision, her awareness of her resiliency, and her ability to harness her inherent resources to make herself well.

As Diane's and Darlene's stories demonstrate, sometimes it *does* take an illness or life-challenging event like cancer or multiple sclerosis to motivate us to make changes in our relationships. For the sake of our well-being, we do what is necessary to take back our life and our power, experience greater joy, and improve our chances of healing.

Attract Relationships That *Are* Healthy.

As you work on spending less time with people who don't contribute to your well-being, focus on nourishing your relationships with individuals who *are* sources of joy and inspiration. Here are some ways to attract positive people into your life:

- **Visualize and expect better relationships.** Remember the Law of Attraction: Like energy attracts like energy. Specific to this context, if you spend time obsessing over the relationships in your life that aren't going so well, you'll end up attracting even more negative people and situations. On the flip side, if you think positive thoughts, you will attract positive things, people, and events into your life. That's why it's so important to be clear about your intentions. You need to decide what a healthy, comfortable relationship looks like for you and keep that picture in your mind.
- **Ask the Universe for the relationships you need.** Send out a simple prayer to God or to the Universe. Specify that you're seeking to be connected to more positive people, and make sure you do so with a sense of expectation and gratitude.
- **Practice positivity.** The Law of Attraction isn't just limited to what you visualize for the future; it also applies to how you're behaving *right now*. Specifically, frequent complaints and negativity breed more of the same. Remember that every morning when you wake up, the ball is in your court in regards to how you want to spend your day. If you exude bitterness, anger, or self-pity, you may be bringing those around you down, too. Indeed, it's possible that some of the people in your life are right and healthy for you, but that you are poisoning the relationship with constant negativity.

Even in the midst of your cancer journey, you can make a conscious choice to surround others with love. By putting a smile on your face and greeting someone else with a cheerful, "Hi! Glad to see you!" you can set the tone for your interaction, as well as change your energy and the energy of those around you.

Confidently Ask Others for What You Need.

Maybe you're the type of person who doesn't want to impose or burden other people with your "problems." If so, you need to ditch that mindset as soon as possible! Remember, one of the reasons we humans were put on this earth is to help each other. Think about it this way: You want to make life easier and better for the ones you love. They feel the same way about you!

So don't hesitate to let your best friends know your situation, and don't feel guilty about letting them assist you, be it through prayer, making a meal or two, a visit, sending you flowers, bringing you gifts, running errands for you, chauffeuring your children, sending you cards, providing a listening ear, accompanying you to appointments, or supporting a favorite cause of yours.

When you allow loved ones to do these things for you, you're giving them a gift, too: The gift of allowing them to feel that they can make a difference in the quality of your healing journey.

Connect with Others Who Understand Your Journey.

Finally, I want to encourage you to consider being a part of a support group that is focused on your type of illness. Individuals who are facing or who have faced similar obstacles will be able to share coping skills, information, and emotional support that may be difficult to obtain from even the most loving and well-intentioned loved ones. Here's an example of what I'm talking about:

For the past few years, along with Dr. Amy Harvey, I have had the honor and privilege of sharing the co-leadership of The GyniGirls, a support group for women with various kinds of gynecological cancers. This is a relatively small group of women who share our sorrows, fears, and joys, including those that many members don't feel comfortable discussing with "outsiders." When we meet, we eat well, laugh a lot, and cry with one another. Each of us looks at our coming together as a safe place to share what is in our hearts, and in which to support one another. We have come to love, trust, and unconditionally accept one another. This is what a support group should be offering you, too.

So, how can you find a support group? In my experience, they are available at most hospitals and treatment centers, so as your doctor for a recommendation. Support can also be found online in the form of chat rooms and at www.carepages.com. My patients (both cancer patients and caretakers) have found these online resources to be especially valuable because they are accessible 24 hours a day. In fact, the friendships made through the years on these sites often endure the test of time and circumstances.

Ultimately, I want you to remember that happiness and health (whether you have cancer or not!) can come only from embracing unconditional love as often as possible. And you can only embrace unconditional love if you are connected in a meaningful way to other people. So even if your instinct is to withdraw and to face cancer with a stiff upper lip, please resist that impulse. In fact, if you focus on attracting and cultivating good relationships, you might look back on this as one of the most rewarding times of your life—a period that was filled with positive growth and increasing joy, even in the midst of physical pain.

"People must believe in each other, and feel that it can be done and must be done: In that way, they are enormously strong. We must keep up each other's courage."

Vincent van Gogh

CHAPTER 17

Understand the Healing Value of Intimacy

"As cliché as it sounds, love and affection with the right person can nurture a healing that reaches beyond your cancer baggage and into the foundation of your well-being. We all have wounds. Once we deal with the upheaval that cancer churns up, those old bruises can finally begin to heal."

KRIS CARR, IN *CRAZY SEXY CANCER TIPS*

Dealing with a diagnosis of cancer (no matter your gender or the kind of cancer you have) or any other life-threatening illness is devastating by itself. What makes your situation even more problematic is that you begin to think thoughts that seem rational, but that may not be so. Do any of the following thoughts sound familiar?

- *Who would want to date or marry me, knowing I have cancer?*
- *How can my husband (wife or partner) and I be intimate while I deal with all the challenges of my treatment and my illness?*
- *Why would my spouse want to be intimate with me, given this situation?*
- *How in the world can I even think of making love when I haven't even got the energy to make dinner or wash my hair?*

The list of things you might be wondering, thinking, and saying to yourself goes on and on. And the truth is, at some point in your cancer journey you may very well feel so impacted by your illness or treatments that you don't have the energy, interest, physical comfort (due to pain), desire, and/or motivation for intimacy.

However, keep in mind that every moment in life is about choice. You, and you alone, have the responsibility to live a life made richer by maintaining or fostering relationships that feed the soul ... and intimacy feeds the soul, as well as your emotional, mental, and physical needs. In other words, intimacy is good for you and has the power to support your immune system.

That's why, in this chapter, I want to dispel the myth that intimacy and cancer aren't compatible. In fact, intimacy can be a powerful way for you to move toward comfort and healing.

First, Understand the Many Definitions of "Intimacy."

Whether you are single or married, dealing with the diagnosis of a life-threatening illness such as cancer is always made less burdensome by loving support, especially the support of one who values and cares for you enough to be a comforting presence during this time.

It is calming and soothing to have your hand held, or to be embraced and hugged, when you most need it. It feels equally comforting to have a loved one accompany you to your doctors' appointments, meals, and treatments. And it can be invaluable to have someone who lays with you at night, cradling you, stroking your hair, holding you tightly, and listening to your fears and concerns—especially when your mind begins playing the *what if* game with a myriad of terrifying thoughts.

Intimacy is so much more than a sexual connection. Yes, it *can* be sexual, but does not have to be—especially for healing. Healing intimacy includes an awareness of a deep connection with another being, a connection that fills your spirit with a sense of warmth, closeness, familiarity, comfort, and safety. When you are ill, you want to feel that you are not alone, that you are valued and cared about, and that you are being supported. After being diagnosed with cancer, you will benefit from feeling an intimate connection with your dear friends and relatives, including your children. Remember, everything is energy—and children are sensitive to energy.

Alice Hoffman, a *New York Times* bestselling author and a survivor of breast cancer, beautifully conveys this message in her exquisitely written, small, and powerful book, *Survival Lessons*. Alice writes that when her beloved sister-in-law, Jo Ann, was dealing with brain cancer, she (Alice) spent time with Jo Ann every day. When Jo Ann bravely admitted one afternoon that she feared dying, Alice quickly, without hesitating, said, "Oh, don't be silly, that's not going to happen." It was not till she was dealing with her own cancer that Alice realized what she needed to have said.

She writes: *"Now I know what she wanted from me on the day she told me she was afraid. It was exactly what I wanted when I had cancer and I thought I was going to die. I should have sat down next to her, put my arms around her, and told her that I loved her. That's all anyone wants. It took me a long time to figure this out. It's a complicated human puzzle. But it's never too late to know that love is all you need."*[1]

Selena's Story: Using Relationships to Heal

Selena, a woman I know and admire, also discovered that intimacy in all its forms can be incredibly beneficial when facing the challenge of cancer. Here is her story.

Selena is an active woman whose appearance belies her age of 63 and whose lifestyle is that of a younger woman. She is a loving wife to her husband, a physician, as well as the mother of two young men. She is passionate about life, her family and friends, and her love of painting.

Selena was unexpectedly diagnosed with renal cancer in January 2012 and immediately had surgery to remove the cancer. She did not have chemo or radiation and was told that she could not do anything more, other than have regular follow-up CAT scans to monitor her health.

When Selena joined our GyniGirls Cancer Support Group, she shared her philosophy regarding her journey forward. "I could either let it [cancer] take over my life or I could deal with it and find something in my life that was and is joyful." And the latter statement is exactly what she did. Specifically, she decided to retire because, in her words, "I wanted to spend the rest of my life doing what I love, which is painting and spending time with my family and friends."

Indeed, Selena has drawn constantly on the healing power of intimacy. She is doing remarkably well and believes the quality of her life has improved immensely since being diagnosed with cancer. Her increased level of contentment is due in part to the intentional decision to see and visit with old friends and spend more quality time with her husband. Before cancer, Selena had experienced trust issues due to painful childhood circumstances. Now, she recognizes that her job is to let go of what does not serve her health, to live in the moment, and to experience great joy with her loved ones!

Given that her diagnosis came so unexpectedly and that she had previously lost friends and family to cancer, Selena now chooses not to put off until tomorrow what she can do today. She feels the need to take advantage of the time she does have to visit or be with those she loves. Selena says that her relationship with her husband (and his with her) has deepened emotionally, and that their marriage is more beautiful and enriched than ever.

While Selena admits that she does experience some anxiety as she approaches each scheduled CAT scan, she has learned the art of "putting it into the background" so that is does not interfere with her quality of life. And since her surgery, each of her scans has shown her to be healthy and cancer free. Selena knows that there are no guarantees, but she intends to focus on what she can control, rather than what she cannot! "It is all about the choices I make, and I choose joy!" she says.

Foster Intimacy in All Its Forms.

Here are some suggestions to foster greater intimacy between you and your loved ones, keeping in mind that intimacy takes many forms:

- **Always communicate to your loved ones what you are dealing with.** This includes your diagnosis, treatment, medication side effects, and any needs (physical, emotional, mental, and spiritual) that you would like to have met, if possible. Additionally, do not hold back in conveying your thoughts and feelings, especially your fears and your worries, so that others can more deeply understand how your cancer journey is impacting you. Finally, do not forget to share your intentions and visions for healing, along with what this looks like to you. Talk about the things that provide you with ongoing hope and pleasure. In return, encourage your loved ones to share their own thoughts and feelings with you.

- **If you are in a relationship, consider sharing your thoughts and feelings as a couple with a third party.** This third party might be, a therapist (such as a psychologist, counselor, or social worker), friend, neighbor, or member of the clergy. He or she may be able to provide you and your partner with a listening ear while helping to nurture and/or restore your sense of connection.

- **Ask your medical team for any help you need.** Consider visiting with your oncologist or specialist if you have concerns related to cancer's impact on your body. Perhaps your physician can offer you something—advice, medications, or tools—to make physical intimacy more comfortable for you.

- **Talk to your loved ones about viewing your situation as an opportunity to grow your soul and spirit.** Remember, you and your loved ones have choices about how you are going to respond to the situation. You can either disconnect completely, or you can collaborate on creative ways to feel one another's love and support. For example, even if you can't go out for an evening, you can come up with an activity that enables you to feel genuine love and understanding for each other; for instance, cooking something special together or playing cards, chess, or a board game.

- **If you are a parent, share your journey with your children.** Depending on your children's ages and what they are able to mentally and emotionally understand and handle, share your journey with them. Remember to *Keep It Simple* (KIS)! Your kids know something is not right, whether or not you share the details of your journey with them. By speaking honestly with them (only what they can handle, please), you take away their fear of the unknown and any irrational sense of responsibility they may erroneously assume for your situation. But, most important, you and your children can and will be sharing an intimate, precious journey in which you all feel deeply connected, valued, and loved—and not alone. All of this enables healing to occur on many levels.

  Do not forget to give and ask your children for hugs, kisses, and embraces, or to hold hands, if they will let you. They may not verbalize it, but your children value you making them a priority when they know you are not feeling your best.

- **When you have extra energy, make appointments to lovingly care for yourself.** For instance, arrange for a manicure, hair appointment, or massage, or make time to buy a new article of clothing, wig, or scarf for your head. These things work wonders for your sense of self, self-confidence, and self-image—all of which can help you desire greater intimacy and feel more intimate.

- **If you are in a relationship with a partner, intentionally carve out time for the two of you to sneak away for an escape.** This could be a romantic dinner, or even a *relaxed* dinner during which the two of you have the time and space to connect over deeper conversation and a glass of wine. It could also be an overnight trip to see a show and visit friends.

If you have children, consider doing the same thing with them. Make time for just you and your child to take a class together, go out to lunch, or visit the park or a museum (or whatever you can handle energetically). This is a great opportunity to share mutual thoughts and feelings and to ease your child's fears and concerns regarding you and your situation. Make your time together special, loving, and joyful, which will be good medicine for both of you.

- **Join a couples' support group.** Look for a group that allows you to talk openly and freely about your intimacy with one another and how your cancer journey affects it. You'll probably be surprised to find that others are in similar situations and that, together, you can find solutions that help to create a sense of greater balance and peace in your lives.

- **Go online.** Use the Internet to inform yourself about cancer and intimacy. You might also be able to connect with others who are interested in the same topic through blogs or chat rooms.

- **Affirm greater intimacy.** Put out the intention that you will find a way to bring in or restore a greater sense of intimacy, and that you will find ways to heal. Affirm: *I am healing and becoming more intimate with my partner. I am finding that cancer* (or whatever illness you have) *is helping us to be even closer than we were previously.*

- **Pray together.** There is intimacy in taking the time to pray with your loved ones. You can gather in your garden to do this, or in the comfort of your family room, living room, or kitchen. This brings many families closer together, providing sensations of warmth, hope, and peace. See in your mind's eye that for which you are praying. And be sure to express gratitude for the fulfillment of your hopes and dreams.

- **Practice the see/feel technique.** In other words, see and imagine what makes you feel better. Actually feel in your body what you see in your mind as you visualize the intimacy you desire with your loved ones. The see/feel technique is a useful tool whether you are trying to improve sexual intimacy with your partner or whether you want to enhance personal intimacy with your family members and dear friends.

- **Talk about potential issues.** If you find that these suggestions are not working, have a discussion with your loved one. Examine what may be going on in the relationship. Cancer has the power to bring preexisting issues to the surface, sometimes disconnecting two beings even more from one another. However, be aware that with an attitude of intentional healing and meaningful discussion, cancer can also contribute to the healing of a relationship. Cancer is a turning point in life because it pushes us to become more responsible for our choices (which can determine our survival)—which is a good thing!

- **Consider developing a loving relationship with a pet, especially a dog or cat.** No, doing so does not mean you are not losing your mind, as some (who are *not* on your cancer journey) might say to you. So many patients with whom I have had the honor of working have shared with me their dependence on their dog or cat during their cancer experience.

  Dogs and cats have the ability to help expedite your healing by means of their presence by your chair or bedside as you manage the impact of your chemotherapy or radiation, or through the unconditional love you receive from them when you feel isolated, different, and terribly frightened. And they do it in the most intimate ways:

Cuddling with you above or below your blanket or stand-
ing, sitting, and sleeping by your feet—or sometimes your
head or heart. And always, always your pet conveys his or
her love and devotion to you. You can't get more intimate
than this.

Because of the bond you *do* have with your pet, it is
important to identify someone (a family member, neighbor, or friend) who can support you in caring for your pet,
even providing him or her with a home if or when you are
unable to take care of his or her needs.

I love what Alice Hoffman writes in *Survival Lessons*
regarding her personal, intimate experience with her Pol-
ish Sheepdog. While Alice was undergoing her chemotherapy, her dog would sit on the window ledge above her
couch and together they would watch the falling leaves.
She writes: *"We both decided nothing was more beautiful or
interesting. I never felt alone when I was with him. Sometimes that's what you need most of all, not to be alone. Sometimes a dog knows that before you do."* [2]

And What if Your Partner Isn't Capable of Sharing the Intimacy You Want and Need?

In *Crazy Sexy Cancer Tips*, Kris Carr writes about being afraid that
no one would want to date her because of her cancer, and of how
hard it was to reveal to those lucky guys interested in her that she
had cancer. She also writes about falling in love with a man who
would not take *no* for an answer when she, wanting to protect
him from the disturbing information she was receiving about her
diagnosis, tried to end the relationship.

Kris writes with refreshing honesty. She says that she knew
she was fortunate to marry her soulmate: One who expedited her
healing and who had the courage not to "bail." While she writes

of her good fortune in marrying someone who was not intimidated by her diagnosis, she advises others who find that their partners are not emotionally, physically, and spiritually available to say goodbye and move on. She advises readers to not be afraid of being alone and of starting life over.

Too often, those with cancer who find that their partners are unable to handle the situation feel trapped and helpless. You are not! I would encourage you to see this as an opportunity to reclaim your power, grab the reins of your life, and redirect your journey to one that feels right for you. In Kris's words, "*Your rejection is God's protection!*"[3]

CHAPTER 18

Do Something Selfless

"It is not a perfect day until you help someone who can't pay you back."

LEWIS KATZ
(REFERENCING A FAMOUS QUOTE BY
UCLA BASKETBALL COACH JOHN WOODEN)

"Helping, fixing, and serving represent three different ways of seeing life. When you help, you see life as weak; when you fix, you see life as broken. When you serve, you see life as whole. Fixing and helping may be the work of the ego, and service the work of the soul."

RACHEL NAOMI REMEN, MD

Throughout this book, I have told you over and over (and over again!) that you must be selfish in order to deal with cancer. And I meant it! You need to care for yourself before you care for others. Perhaps for the first time in your adult life, your own needs and well-being must take first priority. One of the greatest lessons cancer has to teach is that you are here on earth to be responsible *only* for yourself, and that others (except the very young and very old) must assume responsibility for their own lives.

However, that doesn't mean that you have to become a modern-day version of Ebenezer Scrooge. As long as the first fruits of your time and energy are channeled inward, using the remainder to help others can actually expedite your own healing!

The Healing Power of Selflessness

One of the secrets to jump-starting your healing journey is finding someone in whose life you can make a difference, or perhaps a meaningful cause that you can help advance. Having a positive impact on the world will feel right to you on a heart level, and in turn, these feelings will set off a chain reaction of happiness and healing in your body. If you're skeptical, consider the following facts presented in a 2007 *New York Sun* article entitled "Why Giving Makes You Happy":

- People who donate to charity are 43 percent more likely to be "very happy" about their lives than non-givers.
- People who give money to others are 68 percent less likely than non-givers to feel "hopeless."
- Volunteers are 42 percent more likely than non-volunteers to be very happy.
- Charitable activity causes the body to release endorphins, producing a feeling comparable to a mild dose of morphine or heroin!

- Helping others lowers stress hormones like cortisol, epinephrine, and norepinephrine.

And it doesn't stop there! When you're actively engaged in helping someone else, you *don't* have the time to dwell on your own situation. Instead of wallowing in a sea of worry, grief, and self-pity, you're channeling your energy toward advancing the greater good. In fact, I've noticed that for many of my patients, getting "outside" of themselves and giving back is essential to maintaining a balanced, healthy perspective. Don't let cancer consume your days and become your world. Whenever possible, it's much better to focus on leaving a meaningful legacy through your actions and priorities.

Essentially, selflessly helping others is an incredibly powerful way to heal your cells and raise your vibrational energy. The so-called "warm and fuzzies" do much more than making you feel good in the moment—they can impact your long-term health and happiness, and they are a vehicle that can enable you to make a positive impact on the world.

An Important Caveat About Service

Plainly, doing something selfless is being of service. However, as physician and author Rachel Naomi Remen notes in the quote at the beginning of this chapter, being of service is not about fixing or repairing another. Rather, being of service has to do with the connection of your soul with another soul.

All of us on this earth are souls seeking connections (relationships) with other souls so that we can fulfill our life's purpose, which includes learning to unconditionally love and accept ourselves and others. When we make connections with others, we give life to them *and* to ourselves because we see those individuals as apart from, yet like us—a member of the same community of humanity, and beyond any pathology (ours and/or theirs).

Only when we can give selflessly and connect with others can we learn that we are all one. It is this awareness that enables us to grow in wisdom and spirit—all of which contributes to the healing of the soul. In order to exist and be healthy, we need our soul connections!

Stories of Selfless Healing

Over the years, I have seen selflessness help many of many of my patients who have battled cancer. For instance, years ago, a patient of mine was experiencing severe bodily pain that could not be explained. She told me that one of the only ways she had found to get through each day was to find other people who needed her help. She loved to drive cancer patients to their treatments, and often made and delivered meals to those who were housebound. She also prayed for those in need constantly. All of these acts enabled my patient to balance the suffering and pain with which she lived.

Specifically, my patients who are dealing with cancer have shared a number of ways to be of service to others with similar challenges. For example, even while going through her own treatments, Rosemary, a breast cancer survivor, needed to know that she could make life easier for other women who were going through their own treatments. She told me that it brought her so much pleasure to be present for them, sharing humorous stories and music.

Another gal, Heather (also a breast cancer survivor and thriver), has told me that she enjoys helping women who are in the throes of losing their hair find peace of mind by going with them to purchase their new wigs, minimizing the grief associated with this loss. Heather also lets her oncologist's office staff know that she is available to help those patients who are struggling with any or all aspects of their cancer journeys.

Donna, who also counts herself among the ranks of breast cancer thrivers, has often shared with me how much she wishes to be of service. She has offered her services to one of the breast cancer groups in the area, and is looking elsewhere to see who can best make use of her accounting and organizational skills.

Carol, also dealing with breast cancer, has told me that she finds it satisfying to have lunch or brunch with newly diagnosed women so that she can help to minimize their fears while giving them hope and inspiration.

Before moving on, I'd like to share one more story—this one a little longer—with you.

Jean's Story: Walking Forward Hand in Hand

There are people we meet in life who, whenever we think of them, make us smile. Jean, a member of our GyniGirls Support Group, is one of these people for me. To look at Jean, you would have no way of knowing that she had been diagnosed with uterine cancer in April of 2012—nor would you know that her son died unexpectedly within the past decade, leaving her in a state of devastation. Yet, throughout her challenge with cancer, she chose to give of herself to help others.

Like so many individuals diagnosed with cancer, Jean initially believed that once you have cancer, you always have cancer—and, of course, you may die from the disease. So, as you can imagine, the news of her diagnosis terrified her. However, Jean, who worked in a full-time position and who was accustomed to walking five miles a day—wasted little time in beginning her treatment.

Jean's regimen consisted of 18 chemotherapy treatments, followed by six weeks of daily radiation treatments. The loss of her hair was emotionally difficult for her to accept. Additionally, she developed problems with her feet, which were made very sensitive by the drugs she had to take. Her anxiety was exacerbated by the whole experience.

Throughout her treatment, Jean grounded herself, coped with her anxiety, and restored her sense of innate power by pushing herself to get back to walking—which she did the very day she returned home from the hospital. She began with a half-mile walk and gradually increased the distance so that by the end of the week, she was back to walking her usual five miles! (In fact, Jean just participated in a 5K race and came in three minutes sooner than several younger relatives!) The point here is that Jean's cancer and surgery did not and could not stop her from doing what she needed to feel like her "old" self. She had the will to push herself to do what was healing for her!

What I especially love about Jean is that she used her strength to help others going through similar challenges. Throughout her cancer journey (and in the present as well), Jean has chosen to walk for worthy causes to aid in fundraising and to help in her own healing. She has participated in walks for a number of illnesses and organizations including Multiple Sclerosis, the American Cancer Society, the March of Dimes, and The Suicide Prevention Group. (Her desire to help those dealing with suicide and to prevent suicide was sparked by a family member who has several times tried to take her own life.) During these walks, Jean feels she can connect with others going through similar challenges and share stories with them. "It helps them," she told me, "and it helps me in my own healing. I always feel better when I do these walks."

But walking isn't the only way Jean helps others. Overwhelmed by meeting the demands of her cancer diagnosis, she intuitively knew she needed to be with others who were going through similar challenges, which is how she found her way to the GyniGirls. While Jean admits that sometimes the stories that others share frighten her, she has nevertheless found that the group supports and helps her. Even more important, Jean has been an inspiration for the rest of our group and for others, like yourself, who are dealing with cancer on some level. Jean finds that sharing her story has made a difference in the lives of fellow group members. Together, she and the other group mutually raise everyone's vibrations. It is a great healing experience for all of us!

Jean has shared with me that it also brings her pleasure and comfort to pray for those who are going through difficult times. It touches the hearts of the women in our support group to know that their fellow group members will take time to pray for them.

One other way Jean gives selflessly and with humility is consciously choosing to bring humor and lightheartedness to those whose stories truly break your heart. She explained: "I do my best to be upbeat and to use humor as often as I can because I know it has the power to help them feel better." This is especially so within the GyniGirls group, though Jean chooses humor in many other areas of her life as well. She listens with her heart and responds with warmth and humor, and also attempts to share some of her story when she feels it can provide hope and inspiration for others.

Jean is a humble soul. She does not think of herself as actually volunteering; doing for others and being of service. Yet, she did give of herself for others during her illness and continues to do so as a natural part of her life. Jean remembers how afraid she was early on in her cancer journey, and strongly feels that she can help other women by sharing the wisdom she has garnered from her travels with cancer. A model of strength, wisdom, and determination, Jean refused to become the diagnosis and, therefore, is an extraordinary role model for women everywhere.

How to Help Others

Perhaps the stories I've shared have inspired you to begin helping others in a specific way. But I want you to know that there are as many ways to help other people as there are, well, people!

That's because engaging in this type of effort is highly personal. Especially as you're facing a life-challenging illness, it's important that helping others feels meaningful to you, and not like "work." Whenever you participate in the activity of choice, you should experience feelings of positivity, connectedness, and healing.

That said, if you are unsure of how to tap into the healing power of selflessness, here are several broad suggestions to help you get started:

- **Tap into a cause.** What do you feel strongly about? What problems would you like to alleviate? For instance, have you always felt strongly about preventing bullying? Is it important to you that your local parks remain clean and free of pollution? Are you consistently called to help communities affected by natural disasters? Are you concerned about making sure that all families in your area have enough to eat? Do you want to help abandoned animals find loving homes? Would you like to support our nation's military?

  You might even find that you most want to help others who are suffering from cancer. If that's the case, you might help organize a fundraiser to help patients pay for the costs associated with treatments, therapies, and required changes in lifestyle. It's always heartwarming to see communities and neighborhoods come together to support families dealing with such challenges—and it is always appreciated.

  This is just a small sampling of the causes you might want to get involved in. Keep in mind that you don't have to devote large chunks of time to a cause to help advance it; a few hours here and there can make a huge difference and leave a strong legacy. The first step is simply identifying and contacting an organization to find out how you can help.

- **Teach.** Whether you consider yourself to be an "expert" or not, your knowledge, talents, and skills can help others. From tutoring an underprivileged student to showing other members of your cancer support group how to knit, teaching others can help you to develop meaningful relationships and raise your vibrational energy. You'll also be making a valuable investment in humanity's future.

  At this point, I would like to note that sharing stories from your cancer journey with others who are walking similar paths is an excellent way to teach. Stories have great power to inform, comfort, and heal. When you are open, honest, and compassionate with other people whose lives have been altered by cancer, you are giving a great gift.

- **Focus on small acts of kindness.** Maybe you simply don't have the time or energy to devote to an overarching cause or ongoing volunteer activity. Or perhaps you simply aren't sure where you'd like to commit your efforts. That's okay! In this case, I recommend starting small. Simply try to do something nice for someone else each day. Smiling at the grocery store cashier counts, as does waving at your neighbor! You might also make a point to compliment your spouse, or buy an extra bag of dog food to drop off at the animal shelter. Remember, what seems insignificant to you may change the course of another person's entire day.

  As I mentioned earlier, you may find that you want to help other cancer patients specifically. Options that fall into the "small acts of kindness" category include volunteering to cook and deliver a meal to a patient's family when he or she cannot do so, or helping a patient's children with their homework.

- **Pray and affirm.** No matter what your schedule looks like or what your energy levels are, you can pray and/or affirm good things for others. And make no mistake: As we have discussed previously, your thoughts are very powerful and can make a tangible impact in another person's life. You can pray and/or affirm on behalf of specific individuals, or for entire groups of people (for instance, others who are suffering from cancer, those who are depressed, those who are struggling financially, those who are unemployed, etc.).

Prayer, for instance, is an expression of Loving Energy and has scientifically been shown to be effective and powerful. Personally, in my many years of research and clinical observations, I have observed that praying for others provides patients, as well as their friends and family members, with a raison d'être; in other words, a sense of purpose. When you tell someone who is ill that you will pray for them and actually do so, know that you are giving a precious gift. I have been on the receiving end as well as the praying end, and while both feel wonderful, knowing that you are the focus of another's prayers is heart-warming and beautiful.

Along the same lines, in offering prayers for others, you experience a quiet personal joy. Your feelings of self-worth and satisfaction are boosted. And you develop an awareness that you are part of a greater field of energy, to which you are attaching and drawing in additional healing power. All of this helps you to shift to a higher vibration, which, in turn, enables your immune system to function at a more productive level. It is in this manner that prayer for others is healing for you! All of this—the shift, the satisfaction, the quiet joy, the self-healing—is always enhanced when the person or persons for whom you have been praying experience their own healing!

Over the years, I have also observed that those doctors who are both highly skilled and who use prayer to assist the healing of their patients often experience greater success in surgery, as well as fewer problems in the healing phases. I remember Lewis Mehl- Madrona, a Native American physician, psychiatrist, and psychologist and author of *Coyote Medicine*, sharing these thoughts in a lecture he gave to medical students.

In his presentation, Dr. Mehl-Madrona spoke of observing a surgeon friend praying with a patient before surgery; asking for the procedure to go well and for his patient to have minimal, if any, healing problems. Dr. Mehl-Madrona noted that this doctor's patients returned to the hospital with post-surgical complaints less frequently than the patients of any of the other physicians who operated there! I was so pleased that Dr. Mehl-Madrona was making the young doctors of the future aware that they could help their patients by integrating prayer into their practice.

Whatever format selfless giving takes for you, I encourage you to make helping others and establishing soul connections a regular part of your healing journey. Just be sure to consciously check in with yourself on a regular basis to make sure that your efforts remain high-vibrational and healing. If any activity begins to feel draining or obligatory, it may be time to gracefully back away.

Once again, remember that no matter how lofty your intentions are, your actions will ultimately be unhealthy if they have a detrimental effect on you. Especially at this time in your life, it's not at all selfish to prioritize your own physical energy and peace of mind above all else.

"When we connect through these soul to soul connections, it is as though we connect most intimately with another's humanity."

JEANNE ACHTERBERG, PhD

CHAPTER 19

Nutrition as Medicine

"Let food be your medicine and medicine be your food."
HIPPOCRATES, FATHER OF MODERN MEDICINE

"Nutrients make medical therapy more toxic to the tumor and less toxic to the patient."
PATRICK QUILLIN, PhD, RD, CNS

The old expression "You are what you eat" is true. And if you are dealing with a health challenge, be it cancer or anything else, there's another adage that should never be far from your mind: "Food is Medicine."

That's right. Your body's 60 trillion cells are depending on you to feed them well—and keep them healthy—at all times. But it's especially important to be vigilant about what you are eating when you're ill, because many illnesses, cancer included, thrive on specific types of foods—while other foods help fight these diseases.

Yes, meeting the challenge of cancer may require interventions such as surgery, antibiotics, or radiation, but the diet you choose to feed your body's cells and immune system can also be crucial. Remember, everything is energy, including the food we eat. It's important to consciously consume nutrients that support your immune system and overall wellness.

In this chapter, I'll explain how nutrition can help you meet the challenge of cancer, and I'll share some specific guidelines regarding what you might (and might not!) want to put on your shopping list.

Why Is Nutrition so Significant in Fighting Cancer?

Food is therapeutic and medicinal for you because it provides you with nutrition. In other words, it enables your body to grow, heal and thrive. But as you know, not all foods care for you in the same manner. Some enable you to achieve wellness, especially if you are ill, while others may be detrimental to your health, even creating an environment in which cancer can emerge and grow.

The good news is, choosing to ingest healthy, healing nutrients can do one or more of the following for your body:

- Assist in enabling chemotherapy and radiation to work more effectively.
- Boost your body's antioxidant levels, making it more difficult for cancer to grow and expand.
- Aid in the elimination of toxins (such as those from chemotherapy) from your body; especially from your liver.
- Block certain hormones from feeding cancer cells.
- Reduce or block the impact of various carcinogens that contribute to breast, colon, prostate, lung, esophageal, and stomach cancers.
- Slow down the growth of cancer cells.
- Lower your cholesterol and reduce spikes in blood sugar levels.
- Preventing and fight infections in the body. (Some cancers actually begin as infections!)
- Stimulate the growth of natural killer immune cells, which increase the immune system's ability to attack cancer cells.
- Stabilize your immune system.
- Reduce the number of physiological vessels that cancer cells can enter; thus fighting metastasization.

Many cancer survivors who have shared their inspirational healing stories say that they experienced a lack of success with traditional therapies including surgery, chemotherapy and/or radiation. After several relapses, they either integrated or turned to more natural ways of treating their illnesses, one of which was making major lifestyle changes in their diets. There are no guarantees, of course, but the information these thrivers have shared with the public—which is often supported by substantial scientific research—has provided hope and inspiration for countless individuals dealing with similar health challenges.

Specifically, research indicates that there are a number of similarities in the diets of cancer survivors and thrivers. Whether or not they choose to undergo treatments of restrained chemotherapy, radiation, and/or surgery, many of those who modify their food choices by following some of the guidelines I'll share in this chapter have generally met with success in shrinking their tumors, and many have even gone into remission.

Principles of a Healing, Cancer-Fighting Diet

The list I share here is not comprehensive, but it does provide a good overview of foods and drinks that will enhance your health as you meet the challenge of cancer (as well as a few things you should avoid). I've explained the basics of why each "works," and in many instances, I've also shared resources that you can use to find out more on your own, if you so choose.

- **Avoid ready-made processed foods and drinks.** The chemicals used in many processed foods and drinks contribute to the development of various cancers. For example, in *Anticancer: A New Way of Life,* Dr. David Servan-Schreiber (who is a brain cancer survivor) cites numerous studies in which phosphate additives (which are found in meat with preservatives, some processed cheeses, many colas and sodas, processed ice cream, and processed frozen foods) encourage the development and growth of some cancers.[1]

  Here's what you need to remember: Practice KIS; in other words, **keep it simple** when it comes to nutrition. Stay with natural foods that come from the earth and avoid processed foods because they are filled with salt, sugar, and fats. Think about this: Our grandparents and great grandparents tended to live off the earth, eating a healthier diet that was grown without pesticides and was devoid of high sugars, unhealthy fats, growth hormones, and antibiotics—all of which contributed to their low cancer rates.

- **When possible, buy and eat organic.** Yes, organic foods are often more expensive. But whenever possible, I encourage you to purchase organic meats, fruits, and vegetables in order to avoid carcinogenic pesticides and antibacterial agents, as well as growth-enhancing hormones. Organic produce is grown without chemicals and with natural fertilizers, and organic meats are often grass-fed and free range, and are free of antibiotics and hormones. Just be sure to wash organic foods in case they have picked up contamination before making it into your shopping bag.

- **Eat your veggies.** Turns out your mother was right when she told you to eat your vegetables. Many vegetables— especially the most colorful ones—are considered to be among the best antioxidants and anticancer foods because they contain the chemicals your body's immune system needs to stay healthy. If you're interested in the science, the pigments in many colorful vegetables contain powerful phytochemicals like bioflavonoids and carotenoids that stimulate your immune system and that can be lethal to cancer cells.)

  These include: dark green and red lettuces, spinach, tomatoes, squash, carrots, pumpkin, sweet potatoes, beets, cauliflower, bok choy, cabbage, Brussels sprouts, broccoli, onions, garlic, leeks, chives, and more. (These veggies are exceptionally powerful, especially when combined!)

- **Keep cancer away with garlic.** Garlic is considered a superfood. When crushed, it can reduce the expansion of breast and prostate cancer cells, thereby limiting the development of cancerous tumors. In her book *The No-Dairy Breast Cancer Prevention Program: How One Scientist's Discovery Helped Her Defeat Her Cancer*, scientist and breast cancer survivor Jane Plant cites numerous studies that validate the healing powers of garlic in countering viruses, bacteria, and fungi. Additionally, garlic is a wonderful source of *selenium*, which is believed to be a player in the health of the prostate.

- **Include seaweed and kelp in your diet.** Kelp and seaweed have long been a part of the diet of those who live near the sea. Seaweed refers to a variety of marine plants and algae that grow deep within the ocean. Seaweed comes in a number of varieties, including kombu, wakame, dulse, and nori. Kelp is actually another subgroup of seaweed; the difference being that it is the largest form of seaweed and forms marine forests. All of these types of seaweed contain iodine and are valuable in diminishing the impact of radiation and x rays on the body. Seaweed also strengthens the immune system's ability to produce more natural killer cells. Once softened, seaweed can easily be added to soups and stews. Kelp is also helpful for clearing out the toxins that invade the gastrointestinal areas of the body.

- **Love your legumes.** Legumes are pea or bean plants whose seeds grow in pods. These include soybeans, kidney beans, and garbanzo beans, all of which have strong cancer fighting abilities.

   Soy in particular is rich in protease inhibitors, phytoestrogens, and isoflavones, which are able to interfere with cancer cell production. A diet rich in soy helps explain the lower incidence of breast cancer among Asian women. And Asian women who *are* diagnosed with breast cancer tend live longer, in part due to their soy-filled diet. Since soy is considered a source of protein, you can substitute soy products such as tofu, tempeh, miso, and soy milk for meat and dairy products in your diet. The nice thing about soy is that it takes on the taste of whatever you are cooking with it. (Personally, I think it is especially delicious when sautéed with garlic and onions.)

   An important caveat: In his book *Anticancer*, Dr. Servan-Schreiber recommends *not* eating soy while undergoing chemotherapy treatments, because soy has an impact on the efficacy of Taxol.[2] Stop eating soy a few days before treatment, and wait until a few days after to resume.

- **Eat more mushrooms.** Mushrooms are an incredibly valuable anticancer food because they provide polysaccharides and lentinian, which are especially helpful in enabling your immune system to produce the cells needed to fight cancer. Varieties you may want to eat include Maritake, Portobello, Cremini, Oyster, Thistle, Enokidake, Reishi and Shitake. Maritake mushrooms in particular are extremely powerful in positively impacting the immune system.

  According to Dr. Servan-Schreiber, studies have demonstrated that Oyster mushrooms are effective in fighting breast cancer cells. Furthermore, he notes that Chinese women reduced their chances of developing breast cancer by 64 percent when they digested the equivalent of 10 grams of mushrooms a day—and that when they ate mushrooms along with a cup (1 gram) of green tea leaves, the risk of breast cancer was reduced by an impressive 89 percent![3]

- **Snack on healing berries.** Berries contain ellagic acid and polyphenols, both of which cause cancer cells to destroy themselves. You can mix berries (aka, bite-sized anticancer agents) into your morning cereal, have a handful as a snack, or eat them for dessert—perhaps accompanied by a piece of dark chocolate! Berries can be frozen without losing their powers, and they do not create huge glycemic spikes in your blood.

- **Savor herbs, spices, and seasonings.** As you reduce your intake of salt, begin to introduce other seasonings that have anticancer value and the ability to stimulate your immune system. Herbs like rosemary, oregano, mint, basil, thyme, ginger, sage, garlic, and cinnamon are rich in essential oils. Additionally, they contain chemicals that have the power to fight cancer cells. In particular, rosemary helps to empower the impact of some chemotherapy treatments.

- **Tune in to turmeric.** A yellow powder that is an ingredient of yellow curry, turmeric is one of the most important and powerful natural anti-inflammatories in today's world. It contributes to apoptosis (programmed death of cancer cells—a good thing!) and also reduces the formation of tumors. Additionally, turmeric supports the effectiveness of chemotherapy. Dr. Servan-Schreiber notes that a great way to use turmeric is to mix ¼ teaspoon of turmeric with ½ tablespoon of olive oil and a pinch of black pepper. This mixture can be added to soups, salad dressings, and vegetables.[4]

- **Root for ginger.** Ginger root is another excellent anti-oxidant and anti-inflammatory. Ginger can be ingested as an infusion tea to help to reduce the effects of nausea due to chemotherapy. But that's not the extent of its benefits—ginger also kills cancer cells. To incorporate it into your diet, grate ginger root into a frying pan or wok while cooking vegetables.

- **Tap into tomatoes.** The "magic" ingredient in tomatoes is lycopene, which has been shown to help prostate cancer patients live longer. Its anticancer properties stimulate the growth of immune cells and aid in the elimination of tumor cells. However, tomatoes need to be cooked in order to release their healing chemicals. I like to cook canned tomato sauce with olive oil or, if I have more time, I make my own tomato sauce by cooking tomatoes with olive oil over low heat and then adding onions, tofu, garlic, and seasonings. One caution: You may want to avoid purchasing canned tomatoes because of the chemicals that are found in some plastic food-can liners. Instead, opt for fresh tomatoes or tomato products sold in glass containers.

- **Recreate the rainbow on your plate.** I've already mentioned the importance of eating colorful fruits and veggies, but I want to reiterate those instructions in a separate bullet. Let your plate resemble a rainbow by filling it with a multicolored assortment of vegetables and fruits. Each holds precious vitamins, minerals, and chemicals that can protect your body from becoming ill and strengthen your immune system so that it successfully shrinks and eliminates your cancer.

- **Be selective about fats.** It's best to stay away from "bad" fats, including those that are hydrogenated, omega 6 fats from soy and corn, and oxidized fats. Absolutely avoid hydrogenated (trans) fats, because these have been linked to cancer. Fortunately, there are several alternatives. You can use any of the following in place of butter or margarine: organic olive oil, canola oil, vegetable oil sprays (such as Pam), a 50/50 mixture of butter and olive oil, or coconut oil or flax oil (not heated). And keep in mind that the following oils are considered therapeutic *good* fats: fish, flax, borage, evening primrose, pumpkin, grape seed, and black currant.

  When cooking, choose unprocessed meats and those that are lower in fats. And if possible, try to steam, broil, bake, or grill meats and fish rather than fry them. Excessive grilling should be avoided as well.

- **Gravitate toward olive oil.** Olive oil is made from olives, which are rich in antioxidants (the black more so than the green). If possible, buy extra virgin olive oil, which has been associated with protection against a variety of cancers. As a rule of thumb, use approximately one-half to one tablespoon daily, either in your cooking or on your salad.

- **Choose cold water fish high in omega 3 fatty acids.**
Omega 3 fatty acids have been found to lower LDL (low
density lipoproteins; aka, the "bad" cholesterol) in the
blood. They also work to slow the progression of cancer in
the body and bolster the immune system.

  In addition to salmon, which is an excellent source of
omega 3 fatty acids, other cold water fish in this category include sardines, mackerel, halibut, haddock, cod, and
bass. Omega 3s are also found in flaxseed oil. (And speaking of fish: Try to avoid swordfish, shark, orange roughy,
tilefish, and red snapper, as these contain higher levels of
mercury, which is a contaminant.)

- **Avoid (or reduce your intake of) refined sugar.** Refined
white sugar is often viewed as "empty calories" with no
nutrients since it has been stripped of its fiber, protein,
and other matter. And to make matters worse, your cancerous cells use the sugar you consume to develop into tumors. *Sugar feeds cancer cells.* This is extremely important
for you to remember—and will hopefully motivate you to
consume less refined sugar, or better yet, eliminate it from
your diet altogether.

  If you're having trouble letting go of refined sugars despite the information I've shared above, consider that the
more sugar you consume, the higher the glucose levels in
your blood. This negatively impacts your immune system's
ability to do its work. If you can lower the level of glucose
in the blood via your diet, you have a better chance of
managing and reducing the growth of your cancer.

  As you begin to weed refined sugars out of your diet,
begin incorporating these natural sugars: organic honey,
raw brown sugar, molasses, fructose, and fruit juice. You
can also use non-caloric artificial sweeteners like Stevia,
Truvia, and Splenda.

- **Eat plenty of whole grains.** You need fiber in your diet in order for your gastrointestinal organs to do their job of digesting, assimilating, and eliminating the nutrients you take in. But the fiber you want is not your standard processed wheat flour, which has had most of the proteins, minerals, and vitamins removed during processing. Rather, you want to eat whole grains, including whole oats, whole barley, rye, brown rice, millet, wheat berries, and quinoa. You can find some of these ingredients in whole wheat bread and whole wheat pasta, for example.

  One of the gifts of whole grains is that since they are not refined, they help to lower the sugar and insulin in your blood. And research has indicated that the choice of whole grains contributes to the formation of fewer cancers.

- **Choose your proteins wisely.** In both *The No-Dairy Breast Cancer Prevention Program* and *Your Life in Your Hands: Understanding, Preventing, and Overcoming Breast Cancer*, Jane Plant also stresses the importance of choosing organic meats and poultry, because nonorganic animals may have been treated with unknown antibiotics and hormones.

  Meat (as well as proteins like egg yolks, snails, oysters, and sesame seeds) is an excellent source of selenium and zinc, both of which are needed by the body for healing and well-being. It was only after many months of cancer treatments and eating a vegetarian diet that Plant realized she was feeling low and depressed because of a deficiency of zinc. You need this trace mineral in order to recover from your cancer surgery, chemotherapy, and/or radiation. It is also invaluable in recovering from burns and in healing the prostate gland.

  Other healthy protein sources include fish (especially cold water fish) and shellfish; preferably those that are

fresh, not smoked, and unfarmed. Seafood in particular is
a valuable source of iodine, and iodine plays a significant
role in the female breast. Nuts, too, are a powerful source
of protein and are especially tasty when boiled and roast-
ed, a process that also cleans them of microorganisms that
create cancer-causing chemicals. Some cereals can even be
sources of protein.

- **Hold the salt!** Yes, you do need salt (sodium chloride) in
  your diet, but probably not as much as you are consuming. Americans use far more salt than they need—probably about ten times more, according to Patrick Quillin
  in *Beating Cancer with Nutrition.* Especially if your body
  is inadequately supplied with magnesium, calcium, potas-
  sium, and/or fluids, excessive salt can prevent cell mem-
  branes from maintaining the correct electrical charge
  needed to maintain your body.[5] If you need to use salt
  in cooking, Himalayan salt and sea salt are recommended
  by nutritionists. Or you can cook without salt and allow
  diners to add their own salt when eating.

- **Back away from dairy.** If you review the literature dealing with anticancer foods and nutrition, there are very
  few recommendations for eating dairy products (low fat
  and nonfat yogurt are exceptions). In fact, the point is
  frequently made that cow's milk is excellent for calves—
  but not so great for humans. Many references are made to
  the difficulties we human beings have with milk products
  (i.e., allergies and various gastrointestinal sensitivities).
  What is most interesting for our purpose is that there are
  some cancer patients who have used dairy-free food plans
  to completely turn around the progression of their cancers.

      Renowned English geologist Jane Plant created her
  own dairy-free program after undergoing a mastectomy,
  three more surgeries, thirty-five radiation treatments,

twelve chemotherapy cycles, and five reoccurrences of breast cancer. Why? She had discovered that Asian women have a far lower incidence of breast cancer—and that they do not consume dairy as part of their diets. Plant began eating meals rich in vegetables, fruits, and whole grains, and removed most dairy products, except for low-fat yogurt, from her diet. But it was not until she totally removed the yogurt that the inoperable cancer tumor in her neck began shrinking. She has been cancer free for more than 19 years.

Plant's success led her to create and write *The No-Dairy Breast Cancer Prevention Program: How One Scientist's Discovery Helped Her Defeat Her Cancer.* In this book and in *Your Life in Your Hands: Understanding, Preventing, and Overcoming Breast Cancer,* she provides evidence that that there is a demonstrable link between dairy products and breast and prostate cancers. (However, I want to note that Plant doesn't place the blame for cancer solely on dairy—she acknowledges that many factors contribute to cancer, including other foods, lifestyle, environmental exposure to toxins, and more.)

- **Filter the water you drink**. Seventy percent of your body is water. It's important to stay well hydrated by drinking water (at least 8 glasses a day—though the more the better). Masaru Emoto's book *The Hidden Messages in Water* reminds all of us of the general healing properties of water. For maximum effectiveness, though, water needs to be pure and uncontaminated, which requires some form of filtering.

The cancer survivors in Kelly A. Turner's *Radical Remission: Surviving Cancer Against All Odds* stopped drinking sodas, sweet fruit juices, and milk, and began drinking plenty of filtered water—but not tap water, which can contain heavy metals, unknown toxins, chloride, and a variety of minerals. Rather, many chose to drink spring water from Bisphenol A-free at-home water coolers. Others chose to drink tap water that had been passed through a home filtration system (using carbon filters or reverse osmosis). And in *The No-Dairy Breast Cancer Prevention Program* and *Your Life in Your Hands*, Professor Jane Plant describes the filtering and purification process she uses to maintain her healing from breast cancer.

The bottom line: no matter what system you decide to use, your water should be filtered for both drinking and cooking purposes.

- **Drink plenty of green tea.** Green tea has wealth of cancer fighting properties. For instance, drinking several cups of green tea (even decaffeinated) a day enables your liver to better detoxify and to release carcinogenic toxins from the body. Green tea also enhances radiation therapy's impact on cancer cells.

  In *Anticancer*, Dr. Servan-Schreiber cites a Japanese study in which women with nonmetastatic breast cancer who drank three cups of green tea a day experienced 57 percent fewer relapses than those who had only one cup per day! Men with prostate cancer who drank five cups per day had a 50 percent reduced risk of their cancer advancing.[6] If you choose to drink green tea, Dr. Servan-Schreiber recommends steeping 2 grams (0.07 ounces) of green tea for 10 minutes, and then drinking the tea within an hour.[7]

I have emphasized numerous times in this book, everything is energy, including your thoughts. Love is among the highest of all energies, and it can be a powerful healer. So when you prepare food for yourself or a loved one, include love in its preparation. Whether you are cutting up vegetables and fruits, cooking beans and rice, or making bread, be conscious of what you're thinking and feeling. Allow your loving energy to merge into whatever you are mixing, sautéing, baking, etc. You can even say a prayer or two while preparing the food, asking that it be blessed with healing energy. Intend for it to carry your love to the lucky recipient.

And if you're dining on food that you have received from a loved one, (say, chicken soup) remember that it was made with love. Allow yourself to feel the loving, caring, compassionate, joyful energy with which it has been created. Give thanks to the chickens and to your Source for the gifts of vitamins, proteins, minerals, etc. that are in the soup—and enjoy every spoonful. This energy is translated into wonderful, powerful chemicals that will support the work of your immune system and restore the needed balance for healing to occur.

General Shopping, Cooking, and Nutritional Guidelines for Fighting Cancer

Above, I shared information about specific foods, drinks, and nutritional groups to help you create a healthy, anti-cancer diet. Here, I'd like to share some general guidelines that I hope will also be of use in helping you make health-supporting nutritional choices:

- **When grocery shopping, concentrate on the outer aisles.** This, rather than the interior of the store, is where natural, fresh foods tend to be, including organic and non-organic vegetables and fruits.
- **Beware of labels that say "*Flavored with natural [Fill in the blank].*"** This phrase is often misleading because the product in question is most likely *not* natural! The slogan is good for marketing, but not for you. As much as possible, stick with *true* natural flavors that come in the form of actual fruits, vegetables, herbs, etc.

- **Trust your intuition.** When eating out, at home, or shopping for groceries, you may find yourself questioning whether to eat or buy a particular food. In such moments, do a check-in with your Higher Wisdom by taking a few deep breaths to quiet yourself and asking, "Is this good for my body's sixty trillion cells and my immune system?" Then listen for a quick yes or no!

- **Eat more meals featuring smaller quantities of food.** The more-but-smaller-meals strategy serves you emotionally as well as physically. When your body is nourished on a more regular basis, it is better able to manage your blood sugar and the production of insulin. You'll have fewer mood swings and will be less likely to encounter problems with weight and the development of diabetes.

- **Enjoy your favorite healthy foods in moderation.** Too much of anything can interfere with your body's balance, disrupting the flow of the energetic value of the nutrients you put into your body.

- **Be wary of plastic containers.** Use Pyrex or strengthened glass to store and heat your food. Research has demonstrated that BPA (Bisphenol A—a chemical used to harden plastic) has the ability to infuse with your food with cancer-promoting chemicals when heated at high temperatures. Drinking water in plastic bottles is also a concern for similar reasons. Stainless steel containers are considered a safer alternative.

- **Periodically, cleanse your body of toxins.** Cleansing the blood, liver, and body of toxins (especially those from chemotherapy and those that come from our environment, including pesticides and chemicals in our water) is essential. Some nutrients, such as prunes and brans, can help you detoxify, as can coffee enemas and other types of enemas. Brief fasts have also been shown to assist with detoxification. In *Radical Remission*, Kelly Turner cited a study in which the effectiveness of chemotherapy was enhanced and its side effects were diminished by going on a brief fast. Simultaneously, cancer cells were starved of sugar because the food sources that provide glucose had been removed.[8] Even fasting for just a day can be beneficial in supporting your body's cancer fighting ability.

- **When possible, rely on whole foods instead of supplements.** Many people take supplements to do what the bottle says: To supplement what they're already eating. That is fine. However, you should strive to make whole foods the main source of your supplements. Yes, your whole foods supply you with your macronutrients—your carbohydrates, proteins, fats, water, and fiber—but they're also full of the micronutrients (vitamins and minerals) that we often see in pill form.

  Jane Plant writes in her books that she normally takes no supplements, because they are found in the foods she chooses to eat. She did, however, take tablets of selenium with vitamins A, C, and E during her chemotherapy. I have found in my own research that taking supplements is an individual matter; some survivors have chosen to do this, and others have not.

  Your blood work may indicate a need to take supplements in the form of pills. Your choice of diet may also necessitate specific supplements. That's okay! Just be sure to discuss with your team of doctors your thoughts, questions, and concerns regarding the recommended supplements. The choice is yours, but you want to make an intelligent decision.

- **Incorporate exercise into your routine.** Exercise enables your body to be oxygenated, and your body needs oxygen to perform the many actions involved in supporting your immune system's healing abilities with good nutrition. Everything is related energetically!

Different Diets; Different Choices

It's entirely possible for you to use the information in this chapter (and in the other resources I've recommended) to design your own health affirming diet. However, you might also choose to follow a prescribed nutritional course. Here, I'll share the basics of several anti-cancer diets you may want to consider. Before starting a prescribed diet, though, always speak to your medical team to ensure that it is safe for you.

- **The Macrobiotic Diet.** The Macrobiotic diet, developed by a 19th century physician to heal his own cancer, is essentially an organic vegetarian diet that is low in fat and high in fiber. It is also rich in whole grains, vegetables, and soy products. The diet helps you to ingest phytoestrogens, which are thought to be especially helpful in reducing the risk of cancer. Those who wish to learn more and engage in the macrobiotic diet can visit www.kushiinstitute.org, or actually visit the Kushi Institute in Becket, Massachusetts.

- **Gerson Therapy.** Gerson Therapy involves a diet similar to the macrobiotic program in that it places the emphasis on natural foods from the earth. The Gerson Diet helps the body heal itself by treating the causes of illness; that is, the body's lack of nutrients and its toxic build-up.

   The full version of this plant-based, organic diet requires you to drink eight to thirteen glasses of fresh greenleaf and raw carrot/apple juices a day—all made from fresh vegetables and fruits. Additionally, you eat three full plant-based meals a day, along with fresh fruit and vegetables for snacks throughout the day. And for every three glasses of juice you do a coffee enema, which assists the liver in releasing the toxins your new diet is driving out of your body. To learn more, visit www.gerson.org.

However—and this is very important!—if you are dealing with chemotherapy, diabetes, kidney damage, or dialysis, or if you have a pacemaker, breast implants, steel plates, or screws in your body, you should proceed with caution. Refer to Charlotte Gerson's book, *Healing the Gerson Way: Defeating Cancer and Other Chronic Diseases*, before starting the program, and consult with your physician as well.

- **Sun Hee's Peace Diet.** One of the most powerful and inspirational stories that I recommend to my patients is *Cancer Healing Odyssey: My Wife's Remarkable Journey with Love, Medicine, and Natural Therapies* by Sarto Schickel. This is a heartwarming and engaging story of perseverance, determination, and hope. Sun Hee, Sarto's wife, was diagnosed with Stage IV ovarian cancer with pleural effusion. In researching this illness, Sarto learned that only one other person with Stage IV ovarian cancer had survived it.

  This dim prognosis did not deter Sun Hee. She developed her own integrative approach to healing. Having learned about the macrobiotic diet soon after diagnosis, and with her husband's guidance and knowledge of the Gerson diet, she chose a protocol that included surgery, alternative diet, and detoxification therapy, as well as seven months of chemotherapy.

  Sarto documented his wife's journey, which began with Sun Hee following a modified version of the Gerson diet from the day of diagnosis. Essentially, she combined a macrobiotic diet with juicing. Just two weeks later, x-rays showed a significant reduction of pleural fluid around Sun Hee's lungs. (The *only* difference in Sun Hee's lifestyle during this two-week period was the modified Gerson diet!)

Sun Hee continued her modified Gerson diet within weeks of her surgery, though she did not do the coffee enemas during her chemotherapy. Eventually, she visited the Gerson Clinic and instituted a full-fledged Gerson diet approach, though still insisting on her daily miso soup. Today Sun Hee is cancer free but continues to eat the diet she created, which indisputably contributed to her being healed of an "incurable" cancer.

Sun Hee and Sarto now call this diet *Paxdieta*, or *Peace Diet*. A full explanation of the diet is included as an appendix in *Cancer Healing Odyssey*. Sun Hee and Sarto have also created the Paxdieta Prevention Plan, which represents a middle of the road approach to both the Gerson and Macrobiotic diets, and is geared toward the couple's own likes and dislikes. I very much recommend that you learn more about these diets. Many of my patients who have researched them say that the diets made them feel comfortable enough to say to themselves, *This is doable for me—I can actually make this happen.*

- **Juicing.** Juicing, which is currently experiencing a surge of popularity, is a powerful and expedient way of getting foods' essential nutrients into your immune system's cells. Essentially, juicing is the pressing of a juice from raw foods. Consuming fruits and vegetables in this way gives your body easier access to food's precious enzymes and make it possible for your body to make use of all the food's nutrients, including vitamins and minerals. If you'd like to learn more about juicing, read Kris Carr's engaging, informative, and valuable book *Crazy Sexy Cancer Tips*. Carr writes about how this diet has enabled her to stop the progression of her rare cancer, which includes tumors on her liver and in other parts of her body.

  You may have noted that juicing is an integral part of the Gerson Diet as well as Sun Hee's diet. Here, I want to point out that you can juice, and still reap many of its benefits, without juicing eight to thirteen times a day (as the Gerson Diet, for example, prescribes). My thinking is that if you are not juicing at all at this point, juicing even three to four times a day would be helpful for your body. You or a loved one might wish to simply make enough juice for the day and keep it in your refrigerator to drink throughout the day.

Remember, You Get to Choose and Consume What Feels Right for You.

When presented with various healing diet and nutrition options, some cancer patients say, "My doctor did not recommend this. Therefore, I am not adding it to my diet."

However, most of those patients are unaware that in general, medical schools do not provide doctors with much education and training on nutrition. Believe it or not, most physicians are not taught to recognize foods that are therapeutically valuable in shifting the body's balance. In fact, many physicians have written of their frustration that they received no more than a week to a few weeks of classes dealing with nutrition.

My point is, your physician—while extremely knowledgeable and capable in other areas—may not be equipped to guide you nutritionally. This is why you need to do some of your own research, and why I have chosen to include this chapter in the book you're reading. I encourage you to inform and educate yourself so that you can make wise nutritional choices for healing your body. You can then take the information you have gathered and discuss it with your team of doctors.

As you consider information dealing with nutrition, know that you do not need to choose an "all or nothing" approach. What's important is that you become informed about some of the nutritional approaches that have helped others, as well as what "the experts" are sharing, and then find a way to blend what you feel *you* can manage into your life. I write this because so often, patients have told me that they chose not to go with one type of diet because the creators plainly indicated that the diet had to be followed in a purist manner. I understand this. However, after becoming familiar with the research, you get to choose what feels right for you—and this may or may not include integrating several approaches.

I have witnessed and read about so many people who have combined elements of different diet recommendations, and who have noticed improvement. (Remember Sun Hee?) Why? Because the diet is only a part of what is causing change. Your intentions for healing are another part, as is your motivation and the hopefulness you experience when you begin this work.

While there are no guarantees, I strongly feel that when you allow healing intentions to make positive changes in what you are feeding your cells, your body will recognize the differences and do its best to improve your health.

"The take home lesson is: You can take a soup bowl full of potent nutrients to fight cancer while you are being treated by the world's best oncologist, but if your mind is not happy and focused on the immune battle that must occur, then the following program of nutrition will not be nearly as effective as it should be."

PATRICK QUILLIN, PhD, RD, CNS

Diane's Story: Diet, Balance, and Healing

About five years ago, Diane was diagnosed with non-Hodgkin lymphoma. Diane, the wife of a physician and a mother of three (two of whom are physicians) went to the Sloan Kettering Cancer

Center where it was determined that her cancer was a slow growing tumor.

At first, Diane feared death and experienced heart palpitations, fatigue, and weakness. Over time, though, she has learned many lessons, overcame her fear, and now views her cancer as a gift. "Cancer changed my outlook on life," she states. Because of her cancer, Diane has actively grown her spirit and has begun working with an Eden Energy Medicine practitioner who has made her more sensitive to her body's energetic needs and intuitive wisdom. For the purposes of this chapter, though, I want to focus on a specific gift cancer brought to Diane: A new knowledge of what her body needs to be healthy, and a heightened appreciation of her nutritional intake.

At Sloan Kettering, Diane began a macrobiotic diet that focuses on eating grains, vegetables, and fruits while eliminating processed foods, sugar, oils, and the majority of animal products—especially dairy and meats. Diane chose to learn more about the diet by subsequently attending and living at The Kushi Institute in Massachusetts for three months. She felt that if she was going to "do" the diet, she wanted to do it "right." At the Kushi Institute she lost forty pounds and initially felt much better.

However, after returning home, Diane began to feel weak and debilitated. She realized that she still did not know all there was to know about what she was doing, and with more guidance and research, came to realize that her blood type required that she still eat some meat. While Diane continues to practice the heart of the diet, she balances it by sometimes eating organic meats and by juicing.

Diane acknowledges that despite these initial struggles, cancer has had a positive impact not only on her own approach to health, but on her entire family's. For one thing, they all eat better. For another, they have been motivated to learn as much as possible about naturopathy, meditation, energy medicine, yoga, and more.

When I asked Diane what she most wanted to share with you, the reader, she said the following: "The body has the ability to heal itself; you just have to let it do this. You must be optimistic and have hope. Say, 'I will not die!' Cancer is a wake-up call for you to realize what you have not yet accomplished in your life and to then make time to do what you have always wanted to do."

Finally, she emphasized, "You and only you are responsible for your own healing, for getting well, and for your body. There are those who don't get this. They go to the doctor and believe it is up to the doctor to fix them, via a pill or some kind of medical treatment. It is up to you to heal your body and yourself."

Nutrition in My Life

As you know, I have dealt with cancer in my life. And within the past year, as I have written this book, I have experienced several major hospitalizations. (Two were for diverticulitis, an inflammation of the "pouches" or diverticula in the wall of the colon.) I have been warned that if I am not more careful regarding what and how I am eating and drinking, I can expect to experience major problems with my colon—and might even need surgery.

Due to my diverticulitis and my history with cancer, I have become more conscious of the food I choose to prepare and eat, in addition to my intake of fluids. I have been researching nutrition not only for this book, but also for myself! I want to live a quality-filled life, and my health, like yours, depends on what I feed my body—as well as how I live my life.

I wish I had known in the past what I know now. (This may be something you are thinking to yourself as well). But I did not, and therefore, now is a good time to begin. If I were to be diagnosed with an illness such as cancer again in the future, I know I would integrate natural alternative choices such as a nutritional therapy and diet into my conventional therapies.

With this awareness, I am, hopefully, making intelligent choices in my nutritional selection. I buy organic vegetables, fruits, meats, and poultry. Yes, this gets expensive at times—but it's worth it, I feel. With the produce I buy, I make green and fruit smoothies to have during my day, and consume far more vegetables and fruits than I previously did. I have significantly reduced my intake of refined sugar (though I do love my raw honey!), and have also cut back on my intake of processed foods and dairy products. Additionally, I make a conscious effort to eat whole grains and a high fiber diet. I am drinking as much water as I can during a normal day (much more than before), and I choose water over other beverages such as iced tea, fruit juices, and coffee. As a result, I feel better, do not feel hungry as often, and find that I have more energy during the day.

My patients who have made similar changes in their diets have had similar experiences. They tell me that they are feeling stronger, more positive, better, and yes, even healthier. One patient with breast cancer smiled when we discussed making changes in her nutrition, reminding me that she had done the same thing ten years earlier when she wished to become pregnant ... and found that it worked! I had forgotten this. Her daughter is now 11.

Remember, your choice of diet is about your spirit as much as it is about your body. Making nutritious choices enables you to feel empowered, to take control of your life, and can help your body heal itself. A healthy diet is about self-love, because you value yourself and your immune system so much that you are willing to let go of old lifestyle patterns that no longer meet your needs ... and simultaneously, you are giving your immune system the tools it needs to begin healing your body. This is a win-win situation for you. As always, the choice is yours.

CHAPTER **20**

Purposefully Care for Your Mind, Body, and Soul

"All that we are is the result of what we have thought. The mind is everything. What we think, we become."

BUDDHA

Because you are an energetic being and your thoughts and feelings are energy, your journey may be compared to an intricately woven fabric. As the weaver of the fabric of your life, you alone decide whether your life will be beautifully intertwined with threads of gold and silver and blended with the colors of the rainbow, or made with strands of straw and cotton in shades of grays, browns, and other dark, heavy colors.

Every moment of this experience we call a physical life is determined by the choices you make in your thoughts, intentions, and actions. Thus, when you choose to experience a thought, image, or activity from a place of loving, joyful, and compassionate intentions for yourself and others, you have the power to weave a lovely fabric that heals your mind, body, and soul. When you choose differently, the fabric you weave may contribute to an experience of suffering and pain in the form of mental, emotional, physical, and spiritual anguish. The choice is always yours.

There are some simple, easily available, and wise choices—all winners!—that you can make in your daily life to brilliantly empower you, fill you with light, and vibrationally shift you to a feel-better place. Chances are, you already engage in many of these high-vibrational experiences without awareness. Now, as you read through the following paragraphs, allow them to be the gentle reminders you need to make conscious choices for healing your body, mind, and spirit.

Cultivate Gratitude for Your Gifts.

Your goal is always, always to focus on what feels good—*especially* while you are meeting the challenge of cancer. Perhaps it is a matter of compassion; perhaps it is a matter of decency, and perhaps it is a matter of just doing the right thing. But whatever the reason, expressing feelings of great appreciation, heartfelt gratitude, and sincere thanks always enable you to vibrate at a genuinely higher level—and this feels wonderful! Even saying a simple "thank you" to someone else can make your day!

One of the best things about gratitude is that it serves both you and the one to whom you are giving thanks. When you share your feelings of being blessed and grateful, not only do you vibrate at higher level, but your expression contributes to an increase in the energy of those around you, and especially serves the individual to whom you have expressed your thanks. The result is that you raise the level of universal well-being by choosing to focus with gratitude on your blessings.

Try the following strategies to tap into the healing power of gratitude on a regular basis:

- **First, brainstorm your blessings.** Many of us have simply never taken the time to *really* think about what we're thankful for. Take some time to consider all of the elements of your life—not just the big things, but the "little" things, too—that enhance your happiness and well-being, for instance: your family, your friends, your home, your job, your backyard, your garden, your dentist, your doctors, your neighbors, your degree, your job, your children, your grandchildren, etc.

- **Then, consider writing those blessings down.** Many years ago, something called the Gratitude Journal became popular. I encourage you to give the practice a try. By choosing to take a few minutes each day to write down your awareness of the gifts or blessings in your life, you'll gradually shift your perspective. Little by little, something almost miraculous will happen, and you will come to view your circumstances from a different vantage point, enabling you to feel different—even better—about everything. And before you know it, you will experience an improved sense of being—or healing!

- **Affirm gratitude.** The simple words *Thank you* or *I am so grateful* create a high vibration for every cell of your body. In Jane Katra and Russell Targ's book *Miracles of Mind: Exploring Nonlocal Consciousness and Spiritual Healing*, the authors share how Russell called on Jane to assist him with healing from Stage 4 cancer. One of the interventions Jane asked Russell to do involved him saying prayers of gratitude for his blessings, especially before meals. Jane knew that this had the power to help shift Russell's internal vibrational energy to a level that could assist his immune system's functioning. While affirming gratitude was only a part of Russell's therapy, it *did* contribute to his eventual—some might say miraculous—cure.

  You can't go wrong by training yourself to focus on every one of your blessings, be they the food or water on your table, the roof over your head, your friends, your family, your doctors, or your faith, and then expressing *Thank you for everything*. Your cells are listening ... and they respond by enabling your body to take better care of you.

  Affirm gratitude *especially* when you feel vulnerable and worried about not having enough of whatever it is that you are blessed to have—or when you are afraid it will all disappear. (This often occurs when you are experiencing great joy!) Affirm: *Even though I feel worried or frightened that my blessing may disappear, I am so grateful for [name of blessing] being in my life right now. I am blessed and grateful for [name of blessing] and for all my blessings.* Such affirmations will help shift you vibrationally from an uncomfortable, unhealthy place to one that feels better and supports your immune system. Essentially, you will be releasing those thoughts and fears that interfere with your gratitude, thus bringing yourself more joy.

If you are interested in learning more about affirmations and gratitude, Brené Brown writes of a similar affirmation strategy you can use, and discusses the impact of fears and scarcity-thinking on living a joy-filled life, in *The Gifts of Imperfection.*[1]

- **Enhance your gratitude with your breath.** Think of what your life would be like without your blessings. Take one person or thing you love, place it in the middle of your heart, close your eyes, breathe in and out, and focus on the joy it gives you.

  Now imagine it disappearing from your heart. Focus on the emptiness and loss you feel without whatever or whomever this is. See yourself living without this blessing and how difficult the loss is for you to sustain.

  Now put the blessing back into your heart and notice the full, rich feelings you experience. Consciously notice how much joy your blessings bring you. Then do the same with another of your blessings.

  By using your breath and your awareness of what you are deeply appreciative of, you have the ability to help your heart establish a rhythmic, comfortable beat and to experience the release of endorphins and hormones that are life sustaining—and that feel good. Now that is power!

There's one more point you might consider here. Given that you live in an energetic universe with the Law of Attraction (like energy attracts like energy) at work, when you choose to be grateful, you are putting forth a high level of energy—one that will be returned to you. Have you noticed that those around you who give so much to others are blessed with an abundance of gifts being returned to them when the need is there? Such is the power of heartfelt gratitude.

Nourish Your Spirit with Uplifting Stories.

At various points in this book, I have written about the importance of reading positive, inspiring stories that provide hope and comfort. Stories have the power to lift us up from pain and suffering. Whether you're reading about healing, near-death experiences, miracles, angels, synchronicities, or something else, stories can help you begin to view your situation from a higher perspective. In turn, this change of mind and heart will lead to the release of healing endorphins and neuropeptides that enhance your immunity.

The uplifting properties of stories are why I have sprinkled them throughout this book—and why I encourage you to seek them out and read them regularly throughout your cancer journey! Among my favorite books with uplifting stories are *From Incurable to Incredible: Cancer Survivors Who Beat the Odds* by Tami Boehmer, *Survival Lessons* by Alice Hoffman, *Remarkable Recovery* by Caryle Hirshberg and Marc Ian Barasch, *Radical Remission* by Kelly Turner, and *Dying to Be Me* by Anita Moorjani.

Immerse Yourself in Nature.

Your body is so wise. It recognizes what it needs to re-establish wholeness and balance. Being that you are a part of the universe, made of the same elements that compose everything else, it is only natural that you would seek to be in a location that could naturally feed and heal your energy. Nature meets this criteria, and it is where you will feel closest to your Source!

By being out in nature, you can be fully present as you focus on the sounds of a running stream, view a family of birds nesting in your birdhouse, watch a family of deer in your back yard, or glimpse a red fox running across your neighbor's property. It's no coincidence that you feel peace and joy when you fully focus on any of these experiences. In fact, healing is occurring because you are genuinely relaxed!

Take full advantage of your yard if you have one. If not, try to take regular trips to a local park or national forest. If you have the space and energy, this might be a great time to grow a small flower or vegetable garden. Even city dwellers can grow container gardens!

And don't forget your pets (if you have them), which are strongly connected to the natural world. Our birds, rabbits, cats, dogs, etc. provide us with another being to focus on which, once again, takes us out of our own problems and low vibrational emotions. If you're feeling sad or angry, play with your cat or take your dog on a walk. Or simply gather your pet up for a therapeutic hug. Many times, I've noticed that my patients' pets became an essential part of their healing therapy, giving them purpose and even the desire to live!

Nourish Your Temple.

As I wrote in Chapter Nineteen, the care you show (or don't show) your body greatly impacts your health. What we eat makes a difference not only in how well we function, but also in how we feel emotionally and in how well our brains work.

But nourishing your body—or your temple—isn't limited to your diet. Your body warns you when anything in your environment is out of balance, and if you choose to disregard those warnings, you will suffer the consequences—consequences that will *not* advance your healing goals. Too much sun, too much stress, too little sleep, listening to sounds that deafen the eardrums, drinking too much, taking addictive chemicals, etc. ... none of these things are in your best interests.

Remember, unconditional love of self is all about treating your body with loving compassion. Now and in the future, mindfully tap into your intuitive wisdom and do what you know is necessary to treat yourself well. Honor your body by listening to it and by caring for it like the temple it is.

Take Regular Shortcuts to the Joy Zone.

"Joy is what happens to us when we allow ourselves to recognize how good things really are."

MARIANNE WILLIAMSON

Some of the fastest ways to align with your heart's wisdom are to play, laugh, and enjoy yourself! Yes, really! We all tend to take life far too seriously. But when you lighten up and release your worries enough to focus on something—anything!—that makes you laugh and feels like play, you feel the greatest joy and peace. This is when you remember who you really are, which can be very powerful in enlisting your body's natural healing forces.

The problem is that we are so stressed out, so busy caring for others, so rushed, and with so little extra time that we fail to integrate fun into our lives. Once we become adults, we abandon our childhood habit of what I call "going to the joy zone," or allowing ourselves to enjoy the small pleasures of life, and exist in a place of happiness, peace, and love.

Trust me—your sweet, mischievous inner little boy or girl yearns to be allowed to have fun. I have found that making opportunities to allow my inner little girl time to enjoy life brings me an immense sense of joy and satisfaction—and honestly, is something that I continue to work on carving into my life. We are at our best when we allow ourselves, as adults, to play for the sake of playing!

"Laughter, song and dance create emotional and spiritual connection; they remind us of the one thing that truly matters when we are searching for comfort, celebration, inspiration, or healing: We are not alone."

BRENÉ BROWN

During your cancer journey, it's especially important that you take regular shortcuts to the joy zone in order to raise your vibrational energy and enable healing. Here are a few simple ways to do that:

- Take the time to call a friend or family member you miss
- Buy yourself a gift you have wanted for a long time but thought was too "frivolous" or not "practical" enough
- Go to a coffee shop for time alone with a good book, a piece of chocolate, and cup of tea
- Sit down for an hour to watch your favorite movie or show
- Take a bubble bath
- Go for a walk on a beautiful day
- Play a musical instrument
- Sing, dance, or go to the theater
- Play with your pets
- Have a meal with a friend
- Seek out something humorous

Actually, I'd like to talk about humor in a little more detail, because humor is a major healing vehicle. I always tell my patients, even those who are deeply grieving, that I want them to balance their pain with something that makes them smile and laugh, because laughing heals the body. The more you laugh, the less pain you experience, and the more your immune system is enhanced and supported.

Just recently, I visited a friend in the hospital. She later shared with me that laughing a lot during our conversation really helped her to feel better—so much so that she asked her children to bring jokes so that she could laugh some more!

As you meet the challenge of cancer, be sure to laugh often and well. Share jokes and humor with your own friends and family. Watch comedies. Search for humorous stories online. And most of all, try to find the laughter in everyday life.

Fill Your Journey with Music.

Listening to your favorite music helps you to experience joy and creates a wonderful, high vibration—just what your body needs. Specifically, music will increase your endorphins, decrease the amount of stress hormones your body produces, and help you to be present in the moment. So fill your journey with music as fully as possible! For instance:

- Sing your favorite songs while you're driving—really belt out the tunes.
- Put your favorite music on while you're cleaning your home or making dinner. Dance along if the spirit moves you. Even tiny steps taken to the beat of a song you love can make you feel good.
- Teach beloved songs to your children or grandchildren.
- Bring your favorite CDs or your mp3 player to your treatments.
- If you play an instrument, practice it as often as you can. Or take lessons and learn a new instrument! Actually, one of the strategies a patient of mine used to survive his life-threatening diagnosis was to give himself permission to engage in two of his life-long passions: taking both

piano and guitar lessons. Today he is healthy, and he continues to use these instruments in his work and his life.

Live Passionately, Expressing Your Joy and Sorrow in Many Ways.

So often, my patients discover their creative talents while seeking ways to express their feelings of fear, doubt, and worry about their experience. That's a good thing, because (as you know) your feelings are linked to the functioning of your immune system. When you have not found a way to express your fears, worries, guilt, anger, etc., blockages develop within your body and impede the work of your immune system.

That being the case, it's no coincidence that meeting the challenge of cancer so often fosters the birth of extraordinary artistry. Books have been written by survivors, talents have been discovered, and lives have been redirected by potential that has been unleashed and fostered. For some of my own patients, paintings and prints become illustrations of inner thoughts. Others have documented their journeys in their daily journals, describing in detail the impact of cancer on their lives. And several have shared with me the gift of their poetry, a literary form that has brought them great comfort and healing.

Judy Lang is a courageous, determined-to-live, two-time survivor of breast cancer. She chronicled her feelings about her journey both in her journal and in a series of poems, and has graciously agreed to share two of these poems with you.

Getting Fine Is Hard

By Judy Lang

"You're going to be fine,"
the doctor said.
"The cure rate is high for early cancer."

The words roll off his lips
to be absorbed by me.
Absorbed? I am repulsed!
Who me? Cancer?
No!

But no is yes
and slowly I must resolve the conflict within.
At first, even the words "cancer" is difficult to say.
But eventually it comes.
Survivors understand: Getting fine is hard.

It is grueling work saving one's life.
Which option do I choose
Which surgery?
Chemotherapy? Radiation?
Try dealing with that one.
Survivors understand: Getting fine is hard.

How do I accept the assault on my body?
The invasion?
How do I handle the peering over me by so many strangers
and I being there alone, so alone?
Survivors understand: Getting fine is hard.

And the waiting for the test results!
Will the lymph nodes be positive or negative?
How far has the cancer spread?
How much longer do I have to wait?
How much more can I tolerate?
Survivors understand: Getting fine is hard.

How do I make sense out of such wicked nonsense?
The doctor tells me about the cancer.
It is left for me to live it.
No, get rid of it!
Survivors understand: Getting fine is hard.

I muster up my strength.
Decide I'll not march to cancer's cadence
or be its duet.
I will fight it!
Just do my best and travel lightly becomes my motto.
Survivors understand: Getting fine is hard.

I ask myself a thousand times
Will I ever be ordinary again?
Then one day, all of a sudden, I am
not ordinary, but extraordinary.
Survivors understand: Getting fine is hard.
Being fine is extraordinary!

One Year Later: A Cancer Survivor

By Judy Lang

So now I've come full circle.
365 days since the cancer.

I end where I began,
forever changed by what I dreaded most.

In spite of everything,
the pain,
the horror,
the fear of one year ago,
Perhaps because of everything,
I'm here today
to celebrate a wonderful, glorious, sweet transformation:
I am victorious conquistador and dancing ballerina
all in one!

I'm bursting inside!
Can't you understand?
I've crossed the chasm from there to here.
I've put behind what always was before.
Now I'm swimming instead of drowning.
No more elusive kite flying aimlessly in the sky.
Moored firmly to my spirit
I am a special child of God.

I must tell you!
Reach out and shake you up!
Learn the lessons of the heart.
Be impatient for life.
Be infectious for life.
Hug life.
Kiss life.
Tickle life.
Do life and be life,
NOW!

If you enjoy writing poetry, I hope that Judy's work inspires you. And if you feel that poetry isn't your medium, I encourage you to find a way to be creative that *does* speak to your soul. It might be artistically (photography, painting, drawing, creating collages, etc.), through writing, through crafting (quilting, scrapbooking, woodworking, knitting, crocheting, etc.), or through culinary arts (baking or cooking), for example—and, of course, through giving back to others.

Find your passion and dare to live passionately. This is one of the most powerful ways of releasing your body's secret weaponry for meeting the challenge of your illness—and for surviving as a victor, and not as a victim.

Speaking of surviving as a victor, I'd like to close this chapter by sharing the story of my friend Eileen. She is a truly incredible human being who has survived over three decades of health challenges by purposefully caring for herself and choosing high vibrational thoughts, actions, and attitudes.

Eileen's Story: The Power of Purpose

Consider the following scenario: You are told by your doctor that you have renal insufficiency, so you make an appointment with your trusted doctor for a biopsy. But after you get to the hospital, a resident informs you that your doctor, Dr. B., will not be doing the biopsy because he is at the dialysis center. Instead, one of his colleagues, Dr. G., will do the job.

While on your hospital gurney, you notice that Dr. G is getting impatient since there is a delay in the schedule. He informs you that he has a lecture to attend. You tell him, "I am more important than your lecture. You need to cancel it and take care of me, your patient." He pays no attention to you and leaves for his lecture. You say to yourself, "This is not good. I should just get up, get dressed and get out of here." But in spite of your intense feeling, you tell yourself, "I have had all the preadmission testing and I do not like to make waves." So you stay, going against the intuitive wisdom of every one of your cells.

Still on your gurney, you see another doctor come in. You do not even recall an introduction. He tells you to roll over, sticks a needle in your back, and leaves. You are rolled into the recovery area—and then all Hell breaks loose. Suddenly, you feel pressure on your bladder, causing you to declare your immediate need for a bed pan. Blood comes gushing out of you, filling your pan. You're terrified. Your heart is beating a mile a minute. You are about to pass out, and you know this is the worst day of your life. And to make matters even worse, your daughter is right there feeling absolutely helpless and horrible.

At that moment, your husband comes rushing in, sees the commotion, and asks the doctor what's wrong. The doctor replies, "Your wife is hemorrhaging! I hope to God we can stop it!" Your husband screams, "I want a hospital administrator now!"

When all is said and done, you end up in the ICU for three days, having blood transfusions and a stat arteriogram. You are treated by two teams: the medical team (who want to send you home while still bleeding) and the nephrologists (who want to keep you in the hospital). Though you are still bleeding, the medical team wins and you are sent home.

After only two hours at home, you begin hemorrhaging and experiencing great pain once again. So back to the ER you go, for what will be the worst night of your life. Because the ER is filled to capacity, you are put on a stretcher and wheeled into a supply room with three others on stretchers next to you. There you stay bleeding clots of blood, in such pain that you do not care that while you are being catheterized, you are exposed to those in stretchers around you.

Finally, you are taken to your own room where you remain for seven days, being treated by a resident who appears insensitive to your pain and finally insists that you go home, even after a night of running a temperature and still bleeding! This time you make it three whole hours at home before you begin to hemorrhage again and experience excruciating pain in your lower back due to a blood clot in your kidney.

When you return to the hospital, you are taken from the ER into surgery. Two stents are placed in your kidney. Eight days later you go home once again with two tubes in your kidney to help it drain, sticking out of your urethra, and tied to your leg.

In the days, weeks, months and even years that follow, you obsess about why you did not listen to your own higher wisdom. Eventually, you recognize that you *did* survive the ordeal and you now have your life back. You make a point to affirm this with statements like, "This is ridiculous. It's over; it's done. I am living my life, a great life now. I am happy. I am a survivor." Attitude is everything!

As you probably suspect, this isn't a hypothetical scenario. This frightening series of events happened to my friend Eileen— and this is far from the only challenge she's had to deal with in her life. Eileen has also overcome a malignant tumor in the same kidney (which her intuition tells her was a result of the trauma the kidney endured). She has endured primary biliary cirrhosis, the removal of her gall bladder, the pain of chronic pancreatitis, thyroiditis, being misdiagnosed with liver cancer, and more. While her pancreatitis has returned and causes substantial pain—enough to require her hospitalization at times—Eileen considers herself to be fortunate and doing fairly well.

But that's not all—Eileen has also been through what she calls "the heartbreak of psoriasis," which began after the death of her mother and lasted seven years. In our interview, Eileen described the horror she experienced when she would get undressed and find the floor covered with her dry, flaky skin. Can you imagine having to wrap your arms in saran wrap (from your wrists to your arm pits) and your legs from your ankles to your hips night after night for many months? Eileen said she got through this by choosing to sing songs such as "I Feel Pretty" from *West Side Story*. That's my friend Eileen's sense of humor. And it is her intentional use of humor that has contributed to her being alive today.

Clearly, Eileen is a walking miracle in action. But what, do you suppose, is responsible for her surviving so many challenging medical experiences with such grace? What has Eileen brought to each of her health challenges? Besides her incredible youthful appearance at 72 years young and her unbelievable energy, how has she managed to survive her life's tests? I believe it's the fact that she purposefully cares for herself in many ways.

Eileen is known to all those who know her as a survivor and thriver, and this is significantly due to the fact that she has chosen to live her life with positive intention. She purposefully and lovingly cares for her mind, body, and spirit by choosing words, thoughts, and attitudes that are only positive, joyful, and loving. The affirmations Eileen chooses to use are all winners. They include: *Someone has to beat the odds and it will be me! No matter what happens in my life, I will be all right.* Believing in destiny, she also says, *If for some reason it is not meant for me to live a long life, then I will be okay.*

Eileen once told me, "I believe in the power of thought. I try to will illness away, using my inner strength to fight it. No matter what happens, I am going to enjoy my life till the day I die. If you give up, you may as well die of the day of your diagnosis."

Eileen also told me that she intentionally uses deep breathing, along with a lot of visualization. She described to me how she would visualize her pain leaving her body. Eileen also uses progressive relaxation to help her sleep. She relaxes her body, starting with her toes and working upward, and then sees herself entering an elevator and going down deeper.

She lives with an awareness of her gifts as a human being. She loves doing for others, including assisting the homeless and disabled in her community. In fact, I have often admired the extent of her compassion for those in need.

Eileen loves to laugh, smile, and offer stories that uplift the spirit. She fills her joy zone by surrounding herself with her family and especially her grandchildren, whether she is at her home by the water in Longport, New Jersey or in her home in Arizona where she can also be near her family and grandchildren. Her passion for traveling endured throughout all her illnesses, and continues to be a love of hers. However, she lovingly has cared for her body by cutting back on traveling until healing has occurred. Every choice she makes is one that is of a high vibration—and which abundantly supports her immune system.

When I asked Eileen what basic lessons she has learned during the past 40 years of medical challenges, she replied: "Enjoy my life as it is. I do not sweat the small stuff. If I get into an argument, I say to myself: 'I am too important to get aggravated and waste my energy on something stupid. I am saving my energy for the big battles of life.'"

I love Eileen's attitude. It is infectious! Those who have shared hospital rooms with her have been positively influenced by her determined positive energy and healing intentions. She sees herself as a fighter. She says, "I am a fighter to the end. I always think there is hope. I believe in miracles."

Except for what may be her destiny, Eileen feels she has control over her life. "I am not a victim and I do not want anyone to pity me. How I live up to my destiny is my doing. I always say there is someone else that is worse than me. And I do not want to trade places with anyone." Finally, she said, "I want to go out with a smile on my face."

We can all learn the art of caring purposefully for our mind, body and soul from this wise and courageous being.

PART THREE

CHAPTER 21

Be Selective in Creating Your Medical Team—And Think Integrative Medicine

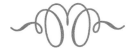

"Radical Remission survivors approach healing from a different perspective, where taking control of your healing is not only considered good but is actually essential for the healing process ... Taking control of your health involves three things: taking an active (versus passive) role in your health, being willing to make changes in your life, and being able to deal with the resistance."

KELLY TURNER, PHD, IN *RADICAL REMISSION: SURVIVING CANCER AGAINST ALL ODDS*

Cancer (or any life-threatening illness) is serious business, and when you receive a diagnosis, you want to be sure you are working with medical professionals who genuinely want what is best for your healing, and whom you can completely trust.

In this chapter, I'll share my insights on identifying the best team and treatment for your particular situation.

Choosing the Right Team Isn't *Just* About Technical Skill—It's Also About Intuition.

Given that you live in the 21st century, you have access to incredible research, treatments, and tools—none of which would have been available to someone in your position several decades ago. Let's face it: Had you been ill in the early part of the 20th century, you would not have had the ability to receive MRIs, ultrasounds, or any number of the sophisticated tests developed to discover possible health concerns. You would not have had access to chemotherapy, radiation, and other effective treatments.

However, the technical aspects of modern medicine are only part of the equation. To some extent, they are only as "good" as the physicians and medical professionals who are utilizing them. It's probably apparent to you that it's important to research the backgrounds of your healers. You want to know that they are well-trained in their specialties, have the appropriate degrees and experience, and come highly recommended by their colleagues and other patients. You want to know that they can answer all of your questions to your satisfaction.

But it's also just as important that you feel intuitively comfortable with your medical team. If that isn't the case, the treatments you receive, regardless of how cutting-edge or skilled they are—will be of limited efficacy. The stress you feel, and its vibrational impact on your body, will counteract your healing. That's why it is important to find doctors with whom you feel you can experience all levels of healing: not just physical, but mental, spiritual, and emotional healing as well. You want to share a similar vision regarding your health and your healing journey with your doctors. You want to be able to trust them.

Over the years, several patients have shared with me that they felt their doctors did not listen to them, took away their hope, were not there for them when they called with questions and concerns, or did not convey a sense of mutual respect. These patients were surprised, deeply angry, and very hurt. But they knew that if they were to survive, they absolutely had to work with doctors who made them feel that they had value and that they mattered as individuals—and not numbers. The patients who felt this way changed doctors, did survive, and are now thriving and happy. Here are two of their stories.

One woman, Ellen, shared with me that after she had finished the protocol for her breast cancer treatment, she met her doctor in the hall of the hospital. In that brief exchange, she felt a sense of lost hope and even betrayal as her doctor told her that it would be wise to go home and put her affairs in order. That was not exactly the message Ellen had hoped to hear. She told me that she did go home and put her affairs in order—by transferring out of that doctor's practice and into another in which she felt the physician was all about hope! Ellen did quite well following this exchange. With her sense of hope intact, her treatments helped her to heal, and she is now enjoying her life.

Another patient, Don, had been diagnosed with non-Hodgkin lymphoma. He told me that the doctor recommended by his oncologist was not returning his calls, and then scheduled an appointment for him too far into the future. Don recognized that none of this felt good to him, so he found another surgeon who came very highly recommended and who was more caring, as well as more sensitive to his needs and concerns. Don is doing very well and feels that by listening to his own intuitive inner voice, he contributed to his improved state of health and well-being.

Remember, you have the power to choose the allies who will help you meet the challenge of cancer. You are also blessed with the gift of your intuitive wisdom, a powerful force that, when listened to, can guide you toward your best interests. (As you know, many of the tools I have shared in this book are designed to help you tap into your inner wisdom so that you can make survival and healing-oriented choices.)

This is your time to TAKE YOUR POWER, and not be intimidated by those in authority. If your intuition does not feel comfortable with what you have heard or treatment you have received, consult with other professionals who are respected in the field. Please do not hesitate to do what you need to do to save your own life. Listen to your own inner guidance.

When Choosing a Treatment Protocol, Think Integrative Medicine.

Keeping in mind that healing encompasses the need to heal your body, mind, and spirit, I believe that the most effective treatments integrate the best offerings of both Western and Eastern medicine. We live in a world in which we are blessed technologically and pharmacologically, but as I have discussed in preceding chapters, when we ignore the energetic aspects of healing, it is often to our detriment.

We are fortunate to live in a time when Eastern medicine is being honored and married with Western medicine, providing you with more alternatives and healing wisdom. Eastern medicine has always honored the relationship of mind, body and spirit. It understands that the energies of the body are tied to the energetic experiences of the mind and the heart, and that the choices we make can lead not just to physical health, but also to our ability to grow and heal the soul.

For the first time, there is within the definition of medicine the understanding that healing involves a team or partnership approach, one that is holistic in enabling you to heal. This approach also recognizes that you are an energetic being and that there are a variety of ways through which you can enhance your ability to restore well-being, harmony, and balance. And the best news is, you have a say in all of this. You are a full partner in the process.

My patients often meet with their oncologists and surgeons, from whom they receive their chemo, radiation, and surgeries, and then combine their treatments with various forms of energy medicine, including Acupuncture, Eden Energy Medicine, Reiki, Therapeutic Touch, Tai Chi, Qigong, and more. Additionally, they often integrate a nutritional program, the use of herbs and supplements, and working with a mental health professional. And as I wrote in the introduction to this book, many of them have experienced physical healing with an improved quality of life.

A Final Note: Keep It Simple (KIS).

When sifting through the number of messages and pages in this book (or any other book), you may find yourself feeling overwhelmed by information, options, and choices. When that happens, take a few deep, calming breaths and remind yourself that your job in meeting the challenges of life is made easier when you choose to keep it simple. What I mean is, create a plan or strategy and then begin to execute it! The more you obsess over an issue, the more complicated things become, and the less you'll be able to accomplish. Not to mention, anxiety lowers your vibrational energy and impedes healing.

When you receive a cancer diagnosis, you may wish to get another opinion, or two, or three—and that is good! But as soon as possible, take action. Meet with your doctors, arrange for your tests, and then decide on your strategy. Love yourself enough to listen to your heart, as well as the "experts." Each of us needs to tune into our own higher guidance (or intuition, or inner wisdom) regarding our individual situations. And what matters most of all is the intention you have for your own healing, as well as the love for yourself and your life that you bring to your situation.

"The winds of grace are blowing; it is you who must raise your sails."
RABINDRANATH TAGORE

CHAPTER **22**

What Your Healers
Want You to Know

"Medicine has its office; it does its share and does it well, but without hope back of it, its forces are crippled—and only the physician's verdict can create that hope when the facts refuse to create it."

SAMUEL CLEMENS (MARK TWAIN)

When you are diagnosed with an illness like cancer, it's likely that you'll feel lost, confused, overwhelmed, and frightened. Odds are, you won't be sure of how to begin your healing journey.

That's why I felt it would be helpful to include in this book the thoughts and feelings of several professional healers who treat those on a journey similar to yours. Each of these individuals brings life experience to his or her work. Each is unique in his or her perspective—and that is a good thing.

While I posed specific questions to these healers, I suggested that each follow his or her heart in choosing to write words of healing wisdom for you. Some answered the specific questions I asked; others chose to share their thoughts on what healing means to them. What they all have in common is their awareness of how important it is for you to create an integrative healing approach. May these healers' words enable you to realize your power in meeting your cancer challenge.

Dr. Peter Yi

Peter Yi, MD, FACP, is an oncologist who trained at Cornell, Harvard, and Sloan Kettering. He has been associated with the Princeton Medical Group in Princeton, New Jersey, for more than 24 years.

The following section presents his thoughts on cancer and medicine. When I approached Dr. Peter Yi, he could not have been more kind and gracious in agreeing to share his thoughts and feelings with you, the reader of this book.

Information and Support Are Key.

If you (or a loved one) were to come to Dr. Yi today, he explained that he would first want you to gain an understanding of the meaning of your prognosis. Information, he feels, is necessary for you to make wise decisions. Such information includes an examination of the possible cause of the disease, what the risk factors may be, and the state of the disease, as well as curability and treatment options. From Dr. Yi's perspective, it might very well be in your best interest to get a second, and possibly even a third opinion.

Dr. Yi is concerned that emotional support be made available to help you navigate such major decisions, especially when you are being overwhelmed by various options.

"It's hard to think straight in such circumstances," he says. "People hear of all sorts of stories on the Internet or from friends, and they become confused. You need to have a team of professionals to help sort everything out and to make your decisions. People need help! Counseling provides such support."

Dr. Yi feels a personal responsibility to enable patients who come in for consultations to feel that all of their questions have been answered by the time they leave. He also strives to help them feel that they have a sense of clarity and direction regarding their treatment options. He has observed that once he has clearly outlined what patients need and ensured that they have clear goals, their anxiety and fears often melt away.

When I questioned him about how he might respond to a patient who resists his suggestions, he admitted, "This is difficult. We do our best to give our very best advice, while, at the same time, trying to gain a genuine understanding of where the patient is coming from. Perhaps their concerns are due to cultural issues; perhaps they have difficulty trusting authority figures. I try to explain as much as is possible about their cancer and how they can treat it.

"For example, if the problem is rooted in cultural differences, I give statistics regarding how many choose chemotherapy in different parts of the world—something with which they can personally identify and, therefore, often helps them feel more comfortable choosing a particular chemotherapy treatment. Some patients feel the need to visit several doctors before deciding. I feel their frustration—and mine, as well. I am disappointed that I was not able to win their trust, and some I just can't help."

Care for the Whole Person, Not Just the Cancer.

Regarding the practice of Integrative Medicine, Dr. Yi explained that he cares for the patient as a whole person—not just the cancer. He spoke of his awareness and sensitivity to the fact that cancer impacts the whole person, stating that it affects patients emotionally, socially, financially, physically, and personally. Some become depressed or have difficulty sleeping, socializing, or being intimate with their partners.

He stated, "As I get to know my patients over time, I gradually and gently recommend therapies that I believe can help them. It may be acupuncture, energy medicine therapy, nutritional counseling, physical exercise, psychological help, or possibly massage. When I share my own personal experience in using these therapies, patients are more inclined to try them."

In an article about Energy Medicine in *U.S. 1*, written by Jamie Saxon in 2010, Dr. Yi shared that while growing up in his home in South Korea, his grandmother would take him to a master acupuncturist, who treated his allergies and knee problems caused by athletic injuries. He and his wife continue get acupuncture.[1]

Eden Energy Medicine Can Be an Extremely Helpful Healing Tool.

One of the primary reasons Dr. Yi refers patients for Eden Energy Medicine (EEM) is because he has seen it spark significant improvement in and have a positive impact on his own patients. He referred to one of his patients in particular who had a rare form of cancer, leiomyosarcoma. This woman had been working with Diana Warren and Geoff White in Kingston, New Jersey, for several years. She had been told that she had six months to live and went on to live another fifteen years, during which she worked with EEM on a weekly basis. Dr. Yi explained that he recalled seeing this woman the day after her treatments and would notice a remarkable difference in her energy and well-being each time.

In the previously mentioned *U.S. 1* article, Saxon wrote about this patient, Janet Lasley, who said that her energy practitioners had been "crucial" in her healing: "They teach my body to use its own immune system, so they do a lot of work with body flow, getting meridians (energy pathways) lined up and connected so your own cells can attack cancers. They have strengthened my liver—I had 60 percent of my liver removed—which in turn strengthens my blood."

In the article, Dr. Yi indicated that after hearing Janet describe how her practitioners had been working on replenishing the energy of her depleted liver, he felt that he needed to try EEM for himself. He strongly felt that if this worked for his patient, it might work for others, too. He stated in the article, "I was intrigued that she was doing so well. I thought that maybe there is something here that I'm not familiar with. As a practicing oncologist you learn a lot from your patients: That's why we call it a practice."

Dr. Yi went on to experience Eden Energy Medicine with White and Warren and came away feeling very positive about the experience. He was impressed with the team's professionalism and ability to measure energy levels throughout the body. As a result, he refers patients who are on chemo and who are open to various forms of integrative medicine to White and Warren.

Dr. Yi has noted that patients who do EEM experience a greater sense of relaxation and feel good that they are taking an active role in meeting their cancer challenge—especially by being positive. Both in the article and in speaking to me directly, Dr. Yi emphasized that he sees no harm in engaging in energy medicine, as long as one is positive, open, and receptive.

Interestingly, Dr. Yi has observed that his patients who engage in various forms of complementary medicine (and especially energy medicine) are more positive, have more energy, and seem to have a better response to their treatment. For example, Dr. Yi's patient, Janet Lasley, also engaged in other forms of complementary medicine, including yoga and meditation. Dr. Yi recognizes that having a highly motivated, passionate, and positive approach to healing plays a major role in one's response to treatment.

"We Need to Not Be Afraid to Go Out of the Box to Help Patients."

When I asked Dr. Yi what he thought was lacking in the training today's physicians receive, he quickly shared his wish to see doctors and nurses receive more training in various types of integrative therapies beyond the traditional chemotherapy and radiation treatments. He feels strongly that more nonscientific training is needed for integrative medicine therapies, including acupuncture, psychology, quality of life issues, energy medicine, psychology, and massage.

He explained, "Unfortunately, you have to be on your own for many years before you learn the implications and value of these treatments. For example, the only psychology I had was part of my six weeks of psychiatry during my training. While it was excellent, it was not enough."

When questioned about what strategy he would use for himself if he were diagnosed with cancer, Dr. Yi replied, "I would take the most conventional approach—and I would combine this with integrative medicine including acupuncture (which I do now for arthritis), counseling, meditation, nutrition, and energy medicine. In other words, I would do everything that might help in my healing."

I ended my interview by asking Dr. Yi what he most loved about his work as an oncologist. He replied, "I love my work. I enjoy being able to help my patients by improving their quality of life. When they come into my office feeling anxious, worried, and frightened, I work to enable them to feel more comfortable, relaxed, and more hopeful by the end of our session—and to have a better perspective than when they came in. I am aware that this carries an enormous sense of responsibility. I know that if I am to help them, I must be respectful of their opinions and careful not to share any biases I might have. I am their healthcare worker and I need to be here for them. And I am aware that at times, we need to not be afraid to go out of the box to help patients."

Dr. Wendy Warner

Wendy Warner, MD, ABIHM, is Board Certified in both Obstetrics/ Gynecology and Integrative Holistic Medicine. She is a past President of the American Board of Integrative Holistic Medicine and a current member of its Board of Directors. After 14 years in a conventional ObGyn practice, she established her own holistic practice, Medicine in Balance, in Langhorne, Pennsylvania in 2004. She teaches physicians and speaks nationally about integrative medicine. She is also the co-author of Boosting Your Immunity for Dummies.

Dr. Warner is passionate about helping people find their right path to vibrant health. She finds that deep listening and compassionate education allows one to find balance and joy in life. She is continually grateful for all that she learns from her patients.

The following section showcases Dr. Warner's responses to my questions:

Susan Apollon: **When someone receives a cancer diagnosis, what course of action would you recommend they take in order to maximize their chances of surviving and thriving?**

Dr. Wendy Warner: The top priority for anyone in these situations is to get past fear. In our society, cancer is feared more than any diagnosis other than dementia. No one can heal adequately working from a place of fear. Ideally, one can reach equanimity regarding the reality of the diagnosis and find a place of acceptance. That doesn't mean you sit back and do nothing; it's just that you strive to reach a place where you aren't attached to the outcome.

I had a friend and colleague, a physician who trained care providers to care for themselves, named Lee Lipsenthal, MD. Lee taught for years that we should live our lives as though each day is a good day to die. He then developed esophageal cancer … and he had the most amazing experience in his last few years! He truly accepted his situation and lived his final years well. Many friends and family thought he had "caved in" and wasn't "fighting" hard enough, but I really think he simply was ok with what was. He wrote a book about it called *Enjoy Every Sandwich* which I suggest to patients when they or a loved one gets a tough diagnosis. You might want to view the trailer for it to get a sense of who Lee was: https://www.youtube.com/watch?v=3UIFbOfWwYE

SA: **How do you respond to a patient who is not comfortable with traditional chemotherapy and radiation?**

WW: This totally depends on the situation. There are some times when science shows that traditional chemo and radiation really do offer the best options long term. In that case, my job would be to help the patient avoid side effects and help the treatments work even better. However, there are other times when what is offered has such a low chance of making any difference that it's best to skip chemo and/or radiation.

Either way, I ask the person to express what it is that makes them uncomfortable. If they simply need more information, sometimes they choose conventional treatment. If their concern is coming from fear, then sometimes they change their stance once they settle into the diagnosis. If their decision is based on the facts plus their personal beliefs, then I'm okay working with them if they choose to avoid traditional chemo/radiation.

A patient's discomfort with chemo and radiation becomes more of an issue if their friends and family are not on board with their decision. Under those circumstances, I do ask the patient to sign a release so the family knows I didn't coerce them in any way!

In general, I wish I had the opportunity to see more people earlier in their cancer journeys. Often, I see them long after treatment has begun, and I have to fight to help them build back up. Most cancers move fairly slowly, so when I begin working with someone soon after diagnosis, there is time to build up the person's reserves prior to instituting chemo and/or radiation.

SA: **Do you feel that you practice what is referred to today as "integrative medicine"?**

WW: Yes, I am board certified in integrative/holistic/functional medicine.

SA: **What do you see as the primary difference between traditional and integrative medicine (and/or the Western approach to medicine versus the Eastern approach)?**

WW: The primary difference between conventional medicine as I was taught versus what I practice now is that in conventional medicine, we are taught to focus on symptom relief and rarely on changing the underlying disease process. In functional/integrative medicine, we look at healing differently: We search for the underlying pathophysiology and work to correct the imbalance. We focus on processes, not diseases.

For instance, the process of inflammation underlies coronary artery disease, autoimmune conditions, Alzheimer's, and hormonal-related weight gain ... and yet none of these things would be listed together in conventional medicine.

In holistic medicine, we focus on the person as a whole, seeking balance for their physical, mental, emotional, and spiritual bodies. We use all appropriate therapies, including body work, energy work, spiritual guidance, and physical treatments such as herbs and supplements. We also use the best of conventional medicine if appropriate.

I actually bristle at the terms "Western" versus "Eastern" medicine. There were holistic practitioners here in the West until the current paradigm ran them out. The eclectic physicians, the midwives and herbalists, the homeopaths—all practiced in a way that would today be called holistic and integrative. It's just that they had to go underground once the Flexner report came out and the AMA took over power. So "Eastern versus Western" really isn't the right paradigm at all!

SA: **What aspects of integrative medicine feel best to you?**

WW: Integrative holistic medicine is what I was born to do; it's why I went into medicine. I just didn't fully understand it at the time. In this medicine, I am partnering with my patients. I am educating them, giving them options, then helping them find how to make their choices work in their lives. Most of the time, I'm asking people to change how they live, not just to take an herb or learn to meditate. I'm usually offering a comprehensive overview of all the ways in which my patients can transform their health … and it usually means changing everything! What I love is that most of the folks I work with are willing to try; they might stumble a lot, but they try. That human interaction is what makes my day.

And this holistic approach works! At my office, it's common for a staffer who has worked in other medical offices to make this statement after working with us for a few months: "This is the only place I've ever worked where people actually get better!"

SA: **If you were diagnosed with cancer today, what approach would you take for yourself?**

WW: I would get opinions from a conventional oncologist as well as from an integrative oncologist/team. Depending on the diagnosis and prognosis, I would probably do a bit of everything:

some conventional treatment, plus a lot of other support. I would slow down, meditate more, and laugh as much as possible. Likely for me, accepting help would be the biggest challenge!

SA: And what approach would you take if your wife or child or best friend was diagnosed with cancer?

WW: I would help them see all their options and then try hard to support whatever decision they made, even if I didn't agree.

SA: What do you feel we are missing today as we help those with cancer to heal?

WW: It's all about the "fight." I think conventional medicine doesn't work hard enough to alleviate fear, since fear is really where most patients are coming from! There is a way of talking that allows people to see that, for instance, hospice isn't about giving up, it's about pain control and comfort. That, however, is not how most folks see it.

I also think we push people too far. I think that many conventional docs have a hard time letting people choose to die peacefully at home; many docs are fairly unrealistic in what they are offering patients, because what they offer is so limited.

Mostly, what we are missing is allowing patients to retain grace and dignity and a sense of themselves. We focus a bit too much on labels like "survivors," when surviving or living with cancer is simply *part* of who they are.

SA: What would you like to see today's doctors learn that you feel is missing or inadequate in their training?

WW: Oh Lord, this a whole book by itself. I think, in short, that *all* care providers need to be trained in functional medicine. I think that *all* care providers need to be familiar with integrative/holistic therapies and thinking.

Most of what I was taught in med school is limited, and much of it is NOT science based. And it's still being used today as "standard of care." Our entire medical education system needs to be overhauled, along with the systems that we've devised to provide care. I always say that before entering med school, I was a lovely, well-rounded individual with a broad liberal arts background; then school was like a crucible, burning me down to my essential abilities to deduct, be analytical, and ignore my intuition. It took me years to find all of myself again. I hate to think that this might still be happening to other docs in training, and I'm pretty sure it is.

SA: **What kind of progress have you noticed in patients who pursue energy-based treatments: acupuncture, energy medicine, tai chi, qigong, etc.?**

WW: Energy medicine can achieve what I often cannot with physical treatments. All pathology is a reflection of damage to the energy body. If we don't fix the energy body, we end up playing "whack the mole," and physical symptoms just keep popping up elsewhere. Essentially, all of my patients get a prescription for energy work, be it acupuncture, HeartMath techniques, Reiki, or shamanic healing. In fact, there are times when I've sent folks to my shaman when I simply wasn't making any progress in what I usually do ... and it almost always has had a huge impact.

SA: **What do you love most about your work?**

WW: Making a connection with those I serve. If I can help someone understand how to balance their own health and remember that their body is designed to be whole and healthy, then I've had a good day.

Also, I teach a lot of docs and other care providers. I'm only one person, so I can only see a limited number of patients each day. But if I can help teach other docs how to do this, and how to transform healthcare, then imagine how many more patients' lives will be impacted!

Dr. Jingduan Yang

Dr. Jingduan Yang is a fifth generation teacher and practitioner of Traditional Chinese Medicine, specializing in acupuncture. He is also a psychiatrist, neurologist, and Chinese medical herbalist. With over 20 years of training in the best of classical Chinese medical knowledge and modern medical science, he has become a leading integrative physician in today's changing healthcare landscape.

He believes that true health comes from an understanding of the whole person, not only from the physical, emotional, and spiritual levels, but also from the person's social and professional contexts.

Dr. Yang currently practices integrative medicine and psychiatry at Tao Integrative Medicine (www.taointegrativemedicine.com), which he founded in 2003. He also teaches Traditional Chinese Medicine and Acupuncture at the Integrative Medicine Fellowship Program at the University of Arizona.

Dr. Yang is the director of acupuncture and Chinese medicine and clinical assistant professor of psychiatry at the Myrna Brind Center of Integrative Medicine, Jefferson University, Philadelphia.

Dr. Yang's "Plan of Attack"

If you have just been diagnosed with a life-threatening illness such as cancer, in addition to seeking second and third opinions, validating the diagnosis, and developing a sensible treatment plan with your doctor, Dr. Yang also advises you to stop and examine what might be causing your symptoms. Dr. Yang recommends that you reflect on what your body is communicating to you by way of your symptoms. Each symptom, he feels, represents a message, even a warning, that you have previously ignored, and to which you now need to listen and pay attention. Take the time to just sit, be, and consider what your message might be.

Specifically, Dr. Yang would have you look at *five major areas* that may have contributed to the creation of your symptoms, including your cancer.

First, consider what you are doing to your body's chemistry. You can do this by checking your exposure to environmental toxins, including chemicals in the air you breathe, in the supplements and medications you take, and even in the foods and drinks you consume. You should also consider whether you may have been exposed to infections and radiation. And, of course, if you are aging or chronically ill, be aware that your body is experiencing physical and chemical changes that impact your immune system's ability to take care of you.

Second, examine your lifestyle. Again, note in particular what types of foods and drinks (and how much of them) you're consuming, as well as the regularity of your dining times. Consider whether you exercise daily and tend to your physical needs, and if you smoke or overuse alcohol. List the activities in which you participate, and determine whether or not you have a relatively regular routine you follow in life.

Third, look at your social support system and your relationships. Ask yourself if you like to socialize more, or if you have difficulty forming and maintaining relationships. Do you like to be alone? Do you feel you are likeable and cared about? Do you care for others?

Fourth, take your emotional temperature. Are you experiencing emotional distress? Ask yourself, "Am I or have I been angry, sad, depressed, resentful, frustrated, or excessively negative, whether recently or for some time—perhaps for an extended period of time?" Think about your emotions regarding your relationships, both personal and professional. Give thought to what you have been focused on and the feelings you've had, but have chosen to not express.

Ask yourself, "Am I feeling stressed? If so, where is this coming from and when do I feel it the most? Where and with whom do I experience significant stress?" In particular, be sure to question yourself regarding feelings you have about your finances, and determine if they are a part of your stress. Ask yourself, "Am I concerned about my job or about being laid off or fired?"

Fifth, reflect upon the spiritual aspects of your life. Ask yourself the following questions: "What am I doing spiritually for myself—if anything? Am I aware of my purpose? Do I feel a connection with my Higher Power? What brings me peace? What might the meanings of the problems and crises I am going through be? Do I have helpful spiritual practices?"

While these five aspects of your life are distinct, *they can and do overlap with one another.* And all of the factors Dr. Yang has asked you to think about can be contributing factors to the evolution of illnesses such as cancer. As I have pointed out multiple times in this book, your cancer may be a wake-up call indicating that certain aspects of your life are unhealthy and need to change. Please don't ignore the messages you may be receiving.

After you have zeroed in on the messages your symptoms might be sending you, it is time to *fine tune your diagnosis.* You will do this with the help of your doctors who practice integrative medicine and Chinese medicine in addition to your oncologist, who will identify the location(s) of your illness, the stage of your illness, and the nature of what is out of balance within the body. (All illness is a function of your body being out of balance, which in turn requires your doctors to determine what is being impacted by the imbalance.) This can be a combination of the stagnation of your qi (energy), phlegm, blood, internal heat, the level of dampness within your body—and more!

After you have determined the causes of your illness, Dr. Yang strongly feels that if your illness has formed structurally (for example, a cancerous tumor), you then need to deal with its removal either surgically or with treatments like chemo and radiation. If you are dealing with inflammation, he recommends starting an ant-inflammation diet.

Other Professionals to Consider in Your Treatment

Because Dr. Yang recognizes that illness results from an energetic imbalance taking place in your body and that your body, mind, and spirit are very much connected, he recommends seeing professionals who can assist you in addressing the physical, emotional, mental, and spiritual concerns that contributed to the evolution of your symptoms and illness. Here are a few professionals he recommends considering in particular:

1. **Nutritionist.** One of the professionals to whom Dr. Yang regularly refers patients is a nutritionist. Most of us fail to recognize that the food we eat has the power to either support or suppress our body's immunity. Nor do we fully understand that we are impacted by when we eat, how we eat, and what we eat. (Yes, these patterns matter!)

   While foods can be healing and medicinal for you, they can also be toxic and chemically unhealthy for you. For example, you may be allergic to seafood, nuts, wheat flour, or milk—any of which can negatively impact your body's ability to energetically care for you. Also, by combining cold drinks, spicy foods, and a lot of red meat, you can and often do exacerbate inflammation of the body's cells. Again, this impacts the healthy flow and balance of your body's energy.

   A nutritionist, Dr. Yang believes, can educate you and make you aware of how you can better choose foods that will boost your immunity and support your healing intentions. Since health-supporting nutrition is not one-size-fits-all, you can benefit greatly from working with a professional who takes into account your particular needs.

2. **Psychotherapist (including a Licensed Psychologist, Psychiatrist, Social Worker, or Mental Health Counselor)** As a psychiatrist, Dr. Yang is especially sensitive to the

traumatic nature of being diagnosed with a life-threatening illness such as cancer. We go through numerous emotionally difficult and even traumatizing events in our lives. Cancer becomes one more such event that has the power to reactivate past traumas—even those for which you have sought help in the past.

When receiving such a diagnosis, you tend to not only experience a reactivation of old traumas but to also lose yourself in questioning the meaning of all that is taking place in the present. You will find yourself asking questions regarding what you have been doing behaviorally, feeling emotionally, and practicing spiritually that could have brought you to your present situation. The past influences the present.

One issue in particular that many patients work through with their psychotherapist is that of grief. So often, your diagnosis represents a perceived sudden loss of your health and well-being. This in turn brings up old losses which reinforce your sense of loss. All of this suppresses the functioning of your immune system. While experiencing grief after a diagnosis *is* normal, Dr. Yang feels that a therapist can enable you to work through these feelings and eventually experience a sense of release and healing. In his own practice, Dr. Yang uses a neuro-emotional technique that involves tapping into energy blockages caused by past trauma.

Another benefit of seeing a psychotherapist is the opportunity to reflect on your life, your relationships, your sense of personal fulfillment, and your spiritual evolution. Talking to a professional enables you to examine your quality of life, to determine what is out of balance, and to express feelings about problematic people and situations in your life. A psychotherapist can provide you with tools to empower and assist you in your personal and spiritual

growth. Your sessions will also enable you to release negative thoughts and feelings that have created the energetic
imbalances leading to your illness.

3. **Classical Chinese Medicine Practitioner.** As an integrative medicine doctor, Dr. Yang views individuals on three
levels: structurally, bio-chemically and energetically. When
any of the three is out of balance, we see this imbalance
manifest physically, biologically, socially, emotionally, financially, and spiritually. This causes problems with the
body's natural flow of energy, leading to disturbances that
impact the working of a healthy immune system.

Therefore, Dr. Yang believes in the value of incorporating classic Chinese medicine, which includes a course of
Chinese herbal remedies and acupuncture, into your healing regimen. Both modalities restore imbalances caused by
aging as well as by your illness and its treatments (such as
chemotherapy and radiation).

Along with the previously discussed recommendations, Dr. Yang believes that you are best able to create
energetic balance by incorporating relaxation techniques
and energy exercises into your routine; for instance, meditation, qigong, tai chi, and energy work. With his own
patients, Dr. Yang recommends Falun Dafa, a Chinese life
cultivation system centered on the goal of becoming spiritually enlightened.

A Closer Look at Herbs and Acupuncture

As noted previously, Classical Chinese Medicine incorporates
herbal remedies and acupuncture. Since neither treatment option
is commonly used in Western medicine, we'll take a closer look at
each of them here.

Herbal Remedies

Dr. Yang views herbs as medicines, not supplements. Herbs are not chemical agents, but energetic agents capable of transforming your body. Given that Classical Chinese Medicine is all about balance, herbs are given to restore balance to the body.

Dr. Yang often uses a formula or combination of herbs that have been proven to be effective for treating specific kinds of illnesses (including cancer) and for promoting general well-being. Herbal remedies differ from traditional western medications in that they do not only work on specific illnesses; they also focus on supporting your system energetically. They work on levels different from those focused on by chemotherapy. Dr. Yang notes that herbs can help shrink, reduce, and remove tumors. That is how powerful they are!

Furthermore, when you develop an illness such as cancer (and even during the normal process of aging), you become deficient in the qi (life force energy) of your kidney, liver, and spleen meridians (pathways through which energy flows). For example, a spleen deficiency may cause symptoms of fatigue, nausea, diarrhea, muscle achiness, and fuzzy thinking. A deficiency in kidney qi can result in hair loss, cognitive loss, tinnitus, hearing loss, a decreased libido, reduced bone density, and emotional fear. And a liver deficiency can cause dizziness, insomnia, depression, anxiety, and joint pain. The use of herbal remedies can shift all of these imbalances and help you heal by restoring your energetic balance.

Dr. Yang believes that the reason doctors in general do not tend to suggest herbal remedies is because they are not taught about them. And without being informed about herbs' healing value, doctors are not likely to recommend them to patients. As part of his work, Dr. Yang takes time to explain to physicians how herbal remedies differ from traditional medicines (that they are not chemicals and that they work with the body's energy systems).

Acupuncture

Acupuncture affects your energy by impacting the energy pathways (the meridians) that are energetically connected to the organs and systems of your body. Unlike pharmaceuticals (which only treat symptoms), this modality works by addressing the root cause of the problem; that is, the energetic imbalance. According to Dr. Yang, acupuncture taps into the body's energetic levels, both past and present, and prepares the body for the future.

Dr. Yang believes it is imperative to begin acupuncture from the first day of your diagnosis. In a presentation to his fellow doctors at Grand Rounds at Jefferson Hospital in Philadelphia, Pennsylvania, on December 3rd, 2013, Dr. Yang explained that acupuncture for cancer opens energy channels that have been blocked, disperses any stagnations of energy, expels phlegm and dampness, clears toxins and heat, and facilitates and strengthens qi—all of which is needed to enable the immune system to function at its best.[2]

In layman's terms, the chief benefits of acupuncture are that it reduces pain and minimizes the side effects of chemotherapy, especially the nausea. It also improves the spleen qi and reduces diarrhea, fatigue, and shortness of breath—all of which are often symptoms of chemotherapy.

If you're interested in learning more about acupuncture (and especially if you're feeling skeptical), I encourage you to read "Is Acupuncture a Deception?," which Dr. Yang wrote for *The Huffington Post*.[3] In the article, he highlights numerous renowned organizations including the American Medical Association (AMA), The World Health Organization (WHO), and National Institute of Health (NIH) that have endorsed acupuncture as a modality of effective treatment for chronic pain with little if any side effects.

Final Thoughts

Whether you are challenged by cancer, any other illness, or aging, Dr. Yang recommends that you consult with a trained integrative medicine doctor to create a plan that will allow you to integrate all healing wisdom with your conventional medical plan.

During our interview, Dr. Yang remarked about the differences between the Eastern and Western approaches to illness. He spoke of conventional medicine being very limited due to the fact that it focuses on the illness as a disease, as well as its symptoms, with the emphasis for treatment being on lab tests, drugs as medications, and specific procedures that involve insurance coverage.

Integrative medicine, on the other hand, views illness as an imbalance of energy and, rather than waiting for you to get sick, chooses to educate patients about well-being and preventative care. Dr. Yang pointed out that Integrative medicine appreciates the mind-body-spirit connection and the impact this has on healing. It saddens Dr. Yang that conventional medicine does not teach medical students enough about subjects like nutrition.

When I asked Dr. Yang how he supports his own wellness, he explained that he follows and adheres to the advice he gives to others. Dr. Yang tries to be sensitive to his own attachments that cause him emotional stress, being mindful so that he can release them. He devotes himself to caring for his spirit and the spiritual aspects of his life. Specifically, he practices Falun Dafa, a life-cultivation system that integrates meditation and qigong in conjunction with following the laws of the universe and leading a truthful, compassionate, and tolerant life. As mentioned previously, its goal is spiritual enlightenment.

Aware of following good nutrition, Dr. Yang rarely drinks caffeinated beverages, except green tea. He does not smoke or drink alcohol, exercises, enjoys his work, and lives his life treating all with respect. In other words, Dr. Yang lives in alignment with his approach to healing the mind, body, and spirit. He practices what he preaches.

Dr. Scarlet Soriano

Scarlet Soriano, MD, is Board Certified in both Family Medicine and Integrative and Holistic Medicine. A graduate of The University of Pennsylvania School of Medicine, Scarlet Soriano is a full spectrum family physician. She recently completed nearly five years of work for the Indian Health Services (IHS) in New Mexico. There, she developed an Integrative Medicine Clinic, focusing on Mind-Body and Energy Medicine techniques. In her words, "I love it when my patients use integrative healing modalities!" She is also an Eden Energy Medicine Clinical Practitioner.

To enable you to better understand why she does what she does as a healer and an Integrative and Holistic Medicine physician, Scarlet wrote the following:

I was awe-struck.

I had expressed my deep desire to serve as an instrument of healing, to go beyond the limitations of biomedicine and, through spiritual practice and harnessing of healing energy, to help a person heal. Her reflection back to me, gentle as it was offered, penetrated deep within my soul. She spoke of a "healing journey." Her wish was not to cure, to perform miracles, but rather to support a soul as it journeyed through the layers of healing, from the physical to the spiritual.

It was a quiet turning point for me. This gentle soul, acupuncturist and Qigong Master, at home in the world of energy, deepened with her words my ability to see illness, wellness, and healing as a profound journey whose ending need not involve resolution of physical ailment or even preservation of life. The soul's integration of its life lessons, its degree of surrender and union with Grace, was, in fact, the miraculous healing, the journey, and the goal at once.

A veil lifted within.

I no longer needed to save.

I needed instead to purify my own inner vessel that I might hold space for Grace to flow through, for unconditional love to manifest within and spread. This was, I now saw, the role of the healer: To, as the amazing energy healer Donna Eden once said, "drop down to soul level." Once there, to offer unconditional love and to kindle and support a process of inner journeying, of releasing the layers of unnecessary weight that bind the spirit and prevent a fuller experience of truth, and joy, and love.

Many, many times we undertake such a powerful journey only when forced out of the comfort of routine, jostled by a harrowing diagnosis into inner exploration and redefinition. There, in the horrendous pain and suffering of a diagnosis that throws the previous trials of daily life out the window, lies ripe terrain for the soul's journey to heal.

How then to support that process? To engage with a dear soul and hold the fear, the anger, the anguish, the unresolved? How to listen with deepest attention, to honor grief, to plant seeds of self-acceptance and inner safety that can lead to reconnection, integration, surrender, and the experience of Grace?

Now, whether working furiously in the ER to support a person's hemodynamic state so that they might live another day or sitting with a patient in clinic, I make an effort to remember that though I will do everything in my power to support life, I must also make every effort to support a deeper process of whole-being wellness that goes beyond the physical and encompasses the mind/body/soul.

I became an Integrative Medicine practitioner in order to best serve this now fuller vision of a healing journey. I see now that the tremendous healing potential hidden beneath the horror of a cancer diagnosis requires that the multiple dimensions of a person's reality be honored, supported, and assisted into a process of releasing the unnecessary and cultivating the life-giving and healing elements within.

Such a journey requires that we mobilize all the positives within the whole of a person's reality, from the quality of the food that goes into the body and the love and prayers that are imbued into the food, to a deepening of spiritual/contemplative connection and community, to balancing of vital energies, to appropriate physical exercise, to a diligent tending of the garden of thoughts that flourishes in the mind. All dimensions of the whole must be supported. All that weighs the mind/soul/body down must be released. No matter how tempting or dramatic, it all must go to make room for healing. A powerful way to support deep inner healing is through the cultivation of Gratitude, and as such it has become a focus of my practice.

Ultimately, the greatest gift I can offer any human being with whom I connect in the path of healing—whether patient or family or friend—is to see them as a soul undergoing deep transformation and to hold and reflect unconditional love for the fullness of their being.

Whatever the ultimate physical outcome, if I can walk through illness with a fellow human and support a process of inner exploration, reconnection with self-acceptance and gratitude, integration of life lessons, and release of resentment and negativity, then I have supported healing. I have served.

Dr. William L. Scarlett

William (Bill) L. Scarlett, DO, FACS, FACOS, FAACS, is an Associate Professor of Plastic Surgery at Philadelphia College of Osteopathic Medicine and Medical Director of Bucks County Aesthetic Center in Bensalem, Pennsylvania. In his private practice in Bensalem, Bill works primarily with women who have been diagnosed with breast cancer and focuses on breast reconstruction. Bill, a respected lecturer and presenter, has developed workshops for cancer patients to better enable them to deal with the psychosocial aspects of cancer. He looks forward to the future publication of his first book, Demanding Compassion. *On a personal note, Bill is a proud father and husband and enjoys competing in Olympic Triathlons.*

Bill graciously agreed to write the following section for this book.

Choosing the Right Doctor and Treatment for You

When facing a new cancer diagnosis, it is important to get referrals and personal recommendations on whom to see and where to go. Great resources can include your primary doctor, the nurse navigator, support groups, friends, and family. However, I would caution you to take treatment recommendations given by friends with a grain of salt. Your friends' intentions are good and of course these individuals want the best for you, but obviously every individual's case is different and must be addressed uniquely. Your next door neighbor or your hair stylist may not be the best person to make surgical recommendations.

I tell my patients that there should be no guilt associated with getting a second opinion. I encourage my patients to get multiple opinions, especially when there are multiple treatment options. This allows for two things to occur: First, you may receive a different treatment option, and second, you will interact with a variety of physicians and staff. I have had patients tell me that they liked a surgeon, but the staff was so rude that they would not return to that practice, knowing that they would need to interact with them on a regular basis. A physician should not take it personally if a patient chooses to get a second opinion. I expect my wife to get three opinions on remodeling the kitchen before making a decision!

After seeking multiple opinions, you will get a feel for whom you want to choose. It may not be something you can put your finger on, but you will probably feel more comfortable and more at ease with a certain person. When getting treated for any illness, you must feel comfortable with and trust your caregiver. If that relationship is not present and healthy, then I would recommend seeking care elsewhere. This doesn't mean that complications and setbacks can't occur, because they can. But if you have a strong working relationship with your physician and you are making decisions together as a team, then you can deal with just about anything.

When my wife and I received her cancer diagnosis, I know my initial reaction was, "When can we get it out of her and how quickly can we get the surgery scheduled? But there was a lot that needed to be done first. There were labs and X-rays, CT scans, and a PET scan.

The reality is that our first reaction is often, "How quickly can we get this taken care of," but the cancer or other illness has probably been there for a while. Doing your homework on the treatments, the procedures, and the physicians is time well spent. Being comfortable with the team that will be caring for you or a loved one, and the plan that is being put in place, is very important. To rush into anything with fear leading the way is never a good medical decision.

Treatment of any serious illness, but especially cancer, is a team approach. There will be multiple physicians and nurses involved in coordinating the care, but the patients and their families must also be involved. It is obvious to most people that family dynamics and schedules need to change in order to accommodate appointments, tests, and still getting the kids to school on time. Having the support of family and friends at the time of diagnosis is paramount, but it may be just as important after recovery.

The Truth About Lifestyle Changes

Recently there have been significant studies that examine cancer recurrence after traditional treatment. They show that lifestyle changes are necessary. We know that with a diagnosis of diabetes, the family needs to help with dietary changes and exercise routines, but we are now seeing both of these things tied to cancer recurrence and metastasis, too. It isn't enough to have surgery, chemotherapy, and radiation, and think that everything is back to normal. The patient and his or her family are now responsible for maintaining a healthy diet and an active lifestyle in order to move forward cancer free.

Lifestyle changes can be viewed as a new beginning for the whole family and a positive influence on all involved. Personally, I know that since my wife was diagnosed with cancer we have changed our diet and our exercise regimen. This has not only put me in the best shape of my life, but has also set a wonderful and healthy example for our two daughters.

The good news is, changing your family's lifestyle doesn't mean that you need to become a vegan, eat only organic, or exercise five times a week. Quitting smoking, losing weight, and exercising regularly are good places to start. Keep in mind, though, that to quit smoking or eat more healthfully while your spouse continues to smoke and eat junk food is a setup for failure. Support doesn't mean just sitting in the waiting room and telling your spouse everything will be okay. The rubber needs to meet the road, and changes need to be made at home.

I tell my patients that this is a partnership to getting them well. I do the smallest part with the surgery. Each of them has the responsibility to make the lifelong changes that will allow them to continue to be cancer free and enjoy their lives and their families.

Recovery vs. Healing: An Important Distinction

Most people understand and expect that there will be a time after surgery that requires them to slow down and take time off from their currently overloaded schedules. During this recovery time the incisions are healing, and you may also be dealing with drains, bandages, and pain pumps. You may be taking antibiotics and pain pills, but the psychological healing has not yet begun. There is a sense of relief that the cancer has been removed, even as you are starting chemo and/or radiation in the future. The abnormality has been removed, you think to yourself, and that is a step in the right direction.

However, true healing doesn't start until treatment is done, when there are no more lists of doctors to see or appointments to keep. It starts when you finally sit down, alone with your thoughts, and say, "What the heck just happened?"

Now the question is, how are you going to move forward and resume life? This diagnosis and treatment have collectively been a disruption of your life, and most likely a wake-up call about your priorities. You may need to reshuffle your daily routine and reevaluate your priorities. This part of healing can be the most difficult.

I work primarily with women who have been diagnosed with breast cancer, and I have noticed that many of them deal with the diagnosis of cancer, or any illness, as a new list of tasks that need to be accomplished. There is often very little emotion involved when I first meet them and we are discussing treatment options. They are on a mission and will tackle whatever needs to be done in order to move forward. It isn't until after the treatment is finished that they "hit the wall." *What happened? Could it come back? What should I be doing moving forward? Do I need to change my lifestyle? Do I need to worry about my daughter?* These questions can be more difficult to handle emotionally than the surgery.

How to Heal? A Few Options I Suggest to Patients

The reality is that a cancer diagnosis is a traumatic event, and healing takes time. Many patients find that support groups are very helpful. A support group is a non-threatening, open environment in which people with similar questions can meet and talk. Unfortunately, some people associate a stigma with support groups—they feel you only go to a support group when you are emotionally unstable and need to cry and have someone hold your hand. Then, when you feel that you are ready to move forward, you stop going. That doesn't reflect reality at all.

Actually, many people who are well through their recovery and have healed continue to participate in support groups and help others. I tell most people that you are going to your support group to help others deal with what you already have. It is much more impactful to listen to someone who has been through the same thing you are going through (or are about to go through) than to have a physician give you statistics on what "most" patients experience.

I was watching a TV special a few years back on trauma patients working with art as a medium for healing. These were abused children, military veterans, and accident victims. The experts were discussing how having a non-threatening, no right-or-wrong answer project allowed these patients to express themselves. I remember thinking that this might be a great way to bring my patients together in a fun, non-threatening, social way. It would also allow them to interact as they wanted to and potentially tell their stories.

So for the last five years my practice has been conducting Art Therapy Workshops. We have invited breast cancer survivors to come and join us for a morning of fun and creativity. We provide bras as a canvas and everything with which to decorate them. We have feathers, beads, pins, and paint. We have a corner with glue guns and another with irons. As the participants move from table to table gathering their materials and working on their creations, they are meeting, mixing, and talking with people who have been through a similar trauma.

At the end of the session, we invite anyone who is interested to share her creation and how it symbolizes her healing journey. This is all a part of the healing. There is usually laughter and tears, but always warm hugs and goodbyes. Often lunch dates are made before parting ways.

After the first two years of this event (which were successes and very well received by the community), I had a patient tell me that she had heard the workshops were wonderful, but "glue guns and feathers really aren't my thing." I had to agree. People heal in different ways, and they need different modalities in which to grow. I was fortunate enough to have a patient whose brother is an accomplished and well-published author, so I approached him about helping me put together a Writing Workshop. The same premise applied: This would be a modality for interaction and sharing.

We now run both of these workshops annually and have had a congressman and other local leaders attend. We have worked with a local non-profit set up by a surgeon that offers painting classes, cooking classes, Zumba classes, and yoga classes to our cancer patients as part of their healing journey.

When patients now ask me, "What do I do now?", I'm glad I have some places where they can start. We may also need to include some psychological counseling as part of various patients' plans, but I feel strongly that creating new friends and fun memories with people who have a common history and a common goal is certainly a step in the right direction.

Integrative Medicine: A Valuable Tool

Some physicians can be opposed to non-conventional therapies due to a lack of knowledge and understanding of the therapy. They may also have the misconception that it will be an alternate treatment, not a complementary treatment. So unfortunately, when patients ask their physicians about non-conventional treatments, their questions are often dismissed, or worse, the patient is labeled as someone who does not want to be treated.

As a patient, you should understand that doctors are trained to evaluate statistics and outcomes. Often, we have not had any formal education in Eastern medicine, and so we really can't comment on treatments that do not have studies for us to review. That said, many non-conventional therapies can still play an important role in the care of patients, but we as physicians need to be educated on how to incorporate them.

Here's my stance: I have had patients ask me about alternative medicine or treatments. My response is that I am not a believer in *alternative* medicine, but rather *integrated* medicine. Alternative means that we are not going to include conventional therapies. I believe that to disregard conventional medicine is just as erroneous as disregarding diet, lifestyle, and Eastern medicine.

Personally, I have found acupuncture, meditation, yoga, Reiki, and massage to be very beneficial. I also am a great believer that diet has a tremendous influence on our disease state and our ability to heal. However, I have had patients tell me that they are not going to undergo chemotherapy for their cancer, but will start eating a raw organic diet. As a vegan, I can applaud them for their dietary changes, but I cannot support their decision to refuse chemo for an advanced tumor. Again, I think that non-conventional treatments need to be complementary, not exclusive.

We are extremely fortunate that in my practice we can offer our patients consultations with acupuncturists, massage and Reiki therapists, dietitians, life coaches, yoga masters, and fitness coaches, all free of charge. By making these therapies available without concerning the patient about the cost, patients are more apt to investigate and participate. We even have pre- and post-surgical programs that have been developed to help people through this difficult time.

As health care providers, we need to educate ourselves and our patients about these non-conventional Eastern therapies. By embracing additional healing modalities, we can help our patients and ourselves become stronger and more whole as individuals.

Dr. Bernie Siegel

Bernie Siegel, MD, is an internationally respected and revered physician, surgeon, speaker. He is the author of numerous books, including Love, Medicine & Miracles. *To learn more about him, please visit his website, www.berniesiegelmd.com.*

Dr. Siegel spoke to me over the phone regarding what he would like patients who have been diagnosed with cancer to know. This section reflects the five major points he made in our conversation, as well as information contained in his book Faith, Hope, & Healing.

Dr. Siegel wants people to feel comfortable enough with him to call him "Bernie," or "Dr. Bernie Siegel." Therefore, I will respectfully refer to him as "Bernie" throughout this section.

Cancer Is a Journey Filled with Choices and Lessons.

If and when you are diagnosed with cancer, keep in mind that this part of your life is a *journey* that is an integral part of the rest of your life, which is also a journey. While your journey will be filled with good and not-so-good days, it will also be filled with lessons that will enable you to grow and heal on many levels: emotionally, mentally, spiritually, and physically. It is not unusual for those challenged by cancer to perceive the lessons they learn as unexpected gifts that come from surviving a life-threatening illness. For example, cancer has the power to teach us to love ourselves and others enough to choose joy and happiness. And in choosing joy, we feel empowered, less fearful, and discover who we really are—all of which contributes to our healing. Yes, it is all a journey—and an amazing one, at that!

In *Faith, Hope & Healing*, Bernie writes, "You have a choice when dealing with the unknown; you can focus on possible disasters or choose to be happy. Optimists live longer, healthier lives even though they may be less in touch with reality than pessimists. When you live one day at a time, you take care of the next five …"[4]

Trust Your Intuition.

If your doctor recommends a specific treatment, be sure to take into consideration that you are here to live each day with pleasure and joy. Do not be afraid to listen to your intuition, and do not be afraid to say no! For example, Bernie shares that when his wife (who also has multiple sclerosis) was diagnosed with breast cancer, the doctors wanted her to undergo a regimen of anti-estrogen therapy that would have impaired her quality of life, making it difficult for her to enjoy her life.

Bernie felt that his wife needed to be treated with female hormones in order to provide her with needed strength and energy, as well as to enhance her quality of life. In his words, "It is not about just dying, but rather it is about having the best day you can—every day." Doctors trained in conventional oncology treatments did not necessarily agree with him. Yet, he intuitively knew that this was and is what his wife needed for life.

The Operating Room Environment is Important.

According to Bernie, you need to be sure your doctors will provide you with the best healing environment during your operating room (OR) experience. He has always felt that the OR needs to be viewed as a place of warmth, safety, and healing—not as one that is cold, dark, and dangerous. (I can attest to the importance of the OR environment myself. During a recent surgery to remove a large benign tumor and my ovaries, my physician held my hand, spoke warmly and lovingly to me, and reassured me that I was safe and being watched over by her and her colleagues. I did feel safe, and the OR was not a threatening place for me. My surgery took place without complications and I healed relatively quickly.)

In particular, Bernie uses music as a tool to shape the OR environment. He explained that many years ago, he began operating on patients, from children to seniors, while playing music on a tape recorder.

Bernie knew that music had the power to assist in healing his patients, and that it would enable him and those working with him to bring their best skills to each patient. He always believed that he could expedite the success of the surgery by creating an environment that felt genuinely safe and comfortable. And he was right. By playing music, he was able to help his patient relax, which in turn helped their bodies respond with greater ease to the surgical intervention and to heal more quickly.

Bernie was one of the first doctors to do this. (He emphasized that it has taken about thirty years for Yale scientists and others to empirically validate the value of playing music in the operating room—not that he needed this proof to know that his approach led to more positive results!)

Express What You Are Feeling—and Consider the Power of Art.

It is important that you find the means to express your emotions rather than holding them deep within you, where they negatively impact your body's immune system. Bernie emphasized the therapeutic value of using drawings. For example, he suggested you draw yourself in the operating room while your surgery is taking place. Then, create a second drawing of how you *wish* to see yourself and your operating team in the OR.

Bernie told me that initially, some patients would draw dark, lonely pictures of themselves in the OR. But when asked to draw how they wished the OR to be, they drew pictures of an OR filled with light, color, warmth, beauty, and music. Here's the best part: If they repeatedly visualized the positive image, things tended to turnout well with all forms of cancer treatments. Bernie's point is that you have the power to determine your own experience. This comes as a result of listening to your own inner guidance and wisdom and combining your intuition with your intentions and desires. This is what a survivor and thriver does!

As a psychologist, I often use art therapy as a healing modality to help patients express, own, and release thoughts and feelings that they have long suppressed. You too can use art to enable you to create what you need for your healing. Remember Albert Einstein's words: *Imagination is more important than knowledge.* In other words, your imagination has the ability to help you create your reality. What you are drawing becomes your focus of attention, which enables you to energetically draw to you similar energy.

You Are Filled with Potential—So Treat Yourself with Love.

Bernie's final message was to remember that you are a being filled with great potential. You are here for so much, and you are capable of so much. You have the potential and the ability to heal and to create what you desire. You were born with this. (As previously indicated, one of the gifts of cancer is that it provides you with opportunities to connect with your potential and to become what you intended to become when you embarked upon this journey.)

What gets in the way of fulfilling our potentials is our fear-driven resistance. This resistance causes us to run from our cancer. It is only when we learn to accept our mortality, stop doing battle with cancer, and go with the flow by nurturing our bodies, minds, and spirits that we are able to harness our healing potential.

In Bernie's words: "I get tired of all the battles and wars people wage against cancer. It is like giving power to the fire if all you do is think about how to control it ... Your body is aware of how much time you spend fighting versus nurturing yourself. The adrenaline response to fight is meant to help you run from the fire as fast as possible, but you can't spend your life running from danger and expect to be healthy."[5]

I agree with Bernie, and would add that the language you use in describing your experience can impact the course of your journey. Rather than thinking in terms of battling, fighting, and killing your cancer, I, like Bernie, encourage you to consider loving, nurturing, and caring for yourself and your body in the most compassionate of ways, all of which empower your immune system to produce the cells needed for healing.

Bernie writes, "I ask you to accept your mortality and live. Surrender to life and find your blessings. Surrendering is not about giving up, but about acceptance and the peace that comes with it. When you surrender, you no longer fight to maintain control, and when you love, you will be free of fear."[6]

By choosing to love yourself enough to surrender your fears to the universe and to your source, and then focusing on your hopes and dreams, you have the power to create your heart's desires, empower your immune system, and expedite your own healing.

As Bernie says,

"When you act out of love, you help yourself to heal and you make your life more meaningful."[7]

Dr. Cynthia R. Aks

Cynthia R. Aks, DO, FACOS, ABIHM, earned her Bachelor of Science in Nursing from Avila University in Kansas City in 1980 and her Doctor of Osteopathic Medicine from the Kansas City University of Medical Biosciences in 1985. After marrying in 1980, she became the first female to complete a General Surgery residency program at St. John's Oakland General Hospital in Detroit in 1990. She chose to become a dedicated breast surgeon in 1997. She gave birth to triplets in 1993 and has had the challenging and exciting role of raising her children as a single parent since 1995.

Cynthia has been a director of a breast program; a consultant; the owner and manager of her own surgical practice; a participant in a myriad of medical, hospital, peer review, and cancer committees; and a part of two medical missions to Nigeria. She is a pioneer in her field as breast cancer surgeon and shares her research and ideas in lectures to her peers and the community. She presently lives in Portland, Oregon where she works with Legacy Health System to provide integrative oncology programs in their hospitals.

Cynthia is also certified as a yoga instructor and has taught restorative/therapeutic yoga. She is also a Reiki Master, a Level I Certified Ayurveda practitioner, a student of nutrition and therapeutic essential oils, and a Diplomate of the American Board of Integrative Holistic Medicine. In Cynthia's words, "I love life and learning ... I live my

*life mindfully, with integrity, kindness, and compassion. What I value
most in my life is my family!"*

*Here, Dr. Aks has written about herself, her philosophy, and her
recommendations for care.*

My Training and Philosophy of Care

I grew up with parents whose core values focused on the importance of love, integrity, humbleness, service, and kindness to
others. My father was an Obstetrician and Gynecologist and my
mother was a lifelong volunteer. As for me, I was fascinated with
the human body and how it worked. This spurred my desire to be
a healer, first as a critical care nurse, then as an Oncologic surgeon.
Throughout my three-plus decades in healthcare, I have seen the
birth of life, the loss of life, acts of man's inhumanity to other
men, as well as acts of incredible kindness and love.

My training as a western physician taught me how to recognize signs and symptoms; how to diagnose and treat. As a surgeon,
I became skilled in the art of surgically removing a disease in order to "fix" a problem. But throughout my journey as a healer, I
came to realize that while western medicine may be good for the
treatment of "acute" care, it falls short of managing chronic illness.
And in the United States, the great majority of healthcare is provided to people who suffer from chronic disease.

To put it differently, conventional medicine focuses on disease
management as opposed to disease resolution. The system must
change. It must begin to identify the underlying causation of disease. Then, and only then, will we be effective in resolving it.

That brings me to my philosophy of care, which focuses on
numerous aspects of a person's life that can result in ill health. Integrative healthcare of this sort stems from the concept of holism,
which is based on the understanding that any one part cannot be
understood or affected separately from the whole. What happens

to the part impacts the whole. This is the root concept of my "Mind, Body, Spirit" approach to healthcare.

As an Osteopathic trained physician, I learned about the interconnectedness of the body. While growing as a healer, I have come to further appreciate holistic care on a much deeper level. As ill health is a result of multiple factors, effective healthcare should be multifaceted.

Life is energy. Our bodies are made up of matter, which is a manifestation of energy. Our thoughts, feelings, behaviors, and actions are all rooted in energetic vibrations, energy fields, and energetic connections. We may have similar "matter" (e.g., anatomic organs and tissues); however, each one of us is energetically unique. Therefore, I believe and have observed that the care of patients is most effective when individualized and undertaken from a holistic approach.

I love what I do because I love touching people's lives and making a difference. I strongly believe in a relationship-centered practice. Healing is enhanced when practitioners can develop a relationship base on trust, empathy and compassion.

I feel that as a physician, I am in partnership with my patients; working with their beliefs and providing factual information so as to develop a treatment plan that they have ownership of. This generates a sense of control, empowerment, and hope. Ultimately, engaging my patients in a treatment plan that works for them is most effective as they are more motivated, trusting, hopeful, and positive in their thinking. This is very powerful! In working with a team of health providers, I believe the best approach is one respectful of a patient's belief system.

In my private practice in Michigan, I built an office specifically with the intention of creating an environment that was nurturing, comfortable, and therapeutic. I utilized elements of the earth, including naturally lit spaces, glass, stone and wood, water fountains, spa-like music, and calming, relaxing aromas with diffusers and eye pillows. Warm blankets were also offered.

I find it important to establish relationships with other healing practitioners (e.g., energy healers, acupuncturists, therapeutic masseuses, reflexologists, art and music therapists etc.) in order to be able to offer patients an avenue to obtain comprehensive, integrative care options. I have had numerous patients return to express their gratitude for introducing them to many of these therapy modalities. The benefits received were not only experienced during treatment but also resulted in an overall improved quality of life when patients continued to practice them.

Each person's healing is unique. Although not everyone is curable, the potential for becoming whole again is possible for all. Each of us has the potential to become a hero or to grow wiser. We need to take care of ourselves, honor what is most precious within us, and at the same time become more forgiving of our own humanity.

What makes cancer a heroic journey is the style in which it is done. I often ask myself, "If I were diagnosed with breast cancer, what would I do?" The answer would be in part dependent on the pathological characteristics of the disease at the time of diagnosis and in part on the additional lifestyle changes I would realistically be committed to. But one thing is for sure: My approach would definitely be an integrative one!

What Causes Cancer?

Simply put, "cancer" is a natural phenomenon. Every cell in the body has the potential to become cancerous, as our cells are continuously exposed to numerous factors that impair their natural balancing and regulatory mechanisms. A cancer cell is one that was once normal in its appearance and the way it "behaved," but at some point it has undergone a process of chaotic, accelerated, and inappropriate cellular growth. It is biologically disordered.

At the microscopic level, it appears disfigured and has abnormal internal elements.

The causation of this type of illness is very complex, multi-factorial, and complicated to uncover. It requires spending a lot of time with our patients getting to know various aspects of who they are, how they think, and how they live their lives. We must understand their nutritional habits, their stresses, the support systems they have, how they view themselves, what their environment is like, and what they believe in. Knowing what is going on in our patients' lives helps us to understand what may be going on in their bodies. These are some key elements of information that, when discovered and evaluated, can open the door to a better understanding of the causation of the patient's illness.

People say, "I am sick because I have cancer." The reality is that they have cancer because they are sick. Their mind and body have been in a long-term state of imbalance.

So what might cause and/or exacerbate this imbalance? While there are endless factors that can facilitate chronic disease, some to try to avoid include:

- Poor air quality
- Drinking or bathing in contaminated water or water that is chlorinated or fluorinated
- Eating nutrient-depleted foods
- Smoking
- Chronic stress
- Negative thought and emotions
- Exposure to microbes, viruses, bacteria, fungus, and parasites
- Blocked detoxification systems
- Exposure to pesticides, herbicides, heavy metals, and industrial toxins
- Excess alcohol use

- Inappropriate use of drugs (prescription, nonprescription, and illicit)
- Immunosuppressive drugs
- Exposure to X-rays, power lines, chronic electromagnetic frequencies, and nuclear radiation

When you really think about the implications of this list, you might feel overwhelmed. After all, we are exposed to so many of these things in our daily lives: the air we breathe; the foods we eat; the water we ingest and bathe in; the products we put topically on our hair, skin, and nails; the clothes we wear; the cleaning products in our home; our furniture and carpets; our vaccines and medications; and the list goes on and on.

Some of the above factors we aren't able to control. However, there can always be a starting point in transforming our lives. I tell my patients to take baby steps. We look to evaluate their lifestyles, nutrition, stresses, etc. and identify a few areas in which to begin making changes. A small change can make a big impact!

Lifestyle Changes to Combat or Prevent Cancer

A new diagnosis of cancer, or any other potentially life-threatening illness, creates feelings of denial, fear, anxiety, depression, anger, and guilt. It often results in a sense of helplessness, unworthiness, and poor self-esteem. I spend a lot of time with my patients in education. The diagnosis of cancer precipitates a tumultuous chain of events. There are tests, surgery, often chemotherapy, radiation therapy and/or hormonal therapy.

Throughout this process, there is often an overwhelming sense of being out of control with one's own mortality. Knowledge is empowering and can alleviate fear and anxiety, as well as create focus, emotional strength, and hope. Explaining what cancer (a chronic disease) is and how it can develop allows us to begin developing a treatment plan. It can also create the opportunity for us to develop lifestyle changes and prevention strategies.

Here, I would like to share and briefly explain beneficial lifestyle changes I often recommend to my patients:

- **Effective breathing.** Life essentially begins with our first breath. Breath, often referred to as "prana" in Sanskrit, is our life force. Breath is one of the primary foundations of health. The breath provides oxygenation to our cells. It also results in the interaction of biochemical and neurologic responses that promote health and wellness. Learning effective breathing methods can help patients reduce anxiety and fear. These methods can also reduce blood pressure and heart rate and create a sense of calm, thus lowering stress. I use breathing techniques with my patients in my office, particularly when I am performing a procedure or in the operating room. I also teach easy breathing techniques to my patients to be used at any time.

- **Adequate hydration.** Adequate hydration is critical for health. Seventy-five percent of the human body is made of water, and therefore water is critical to our health. When we are not properly hydrated, our metabolic and thought processes are reduced. Toxins cannot effectively be eliminated, and therefore they accumulate in various tissues. Of course, quality water is important for obvious reasons. We can be adequately hydrated with water that contains harmful contaminants which contribute to poor health. Much research about how to obtain quality water has been published and is readily available to the public. Properly structured, water acts as an antioxidant and is also rich in minerals that are critical for proper functioning of the body.

- **A healthy immune system.** The immune system is very complex. It has been documented that more than 70 percent of our immune cells reside in the lining of the intestinal tract. It is no wonder that all of the antibiotics in our food or those that we are liberally prescribed impair our immune cell function. I recommend cautious and appropriate use of antibiotics as well as the use of probiotic foods or supplements. Chemicals and toxins in our foods also create a situation in which our immune cells have to work overtime, causing a weakened state. I refer to this as "immunologic stress." Our immune cells are our body's army. If we want to win a battle, we want our army of soldiers to be strong.

- **Quality nutrition.** Nutrition has become a hot topic in the last few decades. Ours is an age of stress, high technology, consumerism, and convenience. Our food industry has learned how to synthesize foods, many of which are nutrient-depleted and laced with toxins. We truly are what we eat. If we nourish our bodies with quality macro and micronutrients, we arm our cells with necessary elements for optimal health. I am a proponent of eating an organic, whole food, plant-based diet if possible. Avoid processed, package and GMO foods. Favor foods that are fresh, organic and preferably locally grown. Fresh foods contain the best quality of nutrients (energy). Avoid frozen, canned, reheated, or microwave foods if possible. (If fresh is not available, frozen is preferred over canned.)

  However, through my Ayurvedic medicine training, I have also come to believe that due to our unique physiologic individualities, one "diet" doesn't fit all. Ayurveda does stress certain universal foundations in regard to nutrition, though. For instance, avoid drinking cold liquids at mealtime because the cold causes a constriction of the blood supply to the intestinal tract, which in turn impairs digestion and absorption of nutrients.

No matter what you eat, cook with love and mindfulness. Eat sitting down so that you are in a more relaxed state. Eat only until there is no hunger, and do not overeat. Sit quietly for a few minutes before returning to your activity. This also contributes to proper digestion and absorption of food.

Much has been researched and written about diets for various chronic illnesses. Most chronic illness is rooted in the inflammatory process. I often counsel patients about trying to follow an "anti-inflammatory" diet: One that is rich in fresh and colorful fruits and vegetables, organic, minimizes dairy (goat and sheep is healthier than cow) and animal products, emphasizes healthy fats, and avoids sugars and refined grains. There are also spices and herbs that reduce the tendency toward inflammation, including garlic, nutmeg, turmeric, cumin, black pepper, basil, clove, cinnamon, cilantro, chamomile, rosemary, cardamom seed, fennel seed, and celery seed.

- **Positive thought.** Emotional connections can have powerful effects on health. The mind is very powerful and controls everything in the body. What nourishes the spirit nourishes the body. Conversely, what drains the spirit drains the body. Our cells react to every thought. Specifically, our emotional and psychological states affect the endocrine system via chemical messengers referred to as neuropeptides. Thus a thought and/or feeling results in a physical sensation.

  In essence, we become what we think. Negative thought results in negative physiologic effects; e.g., a lowered immune system. The mind can create healing energy by the use of prayer, meditation, guided imagery/visualization, Reiki, and practicing the power of positive thinking.

- **Adequate sleep.** Quality sleep improves health in many ways. When we're asleep, our cells undergo repair and restorative processes. Sleep improves our mood and memory, lowers stress and inflammation, spurs creativity, improves physical and mental performance, aids in weight management, and improves longevity.
- **Regular movement.** Movement improves the flow of vital body fluids (e.g., blood and lymph); lubricates our joints; oxygenates our tissues; improves our cardiopulmonary system; aids in digestion and elimination processes; improves muscle tone, strength and balance; and aids in weight management. Movement is yet another tool to enhance the immune system and optimize health.

    There are a variety of ways to achieve some of the previously mentioned health benefits. Engage in activity daily, whether that's by going for a walk; taking the stairs instead of the elevator; parking in the furthest as opposed to the closest parking spot; dancing; practicing yoga, qigong, or tai chi; swimming; riding a bike; going bowling; or even getting a massage. Finding any way where movement can be added throughout the day will provide health benefits.
- **Essential oils.** I use daily and recommend the use of certified pure therapeutic essentials oils. These can be used internally, topically, and aromatically. My favorites are Frankincense, Myrrh, Lavender, Eucalyptus, Roman Chamomile, Rosemary, Wild Orange, Oregano, Melaleuca, Helichrysum, Peppermint, and Lemongrass.

More and more people are recognizing the shortfalls of conventional western therapies and are wanting more. I believe we are coming back to an age of "mind, body, spirit" medicine—functional medicine—integrative medicine. I am confronted more and more often with patients coming in for their visits armed with research they have done regarding a variety of therapeutic modalities. I find it refreshing and welcome the opportunity to have a dialogue about integrative therapies. I look forward to collaborating with my patients to provide the kind of care they feel most comfortable with.

So, how do you decide what's right for you? Decisions are best made collaboratively with your medical team, with intellect and intuition, a healing attitude and positive viewpoint.

I continue on my own health journey utilizing many of the tools mentioned above. I have been fortunate to enjoy good health; however, my life experience has not been without losses, trauma, hardships, and grief. These tools have given me the strength to overcome my fears and sense of powerlessness, to become a warrior and survivor, and to find harmony in my life. My personal healing journey has resulted in becoming an integrative focused physician, certified yoga instructor, Reiki Master, and student of Ayurveda medicine and nutrition. I practice daily gratitude, mindfulness, kindness, and compassion. This keeps me centered and open to extraordinary possibilities.

In Summary:

- Partner with a team of healthcare providers who are supportive, open minded, and collaborative. Do your research and be clear about what you want.
- Think of food as medicine.
- Be fully present.
- Eliminate toxins from your life. Small changes can result in huge outcomes.
- Breathe and relax, meditate, and make movement a part of your daily routine.
- Release the negativity in your life. Let go of things and people you cannot change or whose presence in your life is not serving you. Accept that which you cannot control.

- Believe in the energy and power of the universe. Know that sometimes the uphill struggles and challenges we face provide the best "view" (learning experiences) for a happier, healthier life.
- Laugh often, sing loudly, and nourish your spirit.
- Be committed and accountable to yourself. Invest in your health—it will pay big dividends!

Namaste,
Dr. Cynthia R. Aks

Dr. William E. Hablitzel

"This man is an Angel disguised as a medical doctor—His words will touch your soul."

WAYNE DYER

After five years of being a firefighter and paramedic, William (Bill) E. Hablitzel returned to school, earning his MD from the University of Toledo College of Medicine in Ohio. Following his residency in Internal Medicine, Dr. Hablitzel joined the faculty at the University of Cincinnati College of Medicine as an Associate Professor. He has also maintained a private practice and runs a free medical clinic for the underserved of the rural communities of the Appalachian Mountains. Dr. Hablitzel has been recognized by the University of Cincinnati College of Medicine for excellence in teaching, and his community service has been honored by the Ohio State Senate and the Ohio House of Representatives.

Dr. Bill Hablitzel is the author of two award-winning books of healing wisdom, Dying Was the Best Thing That Ever Happened to Me *and his newest book,* It Was Only a Moment Ago. *Both books emphasize the healing value of energy, especially the energy of love and compassion, and the need to heal the soul as well as the body. Dr. Hablitzel recognizes that the most powerful lessons he has learned come from his greatest teachers, his patients. When not caring for patients, writing, or speaking, his pleasures include time spent at his home in the hills of rural Ohio, where he can be with his dogs, out in nature, meditating, and enjoying the birds and wildlife.*

Dr. Hablitzel graciously agreed to write the following section for this book:

As a physician trained in Western medicine and with a medical school faculty tenure spanning more than two decades, if a friend or family member were diagnosed with cancer, my first impulse would be to direct that person to the best specialist I could find at the largest university medical center available. It is here where the best and the brightest of our profession dedicate their lives and live out the traditions that have become modern medicine. If a cure is to be found, most likely it will be found in this place.

Such an impulse would not be wrong, and it is most certainly happening every day in physicians' offices all over the world. The contribution of modern medicine to the human condition is without dispute. Eighteen percent of male infants born in 1900 would die before reaching their first birthday. Today, it takes 62 years of life before men experience a cumulative mortality of 18 percent. The 45-year life expectancy of a child born in 1900 is now over 78 years; an unprecedented advancement in the history of humanity. Innovation in the management of heart disease, the discovery of once-impossible gains in cancer care, and the development of preventative medicine have been nothing less than miraculous—but only if we take advantage of it.

The rigors and traditions of medical education are all about *curing*, and it was with more than a little surprise upon completing my training that I discovered I knew little about *healing*—and that there was a profound difference between the two. It was the point at which my education truly began and I encountered my greatest teachers—the patients who invited me into their lives. Hippocrates wrote, "Natural forces within us are the true healers of disease." It is a truth that has survived the millennia. Physicians do not heal—at our best we can help others find healing.

Those natural forces within us—that healing energy—can be found and put to use in a multitude of ways. Healing touch, acupuncture, massage therapy, and intuitive healing are but a few of the many paths that can lead us there. Perhaps the simplest is also the most powerful. Learning to embrace silence and to be alone with our thoughts—whether we call it prayer, meditation, or reflection—provides an intimate relationship with the energy that can heal. It is there that patients often find the comfort and hope that may be missing in their physician's office, or hear the soft voice and the gentle pull of intuition that guides them in the difficult decisions that modern medicine can insist upon.

For my family and best of friends I offer the best of both worlds: the finest that modern medicine has to offer tempered with the wisdom passed down through the ages, sometimes in the form of a book, an audio tape, a website address, or even a referral to a holistic practitioner. It is a powerful blend of the marvels of cure and the miracles of healing. With my teachers has come a special epiphany, that as we help others find healing, we too are healed. For in each of my patients I have found family, and the best of friends.

Dr. Amy Harvey O'Keeffe

Recognized by Philadelphia Magazine *as a Top Doc in the Greater Philadelphia area, Dr. Amy Harvey O'Keeffe is a Board Certified Gynecologist and Obstetrician. She received her MD from Temple University School of Medicine in Philadelphia, Pennsylvania, where she also completed a residency in Gynecology and Obstetrics. She is in private practice at the Center for Women's Health in Langhorne,*

Pennsylvania, and holds an attending hospital staff position with St. Mary Medical Center and Capital Health Medical Center in Hopewell, New Jersey.

A Master Level Reiki Practitioner, Dr. Harvey O'Keeffe regularly recommends complementary forms of medicine to her patients, including massage, meditation, acupuncture, yoga, Reiki, and nutritional counseling. Joined by her husband Jim, she has been a co-medical director of a medical mission to the Dominican Republic for nine years. Additionally, she established a cancer support group for women with gynecological cancers, The GyniGirls. It has been an honor for me to share with Amy the co-leadership of this amazing group of women. She is also an Advisory Board member for the Teal Tea Foundation for ovarian cancer.

Dr. Harvey O'Keeffe brings love and compassion to her work as a healer. The following section is written in her own words:

So, I must confess. I am scientist—a biologist, actually. I am a physician who uses surgery, medicines, and all the treatment options of conventional western medicine. For me and my physician colleagues there is no twelve step program. Luckily, we have patients to help us.

Over the years my patients have provided endless guidance and much encouragement. These gifts have allowed me to grow both intellectually and spiritually. I call it the ripple effect, like throwing a pebble into the pond. I ask my patients, colleagues, and students regularly to play their part by adding ripples any way they can as they journey through life.

Truthfully, I believe I have practiced integrative medicine long before I knew it even had a name. Like many of my colleagues, during the infancy of my medical career I saw patients who were searching for more, something beyond what traditional or conventional medicine could provide. So my patients were my teachers on my journey to my very own integrative medical practice.

The list of therapeutic modalities I recommend has grown over the years. There are some therapies that I have personally mastered, and some I have just simply tried to practice. My goal is to educate my patients on what may best suit their own individual needs. And although all of the therapies may provide benefits to a patient, I most often recommend Thai or traditional massage, Reiki, acupuncture, yoga, tai chi, and vitamin and herbal therapies. I make a special mention of meditation, deep breathing, and prayer, which I believe are beneficial to everyone. These are always at the top of my list of recommendations for my patients.

My understanding of how these therapies can help each of us came from a multitude of experiences with my patients, my friends, and my family. I, like all of us, have been blessed with a group of what Susan calls Earth Angels. I think of Earth Angels as those beings that we meet here in this life who help us make giant leaps on the journey of spiritual growth. My dear friend Lauren, who dug in deep to find her strength to battle brain cancer, has been a guide and inspiration for all those she touches, but especially to me. And Chris, our friend who fought ALS with dignity and grace, remains an angel to many of us from the spirit world. And then there is Susan ... a kind and gentle soul who helps so many by showing that love and hope are the only paths worth taking. Along with all of her other responsibilities, she is our fearless leader of the GyniGirls, a support group we founded for women who have been diagnosed with a gynecological cancer.

So, what can I offer to a friend or loved one who is diagnosed with cancer? Remember, I am a scientist. So from that perspective, here's my advice: You find a physician who is known for being the best in whatever you need for your care. You research, you get a second opinion when it feels right, you listen to what is said and not said. And you trust your instinct. You listen to your inner wisdom and your intuition. Don't be afraid to ask questions, and don't be afraid to move on if you are not getting what you feel you deserve. Then, you make a plan and you continue to surround yourself with a medical team that has your best interests at heart.

And then comes the next step: dealing with the fear that comes with a diagnosis of cancer. You start with baby steps and take it a day or a minute at a time. And you breathe, allowing peace to come in any way and in any amount that it can. And then you breathe again. And then you lean on your friends and those who care deeply for you. It is their gift to you. You give a bigger gift to them when you let them nurture you in whatever way you need. This is the time to open yourself to receive all that will help you be at peace and find the strength to take that next baby step.

Also, you learn to accept that which has a purpose to your highest good, and you discard that which doesn't. By surrounding yourself with those who will be your pillars, you will have all the strength you need to take that next step. This includes your friends, your family, and your medical team. And you breathe again.

On my journey as a physician, I have treated patients who declined a traditional therapy regimen of chemotherapy or radiation, in spite of the scientific evidence showing a potential good. As a physician and scientist who is trained in modern medicine, I found this most challenging the first time a patient declined a suggested therapy. But I have come to understand that we each travel our own journey and we must choose that which we believe is in our best interest. And, as a physician, I am there to guide each patient along their journey and always within the boundaries of what they can or cannot accept. The Latin origin of the word doctor means "to educate." As physicians, we educate our patients as to what we know may help them, but the ultimate choice is in their hands.

We always hope that a patient will be cured of their cancer. But we must always remember our highest goal is to help them on their journey of healing. Any illness, but especially cancer, provides us with an opportunity to grow spiritually. We have all had patients who tell us that their diagnosis of cancer was "a gift." The ability to use a cancer diagnosis as a life lesson is echoed by many thrivers. When we as physicians help a patient on their journey, we help them find peace with themselves and with those around them. And this is the greatest gift we can offer: teaching our patients to be at peace and have unconditional love for themselves.

The physicians of tomorrow are learning highly complex surgical procedures and using technology in every aspect of their medical practice, all with the hope of providing better and safer care. But during their medical education, there is little time devoted to learning how to tell a patient they have a terminal condition such as a diagnosis of cancer. There are few teachers who help medical students learn how they can best support a patient who just lost a child, or their mother, or their spouse.

Putting humanity back into the education of our physicians will not make them less skilled or less knowledgeable, but it *will* make them better doctors. It will make them more fully present for their patients and for themselves in their own lives. Teaching medical students how to connect to patients will help them on their journeys, no matter what area of specialty they choose. And whatever we can do to keep good physicians practicing for years because they love what they do will improve care for us all. Physicians who feel rewarded by their daily practice of medicine are better doctors.

As we know, with age comes wisdom. And with time, we learn the value of life and the value of the relationships we have with those closest to us: our families, our friends, and our patients who trust us to guide them on their journey to healing. The deep connections I make with my patients is one of life's greatest gifts. It is through our relationships—those deep connections with each other—that we become complete and whole once again. My journey as a physician is one of growth and healing, and it is my patients who allow me to do my greatest work.

Final Thoughts

*"Sometimes the illness is meant to serve a higher function
in our lives. Sometimes the point is not the alleviation of illness,
but finding the grace to allow the furnace of suffering to separate
out the gold from the dross so that we become more aware
of who we are ..."*

CASH PETERS, IN *A LITTLE BOOK ABOUT BELIEVING: THE
TRANSFORMATIVE HEALING POWER OF FAITH, LOVE, AND SURRENDER*

I wish I could promise you that reading this book would enable you to experience healing. But no one can promise this to another being. However, knowing that I wrote this book in order to provide you with awareness, information, and tools born of helping many patients in situations similar to yours, I do believe that you are better prepared to enlist your own healing resources (and you have many!) to meet your challenge.

This journey has the power to bring miracles into your life, as I have written about in *Touched by the Extraordinary, Books One and Two*. Research, my clinical work, and my own life have taught me that miracles are a function of love and of changing your perspective.

Whether your journey with your unwelcome visitor is relatively short or prolonged, you will find yourself transformed by the process. Apart from the physical impact it has on you, it will contribute to an amazing spiritual transformation. Yes, your journey with this formidable opponent has the power to wear you down emotionally and mentally, but ironically, to also strengthen you spiritually. And this is significant.

To grow spiritually is to grow your soul and your spirit by *being* love; that is, discovering, valuing, and loving yourself at the deepest level of your core. Remember, healing is an inside job. It begins deep within you, and it always, *always* begins with compassionate, unconditional love. Healing is learning (albeit the hard way) that you are a magnificent, powerful being who is not only love, but who is dearly loved and certainly never alone. Once you come to realize this, you impact all humanity.

In the words of author and researcher David R. Hawkins, MD, PhD, "*Out of all-inclusive, unconditional compassion comes the healing of all mankind.*"

Somehow, you learn all this due to the paradox inherent in experiencing cancer. The more fatigued and exhausted you are by the treatment or the diagnosis, the more you recognize how resilient and powerful you are. You see this in your determination to persevere and to do whatever you need to do to be healthy again. You begin to realize that the key to your power is your willingness to trust, to let go, and to surrender to your own Higher Power. In relaxing and trusting, you find peace. Your immune system is better able to lovingly care for you—a winning payoff in the end! But all of this is up to you and the choices you make in response to your diagnosis. Once again, remember that healing is an inside job.

In the simple but eloquent words of Camus, *"Life is the sum of all your choices."* My hope is that reading this book enables you to love yourself enough to choose to *be love* and to find the courage to change your perspective about your healing powers. Know that I believe in your ability to be love, your wisdom and your essence. Bottom line: I believe in you.

I leave you with two final gifts. The first was written by a gentle and extraordinarily wise and courageous soul who has met multiple challenges during his journey. It was during a particularly difficult period in his life that he found solace in writing poetry that perfectly articulated his awareness of his own transformation. You and he share similar gifts. You are a treasure in all ways, and his poem, *Treasures*, is as applicable to your life as it is to his. May you always remember how exquisite, extraordinary, and precious you and your life are for all humanity.

Treasures

By Tom Kocubinski, December 11, 2011

the morning beach is strewn with sunlit broken shells ... some recognizable, many are not

some are freshly broken but most are old warriors—etched and worn by sea, sun and time

each is different and unique ... but all are beautiful, interesting and valuable despite their appearance and damage ... they have remained, they have survived

are we no less special with our broken lives and dreams cast upon the beach?

The second selection I'd like to share with you was written by Josi Feit, a beautiful healer in her own right who navigated the challenge of metastatic breast cancer. The lines she has written are, I feel, more powerful than stories of many pages. They succinctly share the secrets to healing on all levels.

Navigating Metastatic Breast Cancer and Beyond

By Josi Feit, January 2015

March 27, 1997 completed a series of surgeries, chemotherapy cocktails, radiation treatments and adjunctive therapies.

The Oncology obstacle course was over, done, finished, behind me. Let it go! Release the Past. Bless the dark gift … THANKFULNESS.

Life is a Gift. I chose to bow, embrace, magnificently embody all that I am. To live fully, freely, completely, creatively, uniquely, passionately, and joyfully as my Self. Be unconditionally present. Let it in! Open, Allow, Receive what is … LOVE

Trust yourself. Totally rely upon Spirit to guide, guard, counsel, and skillfully maneuver what is next. Be gentle with yourself. Accept yourself without judgment, criticism, corrections, improvement, editing or self-imposed limitations. Unconditional love. Let it be. Relax …
COMPASSION

May you find the peace that you desire.
With blessings of love and peace,
Susan

Appendix:
Further Resources
for Reading, Listening,
Education, and Support

Achterberg, Jeanne, Dossey, Barbara, and Kolkmeier, Leslie. (1994). *14 Rituals of Healing: Using Imagery for Health and Wellness*. New York: Bantam.

Aldrich, Joni James. (2009). *The Losing of Gordon: A Beacon Through the Storm Called "Grief"*. Cancer Lifeline Publications.

Aldrich, Joni James. (2009). *The Saving of Gordon: Lifelines to W-I-N Against Cancer*. Cancer Lifeline Publications.

Aldrich, Joni James, and Peterson, Neysa M. (2010). *Connecting Through Compassion: Guidance for Family and Friends of a Brain Cancer Patient*. Cancer Lifeline Publications.

Alexander, Eben. (2012). *Proof of Heaven: A Neurosurgeon's Journey into the Afterlife*. New York: Simon & Schuster.

Altea, Rosemary. (2000). *You Own the Power: Stories and Exercises to Inspire and Unleash the Force Within.* New York: William Morrow.

Apollon, Susan Barbara. *Creating Miracles in Your Life: Extraordinary Stories of Cancer Survivors.* Audio CD and MP3. Yardley, PA: Matters of the Soul.

Apollon, Susan Barbara. *A Guided Meditation for Peace, Healing, and Empowerment.* Audio CD and MP3. Yardley, PA: Matters of the Soul.

Apollon, Susan Barbara. *Healing Loving Imagery to Comfort and Soothe the Soul Challenged by Cancer.* Audio CD and MP3. Yardley, PA: Matters of the Soul.

Apollon, Susan Barbara. *A Healing Meditation to Successfully Meet the Challenge of Cancer.* Audio CD & MP3. Yardley, PA: Matters of the Soul.

Apollon, Susan Barbara. *The Healing Power of Love.* Presented at DSI Hospital in Bucks County, PA. Audio CD and MP3. Yardley, PA: Matters of the Soul.

Apollon, Susan Barbara. (2005). *Touched by the Extraordinary: An Intuitive Psychologist Shares Insights, Lessons, and True Stories of Spirit and Love to Transform and Heal the Soul.* Yardley, PA: Matters of the Soul. Also on audio CD.

Apollon, Susan Barbara. (2010). *Touched by the Extraordinary, Book Two: Healing Stories of Love, Loss, and Hope.* Yardley, PA: Matters of the Soul. Also on audio CD.

Apollon, Susan Barbara. (2013). *Affirmations for Healing Mind, Body, and Spirit.* Yardley, PA: Matters of the Soul.

Apollon, Susan, and Maniates, Yanni. (2008). *Intuition Is Easy and Fun: The Art and Practice of Developing Your Natural Born Gift of Intuition.* Morrisville, PA: Intuitive Wisdom. Also on audio CD.

Barghout, Vicki, and Kim, Victoria. (2013). *Reduce Your Risk of Cancer: Viver Pocket Health Guide.* Morristown, NJ:

Viver Health, LLC, in partnership with Healing Consciousness Foundation, Bucks County, PA.

Benson, MD, Herbert. (1975, 2000). *The Relaxation Response* (reissue ed.). New York: HarperTorch.

Boehmer, Tami. (2010). *From Incurable to Incredible: Cancer Survivors Who Beat the Odds.* Createspace.

Borysenko, Joan. (1994). *Fire in the Soul: A New Psychology of Spiritual Optimism* (reprint ed.). New York: Grand Central.

Borysenko, Joan. (1994). *Pocketful of Miracles: Prayers, Meditations, and Affirmations to Nurture Your Spirit Every Day of the Year* (reprint ed.). New York: Grand Central.

Borysenko, Joan. (2006). *Meditations for Self-Healing and Inner Power.* Audio CD. Carlsbad, CA: Hay House.

Borysenko, Joan. (2007). *Minding the Body, Mending the Mind* (revised ed.). Boston: DaCapo.

Borysenko, Joan. (2009). *It's Not the End of the World: Developing Resilience in Times of Change.* Carlsbad, CA: Hay House.

Brennan, Barbara Ann. (1988). *Hands of Light: A Guide to Healing Through the Human Energy Field* (reissue ed.). New York: Bantam.

Brown, Brené. (2010). *The Gifts of Imperfection: Let Go of Who You Think You're Supposed to Be and Embrace Who You Are.* Center City, MN: Hazelden.

Burch, Wanda Easter. (2003). *She Who Dreams: A Journey into Healing Through Dreamwork.* Novato, CA: New World Library.

Burley, Philip. (2010). *Heart's Healing: Comforting Words about Life after Death.* Phoenix, AZ: Mastery.

Byrne, Lorna. (2011). *Angels in My Hair: The True Story of a Modern Day Mystic.* New York: Harmony.

Byrne, Lorna. (2011). *Stairways to Heaven.* Great Britain: Coronet.

Callanan, Maggie, and Kelley, Patricia. (1992, 2012). *Final Gifts: Understanding the Special Awareness, Needs, and Communication of the Dying* (reprint ed.). New York: Simon & Schuster.

Campbell, T. Colin, and Campbell, Thomas M. II. (2006). *The China Study: The Most Comprehensive Study of Nutrition Ever Conducted and the Startling Implications for Diet, Weight Loss, and Long-Term Health*. Dallas, TX: BenBella.

Carr, Kris. (2007). *Crazy Sexy Cancer Tips*. Guilford, CT: Skirt!

Chance, Sue. (1992). *Stronger Than Death: When Suicide Touches Your Life: A Mother's Story*. New York: W.W. Norton.

Childre, Doc, and Martin, Howard. (1999). *The Heartmath Solution*. New York: HarperCollins.

Chodron, Pema. (1999). *Good Medicine: How to Turn Pain into Compassion with Tonglen Meditation*. Audio CD. Boulder, CO: Sounds True.

Chopra, Deepak. (1990). *Quantum Healing: Exploring the Frontiers of Mind/Body Medicine*. New York: Bantam.

Chopra, Deepak. (2007). *The Essential How to Know God: The Soul's Journey into the Mystery of Mysteries*. Essential Deepak Chopra. New York: Harmony.

Craig, Gary. (2009). EFT *for PTSD*. EFT Emotional Freedom Techniques Paperback. Santa Rosa, CA: Energy Psychology.

Cumming, Heather, and Leffler, Karen. (2007). *John of God: The Brazilian Healer Who's Touched the Lives of Millions*. New York: Atria/Beyond Words.

Derosier, Cynthia Y.H., and Anshutz, James. (2008). *The Survivor Spirit: The Beauty, Passion, and Power of Breast Cancer Survivors*. Kailua, HI: Good Juju.

Dossey, Larry. (1993). *Healing Words: The Power of Prayer and the Practice of Medicine*. New York: HarperCollins.

Dossey, Larry. (1997). *Prayer Is Good Medicine: How to Reap the Healing Benefits of Prayer*. San Francisco: HarperSanFrancisco.

Dossey, Larry. (1999). *Reinventing Medicine: Beyond Mind-Body to a New Era of Healing*. New York: HarperCollins.

Dossey, Larry. (2013). *One Mind: How Our Individual Mind Is Part of a Greater Consciousness and Why it Matters.* Carlsbad, CA: Hay House.

DuPree, Beth Baughman. (2008). *The Healing Consciousness: A Doctor's Journey to Healing.* Boulder, CO: Woven Word.

Dyer, Wayne W. (2005). *The Power of Intention: Learning to Co-create Your World Your Way.* Carlsbad, CA: Hay House.

Eadie, Betty. (1994). *Embraced by the Light.* New York: Bantam.

Eden, Donna, and Dahlin, Dondi. (2012). *The Little Book of Energy Medicine: The Essential Guide to Balancing Your Body's Energy.* New York: Tarcher.

Eden, Donna, and Feinstein, David. (2008). *Energy Medicine: Balancing Your Body's Energies for Optimal Health, Joy, and Vitality.* New York: Tarcher.

Eden, Donna, and Feinstein, David. (2008). *Energy Medicine for Women: Aligning Your Body's Energies to Boost Your Health and Vitality.* New York: Tarcher.

Eden, Donna, and Feinstein, David. (2014). *The Energies of Love: Using Energy Medicine to Keep Your Relationship Thriving.* New York: Tarcher.

Emoto, Masaru. (2004). *The Hidden Messages in Water.* Hillsboro, OR: Beyond Words.

Estés, Clarissa Pinkola, and Myss, Carolyn. (2003). *Intuition and the Mystical Life.* Audio CD. Boulder, CO: Sounds True.

Feinstein, David. (2004). *Energy Psychology Interactive Self-Help Guide.* Ashland, OR: Innersource.

Foundation for Inner Peace. (2008). *A Course in Miracles.* Mill Valley, CA: Foundation for Inner Peace. Originally published in 1976.

Frankl, Viktor E. (2006). *Man's Search for Meaning.* Boston: Beacon. Originally published in 1959.

Gawande, Atal. (2014). *Being Mortal: Medicine and What Matters in the End.* New York: Metropolitan.

Gellman, Marc. 2002. *And God Cried, Too: A Kid's Book of Healing and Hope.* New York: Harper Trophy.

Gerber, Richard. (2001). *A Practical Guide to Vibrational Healing: Energy Healing and Spiritual Transformation.* New York: Quill.

Gibbs, Nancy. (1993). Angels Among Us. *Time,* December 27, 56-65.

Guggenheim, Bill, and Guggenheim, Judy. (1997). *Hello from Heaven: A New Field of Research-After-Death Communications Confirms That Life and Love Are Eternal* (reprint ed.). New York: Bantam.

Hablitzel, William E. (2006). *Dying Was the Best Thing That Ever Happened to Me: Stories of Healing and Wisdom Along Life's Journey.* Blue Creek, OH: Sunshine Ridge.

Hablitzel, William E. (2008). *12 Secrets for Healing: Sacred Wisdom to Enrich the Healing Life.* Blue Creek, OH: Sunshine Ridge.

Hablitzel, William E. (2011). *It Was Only a Moment Ago: More Stories of Healing and Wisdom Along Life's Journey.* Blue Creek, OH: Sunshine Ridge.

Halberstam, Yitta, and Leventhal, Judith. (2002). *Small Miracles for the Jewish Heart: Extraordinary Coincidences from Yesterday and Today.* Avon, MA: Adams Media.

Harricharan, John. (2009). *When You Can Walk on Water, Take the Boat* (revised ed.). New York: New World.

Hawkes, Joyce Whiteley. (2010). *Cell-Level Healing: The Bridge from Soul to Cell* (reprint ed.). New York: Atria.

Hawkins, David R. (2014). *Power Versus Force: The Hidden Determinants of Human Behavior* (reprint ed.). Carlsbad, CA: Hay House.

Hay, Louise. (1984). *You Can Heal Your Life.* Carlsbad, CA: Hay House.

Hay, Louise. (2005) *You Can Heal Your Life Study Course.* Audiobook. Carlsbad, CA: Hay House.

Hay, Louise, and Richardson, Cheryl. (2013). *You Can Create an Exceptional Life*. Carlsbad, CA: Hay House.

Hay, Louise L., and Schulz, Mona Lisa. (2014). *All Is Well: Heal Your Body with Medicine, Affirmations, and Intuition*. Carlsbad, CA: Hay House.

Hicks, Esther, and Hicks, Jerry. (2004). *Ask and It Is Given: Learning to Manifest Your Desires*. The Teachings of Abraham. Carlsbad, CA: Hay House. Also on audio CD.

Hicks, Esther, and Hicks, Jerry. (2006). *The Law of Attraction: The Basics of the Teachings of Abraham*. The Teachings of Abraham. Carlsbad, CA: Hay House. Also on audio CD.

Hicks, Esther, and Hicks, Jerry. (2007). *The Astonishing Power of Emotions: Let Your Feelings Be Your Guide*. The Teachings of Abraham. Carlsbad, CA: Hay House. Also on audio CD.

Hirshberg, Caryle, and Barasch, Marc Ian. (1995). *Remarkable Recovery: What Extraordinary Healings Tell Us About Getting Well and Staying Well*. New York: Riverhead.

Hoffman, Alice. (2013). *Survival Lessons*. Chapel Hill, NC: Algonquin Books of Chapel Hill.

Jampolsky, Gerald G. (2000). *Teach Only Love: The Seven Principles of Attitudinal Healing* (expanded ed.). New York: Atria/Beyond Words.

Jampolsky, Gerald G. (2010). *Love Is Letting Go of Fear* (third ed.) Berkeley, CA: Celestial Arts.

Journal of Near-Death Studies. Durham, NC: International Association for Near-Death Studies. iands.org.

Kabat-Zinn, Jon. (2005). *Wherever You Go, There You Are: Mindfulness Meditation in Everyday Life*. New York: Hyperion.

Kabat-Zinn, Jon. (2013). *Full Catastrophe Living: Using the Wisdom of Your Body and Mind to Face Stress, Pain, and Illness* (revised and updated ed.). New York: Bantam.

Kane, Dave. (2006). *41 Signs of Hope*. Johnston, RI: Nicky's Counting.

Kessler, David. (2007). *The Needs of the Dying: A Guide for Bringing Hope, Comfort, and Love to Life's Final Chapter* (tenth anniversary ed.). New York: Harper Perennial.

Kircher, Pamela M. (2013). *Love Is the Link: A Hospice Doctor Shares Her Experience of Near-Death and Dying* (second ed.). Pagosa Springs, CO: Awakenings.

Kirven, Robert H. (1994). *Angels in Action: What Swedenborg Saw and Heard.* West Chester, PA: Chrysalis.

Kubler-Ross, Elisabeth. (1983). *On Children and Death.* New York: Macmillan.

Kubler-Ross, Elisabeth. (1991). *On Life After Death.* Berkeley, CA: Celestial Arts.

Kubler-Ross, Elisabeth. (1995). *On Life, Death and Life After Life.* Barrytown, NY: Station Hill.

Kubler-Ross, Elisabeth. (1999). *The Tunnel and the Light: Essential Insights on Living and Dying.* New York: DaCapo.

Kubler-Ross, Elisabeth. (2014). *On Death and Dying: What the Dying Have to Teach Doctors, Nurses, Clergy, and Their Own Families* (reprint ed.). New York: Scribner.

Kubler-Ross, Elisabeth, and Kessler, David. (2014). *Life Lessons: Two Experts on Death and Dying Teach Us About the Mysteries of Life and Living* (updated ed.). New York: Scribner.

LeShan, Lawrence. (1974, 1995). *The Medium, the Mystic, and the Physicist: Toward a General Theory of the Paranormal.* New York: Penguin.

LeShan, Lawrence. (1994). *Cancer as a Turning Point: A Handbook for People with Cancer, Their Families, and Health Professionals* (revised ed.). New York: Plume.

Lesser, Elisabeth. (2005). *Broken Open: How Difficult Times Can Help Us Grow* (reprint ed.). New York: Villard.

Lesser, Elisabeth. (2007). *Broken Open: Overcoming Our Fear of Change, Loss, and Death.* Recorded during Being Fearless Conference of Omega. Audio CD. Omega.

Lipton, Bruce. (2007). *The Biology of Belief: Unleashing the Power of Consciousness, Matter, and Miracles.* Carlsbad, CA: Hay House.

McTaggart, Lynne. (2008). *The Field: The Quest for the Secret Force of the Universe* (updated ed.). New York: Harper.

McTaggart, Lynne. (2008). *The Intention Experiment: Using Your Thoughts to Change Your Life and the World* (reprint ed.). New York: Atria.

Maniates, Yanni. (2004). *Peace of Mind Is a Breath Away: Breathing Free Meditations.* The Life Mastery Institute. learnmastery.com.

Maniates, Yanni. (2004). *Peace of Mind Is an Image Away: Visualization Meditations.* The Life Mastery Institute. learnmastery.com.

Maniates, Yanni. (2004). *Peace of Mind Is a Thought Away: Mastery Meditations.* The Life Mastery Institute. learnmastery.com.

Maniates, Yanni. (2007). *Magical Keys to Self-Mastery: Creating Miracles in Your Life.* Morrisville, PA: Mentor with the Masters.

Manning, Doug. (1984). *Don't Take My Grief Away: What to Do When You Lose a Loved One.* New York: HarperOne.

Mehl-Madrona, Lewis. (1998). *Coyote Medicine: Lessons from Native American Healing.* New York: Fireside.

Mendes, Dena. (2011). *A Survivor's Guide to Kicking Cancer's Ass.* Carlsbad, CA: Hay House.

Moody, Raymond. (1975, 2001). *Life After Life: The Investigation of a Phenomenon: Survival of Bodily Death.* San Francisco: HarperSanFrancisco.

Moorjani, Anita. (2014). *Dying to Be Me: My Journey from Cancer to Near Death to True Healing.* Carlsbad, CA: Hay House.

Morse, Melvin L., and Perry, Paul. (1991). *Closer to the Light: Learning from the Near-Death Experiences of Children* (reprint ed.). New York: Ivy.

Morse, Melvin L., and Perry, Paul. (1992). *Transformed by the Light: The Powerful Effect of Near-Death Experiences on People's Lives*. New York: Villard.

Morse, Melvin L., and Perry, Paul. (2001). *Where God Lives: The Science of the Paranormal and How Our Brains Are Linked to the Universe*. New York: HarperOne.

Mukherjee, Siddhartha. (2011). *The Emperor of All Maladies: A Biography of Cancer* (reprint ed.). New York: Scribner.

Myss, Caroline. (1998). *Why People Don't Heal and How They Can*. New York: Harmony.

Myss, Caroline. (2012). *What Makes Us Healthy: Understanding Mystical and Your Parallel Reality*. Audio CD. Carlsbad, CA: Hay House.

Naparstek, Belleruth. (1991). *A Meditation to Help You Fight Cancer*. Audio CD. Health Journeys.

Naparstek, Belleruth. (1991). *A Meditation to Help You with Chemotherapy*. Audio CD. Health Journeys.

Naparstek, Belleruth. (1992.) *Meditations to Ease Grief*. Audio CD. Health Journeys.

Naparstek, Belleruth. (1992.) *Meditations to Promote Successful Surgery*. Audio CD. Health Journeys.

Naparstek, Belleruth. (1995). *A Meditation to Help Ease Pain*. Audio CD. Health Journeys.

Naparstek, Belleruth. (2006). *4 Meditations for Unlocking Intuition*. Audio CD. Health Journeys.

Naparstek, Belleruth. (2009). *Your Sixth Sense: Unlocking the Power of Your Intuition* (reprint ed.). New York: HarperOne.

Naparstek, Belleruth. (2010). *Guided Imagery for Connecting with Your Spiritual Guide*. Audio CD. Health Journeys.

Northrup, Christiane. (2008). *The Power of Joy: How the Deliberate Pursuit of Pleasure Can Heal Your Life*. Audio CD. Carlsbad, CA: Hay House.

Northrup, Christiane. (2010). *Women's Bodies, Women's Wisdom: Creating Physical and Emotional Health and Healing* (revised and updated ed.). New York: Bantam.

Orloff, Judith. (1996, 2010). *Second Sight: An Intuitive Psychiatrist Tells Her Extraordinary Story and Shows You How to Tap Your Own Inner Wisdom* (reissue ed.). New York: Harmony.

Orloff, Judith. (2000). *Dr. Judith Orloff's Guide to Intuitive Healing: 5 Steps to Physical, Emotional, and Sexual Wellness.* New York: Times.

Orloff, Judith. (2004). *Positive Energy: 10 Extraordinary Prescriptions for Transforming Fatigue, Stress, and Fear into Vibrance, Strength, and Love.* New York: Harmony.

Ortner, Nick. (2014). *The Tapping Solution: A Revolutionary System for Stress-Free Living.* Carlsbad, CA: Hay House.

Pearsall, Paul. 2001. *Miracle in Maui: Let Miracles Happen in Your Life.* Makawao, Maui, HI: Inner Ocean.

Peters, Cash. (2011). *A Little Book About Believing: The Transformative Healing Power of Faith, Love, and Surrender.* Beverly Hills, CA: Penner.

Pert, Candace B. (1997). *Molecules of Emotion.* New York: Touchstone.

Plant, Jane. (2001). *The No-Dairy Breast Cancer Prevention Program: How One Scientist's Discovery Helped Her Defeat Her Cancer.* New York: Thomas Dunne.

Plant, Jane. (2001). *Your Life in Your Hands: Understanding, Preventing, and Overcoming Breast Cancer.* New York: Thomas Dunne.

Quillin, Patrick. (2005). *Beating Cancer with Nutrition* (fourth ed.). Carlsbad, CA: Nutrition Times.

Quindlen, Anna. (2000). *A Short Guide to a Happy Life.* New York: Random House.

Radin, Dean. (2009). *The Unconscious Universe: The Scientific Truth of Psychic Phenomena* (reprint ed.). New York: HarperOne.

Rando, Therese A. (1991). *How To Go On Living When Someone You Love Dies*. New York: Bantam.

Remen, Rachel Naomi. (2006). *Kitchen Table Wisdom: Stories That Heal* (tenth anniversary ed.). New York: Riverhead.

Remen, Rachel Naomi. (2001). *My Grandfather's Blessings: Stories of Strength, Refuge, and Belonging*. New York: Riverhead.

Remen, Rachel Naomi. (2001). *The Will to Live and Other Mysteries*. Audio CD. Boulder, CO: Sounds True.

Rinpoche, Sogyal. (2012). *The Tibetan Book of Living and Dying* (revised ed.). San Francisco: HarperSanFrancisco.

Rodegast, Pat, and Stanton, Judith. (1987). *Emmanuel's Book: A Manual for Living Comfortably in the Cosmos*. New York: Bantam.

Rodegast, Pat, and Stanton, Judith. (1989). *Emmanuel's Book II: The Choice for Love*. New York: Bantam.

Rodegast, Pat, and Stanton, Judith. (1989). *Emmanuel's Book III: What Is an Angel Doing Here?* New York: Bantam.

Ruiz, Don Miguel. (1997, 2012). *The Four Agreements: A Practical Guide to Personal Freedom*. San Raphael, CA: Amber-Allen.

Schickel, Sarno. (2012). *Cancer Healing Odyssey: My Wife's Remarkable Journey with Love, Medicine, and Natural Therapies*. Paxdieta.

Schulz, Mona Lisa. (1999). *Awakening Intuition: Using Your Mind-Body Network for Insight and Healing*. New York: Three Rivers.

Sams, Jamie, and Carson, David. (1999). *Medicine Cards: The Discovery of Power Through the Ways of Animals* (revised ed.). New York: St. Martin's.

Sanders, Catherine M. (1992). *Surviving Grief ... and Learning to Live Again*. New York: John Wiley & Sons.

Schwartz, Gary E. (2007). *The Energy Healing Experiments: Science Reveals Our Natural Power to Heal*. New York: Atria.

Schwartz, Morrie. (1996). *Letting Go: Morrie's Reflections on Living While Dying*. New York: Pan.

Servan-Schreiber, David. (2009). *Anti-Cancer: A New Way of Life*. New York: Viking.

Sheldrake, Rupert. (2011). *Dogs That Know When Their Owners Are Coming Home* (updated and revised ed.). New York: Three Rivers.

Siegel, Bernie S. (2013). *The Art of Healing: Uncovering Your Inner Wisdom and Potential for Self-Healing*. Novato, CA: New World Library.

Siegel, Bernie S., and Sander, Jennifer. (2009). *Faith, Hope, and Healing: Inspiring Lessons Learned from People Living with Cancer*. Hoboken, NJ: John Wiley & Sons.

Siegel, Bernie S. (1998). *Love, Medicine, and Miracles: Lessons Learned About Self-Healing from a Surgeon's Experience with Exceptional Patients*. New York: William Morrow.

Silberstein, Susan. (2005). *Hungry for Health*. Conshohocken, PA: Infinity.

Siles, Madonna. (2006). *Brain, Heal Thyself: A Caregiver's New Approach to Recovery from Stroke, Aneurysm, and Traumatic Brain Injuries*. Charlottesville, VA: Hampton Roads.

Smith, Penelope. (1999, 2008). *Animal Talk: Interspecies Telepathic Communication*. New York: Atria/Beyond Words.

Targ, Russell, and Katra, Jane. (1998). *Miracles of Mind: Exploring Nonlocal Consciousness and Spiritual Healing*. Novato, CA: New World Library.

Temes, Roberta. (2006). *The Tapping Cure: A Revolutionary System for Rapid Relief from Phobias, Anxiety, Post-Traumatic Stress Disorder and More*. New York: Marlowe.

Tittel, Joseph. (2007). *Messages from the Other Side*. BookSurge.

Turner, Kelly A. (2014). *Radical Remission: Surviving Cancer Against All Odds*. New York: HarperOne.

Urheber, Michael. (2014). *Bava's Gift: Awakening to the Impossible*. Princeton, NJ: ICRL.

Van Praagh, James. (1999). *Reaching to Heaven: A Spiritual Journey Through Life and Death* (reprint ed.). New York: Signet.

Van Praagh, James. (1997). *Talking to Heaven: A Medium's Message of Life After Death* (reprint ed.). New York: Signet.

Virtue, Doreen. (1998). *Divine Guidance: How to Have a Dialogue with God and Your Guardian Angel.* Los Angeles, CA: Renaissance.

Virtue, Doreen. (1999). *Healing with the Angels: How Angels Can Assist You in Every Area of Your Life.* Carlsbad, CA: Hay House.

Virtue, Doreen. (2005). *Saints and Angels Cards.* Carlsbad, CA: Hay House.

Virtue, Doreen, and Virtue, Grant. (2010). *Angel Words: Visual Evidence of How Words Can Be Angels in Your Life.* Carlsbad, CA: Hay House.

Wakefield, Dan. (1995). *Expect a Miracle: The Miraculous Things That Happen to Ordinary People.* New York: HarperCollins.

Walton, Charlie. (1996). *When There Are No Words: Finding Your Way to Cope with Loss and Grief.* Ventura, CA: Pathfinder.

Warner, Wendy, and Pettruchi, Kellyann. (2013). *Boosting Your Immunity for Dummies.* Hoboken, NJ: John Wiley & Sons.

Weil, Andrew. (1999). *Breathing: The Master Key to Self-Healing.* The Self-Healing Series. Audio CD. Boulder, CO: Sounds True.

Weil, Andrew. (2000). *Spontaneous Healing. How to Discover and Embrace Your Body's Natural Ability to Maintain and Heal Itself.* New York: Ballantine.

Weiss, Brian. (1988). *Many Lives, Many Masters: The True Story of a Prominent Psychiatrist, His Young Patient, and the Past-Life Therapy That Changed Both Their Lives.* New York: Fireside.

Wood, Eve A. (2004). *There's Always Help; There's Always Hope: An Award-Winning Psychiatrist Shows You How to Heal Your Body, Mind, and Spirit.* Carlsbad, CA: Hay House.

Yogananda, Paramahansa. (1972, 1998). *Autobiography of a Yogi* (reprint ed.). Los Angeles: Self-Realization Fellowship.

Zukav, Gary. (1989, 2014). *The Seat of the Soul* (twenty-fifth anniversary ed.). New York: Simon & Schuster.

Musical CDs: Favorites for Stress Management, Healing, and Meditation Work

All beautiful!

Drucker, Karen. *Songs of the Spirit, I, II, and III.* Tay Tunes Music BM.

Gass, Robert, and On Wings of Song. (1996). *Songs of Healing.* Boulder, CO: Spring Hill Music.

Kaur, Singh, and Robertson, Kim. *Crimson Collection, Volumes 1 & 2.* Phoenix, AZ: Invincible Productions.

Kaur Singh, Robertson, Kim, and Mosaic. *Crimson Collection, Volumes 5 & 6.* Phoenix, AZ: Invincible Productions.

Maxwell, Michael. (1998). *The Elegance of Pachebel.* CD or MP3. Ontario: Avalon Music.

Premal, Deva and Miten. (1998). *The Essence.* White Swan Records.

Premal, Deva. (2002). *Embrace.* White Swan Records.

Premal, Deva and Miten. (2013). *A Deeper Light.* White Swan Records.

Resources

Many are self-explanatory.

baldisbeautiful.org

beatcancer.org

breastcancer.org

> Established by oncologist Marisa Weiss, yields volumes of valuable information for women diagnosed with breast cancer.

berniesiegelmd.com

> This site shares the healing wisdom of physician and author Bernie Siegel and provides women with resources for healing mind, body, and spirit.

cancer.org

> The official site of The American Cancer Society. Provides numerous resources and help for dealing with all types of cancers.

cancer101.org

> A site intended to provide information, guidance and support to empower and provide a sense of control to meet the challenge of cancer.

cancercare.org

> Created by a dedicated social worker, this site provides free counseling, guidance, information and stories of hope to inspire cancer patients and their caretakers.

crazysexycancer.com

> Kris Carr shares tips, education, and valuable resources for young cancer patients.

dfhcc.harvard.edu

> This site shares research findings for fighting cancer, gathered from the DanaFarber/Harvard Cancer Center (one of the largest cancer centers in the world).

gutwisdom.com

> Alyce Sorokie, colon therapist, founder of Partners in Wellness, created this site to educate and support those dealing with colon issues.

gildasclubnyc.org

> Here you will find a community of those challenged by cancer, as well as programs, classes, and activities to support , comfort, inspire, and guide you on your journey. (Note: Gilda's Clubs can be found in numerous cities in the United States.)

iands.org

> One of the most important websites. Sponsored by the International Association for Near-Death Studies, which contributes to increased understanding and research of the near-death experience.

locksoflove.org

melvinmorse.net

Melvin Morse is a renowned pediatrician, researcher of near-death experiences, and author of books dealing with NDEs. His site provides anecdotal and scientific findings regarding those who have experienced the Light.

pregnantcancer.com

For women who are pregnant and who have cancer, a community of support!

rachelremen.com

Renowned physician, author, teacher, and healer Rachel Naomi Remen has created a beautiful newsletter of stories of healing wisdom.

stupidcancer.org

A great site that encourages the expression of legitimate feelings associated with this diagnosis. It also provides needed education and guidance for young people.

thehealingconsciousness.com

This is the site of The Healing Consciousness Foundation, established by breast surgeon Dr. Beth DuPree, to assist those dealing with breast cancer. The Comprehensive Breast Care Surgeons include Beth DuPree, MD, Stacy Krisher, MD, Catherine Carruthers, MD, and Amanda Woodworth, MD — an extraordinary team of breast surgeons who are affiliated with Holy Redeemer Hospital in Meadowbrook, PA. Dr. DuPree is also the author of *The Healing Consciousness: A Doctor's Journey to Healing.*

touchedbytheextraordinary.com

Psychologist Susan Apollon shares valuable information, inspiration, and resources for better managing a diagnosis of cancer, loss, energy, and healing. Her newsletter includes *Seeds for the Soul,* inspirational messages.

ulmanfund.org

The site describes great resources for educating young people and their families about cancer and cancer prevention.

Also be sure to check out ulmanfund.org/get-informed/. Doug
and Diana Ulman wrote *No Way, It Can't Be!: A Guidebook for
Young Adults Facing Cancer.*
vitaloptions.org
Promotes communication and advocacy for those with cancer
at the international level.
wigsite.com
y-me.org
Support for those diagnosed with breast cancer.
youngsurvival.org
For women age 40 and under, this site yields a wealth of resources and a community with which to share unique experiences.

Information About Alternative Therapies

Center for Advanced Cancer Education: Susan Silberstein, PhD,
established this organization following the early death of her
husband due to a rare form of cancer. Valuable articles, information, and guidance for preventing as well as treating cancer!
300 E. Lancaster #100, Wynnewood, PA 19096, (610) 642
4810, beatcancer.org.
Commonweal Cancer Help Program, Box 316, Bolinas, CA
94924, (415) 868 0970, commonweal.org. This organization
offers outstanding educational and creative programs designed
for healing individuals who are dealing with cancer and learning to care for themselves.
National Foundation for Alternative and Integrative Medicine,
1629 K St. NW, Suite 402, Washington, DC 20006, (202)
463-4900, nfam.org. Their mission is to identify complementary and alternative therapies as well as to research and inform
the public of their effectiveness.

The Center for Mind-Body Medicine, 5225 Connecticut Ave. NW, Suite 414, Washington, DC 20015, (202) 966-7338, cmbm.org. The Center combines science with the wisdom of various healing traditions, concentrating on the impact of emotional, mental, spiritual, and social factors on the body. It promotes the teaching of a medical model that integrates various types of mind-body medicine (meditation, biofeedback, yoga, guided imagery, acupuncture, etc.).

Chapter Notes

Chapter 12:

1. Caryle Hirshberg and Marc Ian Barasch, *Remarkable Recovery: What Extraordinary Healings Tell Us About Getting Well and Staying Well* (New York: Riverhead Books, 1996), 198.

Chapter 15:

1. Neal Conan and Greg Smith, "Do You Believe in Miracles? Most Americans Do," *NPR*, 23 February 2010, accessed 02 September 2014, http://www.npr.org/templates/story/story.php?storyId=124007551.

Chapter 17:

1. Alice Hoffman, *Survival Lessons* (Chapel Hill, NC: Algonquin Books, 2013), 28-29.

2. Hoffman, *Survival Lessons*, 62.

3. Kris Carr, *Crazy Sexy Cancer Tips* (Augusta, GA: Morris Publishing Group, 2007), 176.

Chapter 19:

1. David Servan-Schreiber, *Anticancer: A New Way of Life* (New York: Viking, 2009), 86-87.

2. Servan-Schreiber, *Anticancer*, 137.

3. Servan-Schreiber, *Anticancer*, 137-138.

4. Servan-Schreiber, *Anticancer*, 134.

5. Patrick Quillin and Noreen Quillin, *Beating Cancer with Nutrition: Combining the Best of Science and Nature for Full Spectrum Healing in the 21ˢᵗ Century* (Carlsbad, CA: Nutrition Times Press, 2001), 155.

6. Servan-Schreiber, *Anticancer*, 111.

7. Servan-Schreiber, *Anticancer*, 133.

8. Kelly A. Turner, *Radical Remission: Surviving Cancer Against All Odds* (New York: Harper Collins, 2014), 26.

Chapter 20:

1. Brené Brown, *The Gifts of Imperfection: Let Go of Who You Think You're Supposed to Be and Embrace Who You Are* (Center City, MN, 2010), 84.

Chapter 22:

1. Jamie Saxon, "Balancing Your Body's Energy for Optimal Health," *U.S. 1*, 3 March 2010, accessed 21 August 2014,

http://www.princetoninfo.com/index.php/component/
us1more/?key=03-03-2010%20Energy.

2. Jingduan Yang, MD, "Chinese Medicinal Diet" (presentation, *Integrative Medicine Lectures, Presentations & Grand Rounds, Jefferson University, Philadelphia, PA, December 3, 2013*). http://jdc.jefferson.edu/jmbcim_lectures/64

3. Jingduan Yang, MD, "Is Acupuncture a Deception?" *Huff-Post Healthy Living*, 8 October 2013, accessed 7 August 2014. http://www.huffingtonpost.com/dr-jingduan-yang/acupuncture_b_3908855.html.

4. Bernie Siegel, *Faith, Hope & Healing*, (Hoboken: Wiley, 2009), 95.

5. Siegel, *Faith*, 89.

6. Siegel, *Faith*, 65.

7. Siegel, *Faith*, 95.

About the Author

Susan Barbara Apollon is a Pennsylvania-licensed psychologist, as well as a cancer survivor and thriver. She has been in private practice since 1991 and specializes in grief, integrative oncology, and trauma. She is also an author, educator, and researcher of consciousness, mind, prayer, intuition, angels, energy, and healing.

Physicians refer their patients to Susan for assistance in healing their grief or meeting their cancer challenge. Susan's roots are in medicine. Her path and her approach, however, have enabled her to develop a unique perspective on healing—one that is based on an understanding that everything is energy and that energy is also medicine. With certification in Eden Energy Medicine and training in a number of energy modalities, as well as Energy Psychology, Susan shares with her patients her research findings concerning the primary factors that contribute to remission and healing. Her intention is to provide them with the wisdom and tools needed to achieve balance and wholeness, as well as to survive and thrive.

Susan is the author of four books: *Touched by the Extraordinary (Book One)*; *Touched by the Extraordinary, Book Two: Healing Stories of Love, Loss & Hope*; *Affirmations for Healing Mind, Body*

& Spirit; and (coauthor) *Intuition Is Easy and Fun*. She is also the creator of several CDs, including: *Guided Meditation for Peace, Healing and Empowerment*; *Healing, Loving Imagery to Comfort and Soothe the Soul Challenged by Cancer*; *A Healing Meditation to Successfully Meet the Challenge of Cancer*; *Creating Miracles in Your Life: Extraordinary Stories of Cancer Survivors*; and *The Healing Power of Love*. Susan hopes this body of work will enable readers and listeners to appreciate the extraordinary spiritual implications of their journey with grief and/or cancer.

Susan loves sharing her passion for healing and the extraordinary (including miracles, the power of prayer, and angels). Her belief in the inherent healing wisdom and power within each of us, along with her unique blend of research and personal anecdotal material and stories, have helped many to shift and grow spiritually.

Her articles have appeared in national publications, including magazines, newspapers, and websites. Additionally, she has been a guest on numerous radio and television shows. She has conducted workshops, taught seminars, led healing retreats, and been asked to be a part of interfaith events.

Susan is honored to co-lead The GyniGirls, along with Dr. Amy Harvey. Being a part of this women's cancer support group nurtures her soul. Additionally, she enjoys speaking and sharing her research, as well as volunteering at a free monthly Energy Medicine Clinic.

Family, friends, and pets mean everything to Susan. When not engaged in research, writing, speaking, and her clinical work, she longs to be out in nature. What she loves most is being with her husband, to whom she has been married for 50 years, her children—especially her new granddaughter—her cherished pets, and dear friends. She knows she is richly blessed.

Index

A

ABCs, 152, 170
    A is for Awareness and Acknowledgment, 109–110, 185–186
    B is for Breath and Breathing out your pain, 110, 186
    C is for Choice and Choosing Thoughts and Images, 110,
        186–187
Acceptance, 42
Achterberg, Jeanne, 255
Acidic diet, 25
Acknowledgment, 109–110, 185–186
Actualization, self, 29
Acupressure, 95
Acupuncture, 13, 40, 48, 95, 309, 316, 322, 328, 330, 341, 362
Adrenalectomy, 58
Adrenaline, 17
Adrenal tumors, 58
Adversity, as opportunity for spiritual growth, iii
Affirmation(s)
    combining with breath, 163–164
    of gratitude, 286–287

harnessing the healing power of positive, 161–164

of healing, 160–161

making constant habit, 163

prayer and, 253–254

putting in writing, 82–84, 163, 194

Aks, Cynthia, vi, 347–358

Aldrich, Joni James, 127

Alexander, Eben, 128

Alignment, 179–195

ABCs in identifying what needs to go, 185–186

finding, through forgiveness and reclaiming power, 191–195

learning to say no, 188–189

moment-by-moment, 187–188

quitting of job and, 182–185

rating long-term levels, 189–191

with values, 46

visualization in, 187

Alkaline diet, 25

Allie Bird, 130

Alternative medicine, 341. *See also specific*

Alzheimer's disease, 319

Angel Cards, 214, 215

Angels, 194

among us, 213–214

in bringing healing, 144–146

earth, 362

Angels in My Hair (Byrne), 149–150

Anger, 19, 167, 175, 177, 228

self, 167

Angotti, Donna, vi

Antibiotics, 260

Anticancer: A New Way of Life (Servan-Schreiber), 260, 262–263, 264, 270

Anticipatory grief, 19

Anti-inflammation diet, 325, 355
Antioxidants, 261, 265
Anxiety, 16, 219
Apoptosis, 264
Apprehension, feeling, 16
Art therapy, 339–340, 345
Asking, gift of receiving and, 214–215
Attention, paying, to feelings, 222
Attig, Thomas, 101
Attraction. *See* Law of Attraction
Autoimmune conditions, 319
Automatic writing, 93–94
Awareness, 109–110, 185–186
Ayurvedic medicine, 354

B
Balance, 38
      being in touch with the Source, 28
      in diet, 25
      fun in your life and, 28–29
      grief and, 48–49
      healing and, 39
      letting go and, 32–33
      in lifestyle, 25–26
      primary relationships and, 27
      quiet zone and, 26–27
      self-love and, 29–31
      social networks and, 27–28
      well-being and, 24
      in work-life, 68
Barasch, Marc Ian, 173, 288
Basil, 263–264, 355
Being love, 41–42
Benson, Herbert, 198–199

Berries in diet, 263
Biofeedback, 198
Bioflavonoids, 261
The Biology of Belief: Unleashing the Power of Consciousness, Matter and Miracles (Lipton), 6, 37
Bitterness, 228
Black currants, 265
Black pepper, 355
Blessings
    brainstorming your, 285
    writing down your, 285
Body
    caring for your, 284–301
    healing of, 65
Boehmer, Tami, 288
Bone infection, 10–11
Boosting Your Immunity for Dummies (Warner), 317
Borage, 265
BPA (Bisphenol A), 272
Braden, Gregg, 149
Brain cancer, 104, 235
Brainstorming blessings, 285
Brain tumors, 8–9
BRCA genes, 192
Breaks, building, into workday, 184
Breast cancer, 58, 146, 192, 212, 214, 215, 218–219, 227, 235, 262, 263, 269, 293, 307
Breathing, 44
    combining affirmations with, 163–164
    deep, 362
    de-stressing with relaxing, 183–184
    effective, 353
    enhancing gratitude with your, 287
    exhalation, 151

inhalation, 151
meditative, 151
mindfulness in, 197–203
relaxing, 183–184
rhythmic, 199, 202
science of, 198–199
of your pain, 110
Brown, Brené, 33, 73, 287, 291
Bruhn, John, 219
Buddha, 283
Byrne, Lorna, 149–150

C
Caisse, Rene, 55
Callahan, Roger, 117
Callanan, Maggie, 129
Campbell, Anna, v
Camus, 367
Cancer. *See also* Tumors
brain, 104, 235
breast, 58, 146, 192, 212, 214, 215, 218–219, 227, 235, 262,
263, 269, 293, 307
as catalyst for growing your spirit, 141–144
cervical, 104
clarity and, 223, 224–226
empowerment and, 144
esophageal, 318
existence of miracles and, 143–144
fear of, 124
gifting of life and, 215–216
gynecological, 227
keeping away with garlic, 261–262
learning from experience with, 52–53
lifestyle changes in combating or preventing, 352–357

looking for hope and, 142–143
low vibrations and, 16
lung, 19
making choices and, 181
miracles and, 207–208
need for help and, 142
ovarian, 18
prostate, 269, 270
renal, 236
seeing, as gift, 55–71, 137
in shifting your priorities, 141
significance of nutrition in fighting, 258–260
in slowing you down, 141
teachings of, 66–69
Cancer cells, 273, 350–351
development of, 17
Cancer diagnosis
approaches to, iii, x
chain of events in, 352
dealing with, 234
fear of, ii, x–xii, 16, 41, 56, 75, 363
getting second opinion on, 10, 309, 335
Cancer Healing Odyssey (Schickel), 275–276
Cancer journey
choices and lessons in, 342–343
energy in, 7–8
guiding principles for, 37–53
The Cancer Support Network, 127
Cardamom seeds, 355
Cardiac situations, 160
Cardiovascular disease, 221
Caregivers in assisting in process of dying, 135–136
Carotenoids, 261
Carr, Kris, 233, 242–243, 276

Cause, tapping into a, 252
Celery seed, 355
Cells
    cancer, 17, 35–351, 273
    macrophage, 21
    natural killer, 21
    T-, 21
Cervical cancer, 104
Chamomile, 355
Chance, Sue, 173–175, 176
Changes, 47–48
    inability to make, 42–43
Chardin, Pierre Teilhard de, 154
Charity walks, 250
Chemotherapy, 9, 192, 264, 330, 363
    platelet count and, 11
    responding to patient not comfortable with
        traditional, 318–319
Chinese herbal remedies, 328
Chocolate, dark, 263
Choice(s)
    choosing thoughts and images and, 110, 186–187
    making, 181
    power of, 65
    that feel good or better, 186–187
Chronic fatigue, 160
Chronic myelogenous leukemia, 62–66
Cilantro, 355
Cinnamon, 264, 355
Clarification, 67
Clarity
    letting cancer sharpen your, 223, 224–226
    of your values, 221–222
Classical Chinese medicine practitioner, 328

Clemens, Samuel, 311

Closer to the Light: Learning from the Near-Death Experiences of Children (Morse and Perry), 128

Cloves, 355

Coffee enemas, 272, 274, 276

Coincidences, 126

Cold water fish in diet, 266

Compassion, 46, 64

Complementary medicine, 316

Confidence, self, 239

Connecting through Compassion: Guidance for Family and Friends of a Brain Cancer Patient (Aldrich), 127

Conscious grieving, 105

Consciousness, 43–44

    research on, 5

Consideration, 46

Coronary artery disease, 319

Cortisol, 17, 247

Counseling, 316

    grief, ii

    nutrition, 13

    one-on-one, ii

Coyote Medicine (Mehl-Madrona), 255

Craig, Gary, 117

Crazy Sexy Cancer Tips (Carr), 242–243, 276

Criticism, self, 32

Cumin, 355

D

Dairy in diet, 268–269

Dark chocolate, 263

Death. *See also* Dying

    fear of, 63, 123–138, 124, 235–236

    grief and, 88

Kübler-Ross on, ix, 123, 128, 136
    making peace with, 137–138
    as a transition, 124–125
Death Is of Vital Importance: On Life, Death, and Life After Death
    (Kübler-Ross), 128
Deep breathing, 362
DeHart, Dottie, v
Demanding Compassion (Scarlett), 335
Denial, 167
Depression, 219
De-stressing, 183–184
Detoxification, 270, 272
DHEA, 21, 156, 199
Diabetes, 160
Diet. *See also* Meals; Nutrition
    acidic, 25
    alkaline, 25
    anti-inflammation, 325, 355
    avoiding refined sugar in, 266
    berries in, 263
    cold water fish in, 266
    dairy in, 268–269
    fats in, 265
    garlic in, 262–263
    Gerson, 274–276
    ginger in, 264
    green tea in, 270
    herbs, spices, and seasonings in, 263–264
    kelp in, 262
    legumes in, 262–263
    macrobiotic, 274, 279
    mushrooms in, 263
    olive oil in, 265–266
    organic foods in, 261

    proteins in, 267–268
    ready-made processed foods and drinks in, 260
    recreating rainbow on your plate, 265
    salt in, 268
    seaweed in, 262
    tomatoes in, 264–265
    turmeric in, 264
    unhealthful foods in, 25
    vegetables in, 261
    water in, 269–270
    whole grains in, 267
Discomfort, hospice in diminishing, 134–135
Diverticula, 280
Diverticulitis, 280
Divine, connecting with, in nature, 150–151
Divine energy, 5, 6, 28, 164, 169, 201
Doctor, choosing right, 335–336
Donne, John, 218
Doomsday thinking, 88
Dossey, Larry, 5, 6
Dr. Seuss, 87
DuPree, Beth Baughman, iv, vii, 8, 103
Dyer, Wayne, 358
Dying. *See also* Death
    caregivers in assisting process of, 135–136
    fear of process, 124
Dying to Be Me (Moorjani), 15, 128, 175, 288

E
Eadie, Betty J., 128
Earth Angels, 362
Eastern medicine, 40, 308, 320, 331
Eden, Donna, 112, 184, 333
    Five Minute Energy Routine, 184

Eden Energy Medicine, 100, 112, 113–115, 134, 309, 314–316
Eger, Edith Eva, 173
Einstein, Albert, 3, 4–5, 216
Ellagic acid, 263
Embraced by the Light (Eadie), 128
Emerson, Ralph Waldo, 60
Emotional Freedom Technique, 117
Emotional healing, 74, 75, 76
Emotional temperature, 324
Emotions
    low-vibrational, 128
    negative, 17–18
    suppressed, 103
Emoto, Masaru, 6, 269
Empowerment, cancer and, 144
Empty calories, 266
Endorphins, 21, 48, 163, 199, 246, 287
Enemas, 272
    coffee, 272, 274, 276
Energy, 3–13
    balancing with Eden Five Minute Energy Routine, 184
    balancing with grief, 95–96
    in cancer journey, 7–8
    defining, 4
    divine, 5, 6, 28, 164, 169, 201
    negative, 117, 186
    positive, 8–13, 186
    science on, 4–6
    vibrational, 6, 7, 28, 40–41, 44, 48, 104, 106, 156
Energy medicine, 40, 279, 316–317, 322
    in providing peace, 134
    in rebalancing and healing, 111–113
Energy Medicine (Eden), 112
Energy psychology, 100, 117

Energy therapy, 20
Enjoy Every Sandwich (Lipsenthal), 318
Epinephrine, 247
Esophageal cancer, 318
Essential oils, 356
Esteem, self, 352
Evening primrose, 265
Exercise
    benefits of, 26
    incorporating into routine, 273
Exhalation breath, 151
Experiences, Law of Attraction in creating negative or positive, 156–157
Extraordinary experiences, opening yourself to, 205–216

F
Face/Embrace/Replace process, 100, 105–109, 152, 158, 170, 176
    FACE your feelings and thoughts, 106
    EMBRACE your feelings and thoughts, 106–107
    REPLACE your feelings and thoughts, 108–109
Faith, Hope & Healing (Siegel), 342, 343
Falun Dafa, 328, 331
Fats in diet, 265
Fear
    of cancer, x–xii, 124
    of cancer diagnosis, ii, x–xii, 16, 56, 363
    of death, 63, 123–138, 124, 235–236
    in driving resistance, 346
    feeling, 16
    stories in coming to terms with, 128–129
Feel-good thoughts, 7
Feelings
    embracing your, 106–107

facing your, 106
    paying attention to, 222
    replacing your, 108–109
    repressing, 106–107
Feinstein, David, 117
Feit, Josi, 368, 369
Fellowship, gift of, 62
Fennel seed, 355
The Field: The Quest for the Secret Force of the Universe
    (McTaggart), 6
Final Gifts (Callanan and Kelley), 129
Fish, in diet, 266
Five Minute Energy Routine (Eden), 112
Flexner report, 320
Flicker, Karen, vi
Forgiveness, 65, 67, 166–177
    case study in, 173–175
    choosing for others, 170–172
    constantness in, 176–177
    finding alignment through, 191–195
    self, 168–170
    for the tough-to-forgive, 172–173
    types of, 166
    as unconditional, 166–168
Friendships, cultivating, 27–28
From Incurable to Incredible: Cancer Survivors Who Beat the Odds
    (Boehmer), 288
Frustration, 19
Fun
    need for, 28–29
    permission to have, 63

G

Gamut, 118, 119

Gandhi, 165

Garbanzo beans, 262

Garlic, 264, 355

    in diet, 262–263

    keeping cancer away with, 261–262

Gerber, Richard, 6

Gerson, Charlotte, 275

Gerson Clinic, 276

Gerson diet, 274–276

Gerson Therapy, 274–275

"Getting Fine Is Hard" (Lang), 294–295

Gift(s)

    of asking and receiving, 214–215

    breath as, 44

    gratitude as, 59–60, 284–287

    imagination as, 44

    intuition as, 44

    seeing cancer as, 55–71, 137

The Gifts of Imperfection (Brown), 287

Ginger in diet, 264

GMO foods, 354

Grad, Bernard, 5

Grape seed, 265

Gratitude, 201–202

    affirmation of, 286–287

    enhancing, with your breath, 287

    gift of, 59–60, 284–287

    value of, 64

Gratitude Journal, 285

Green tea, 270, 331

Grief, 177

    allowing, 87–101

anticipatory, 19
association with death, 88
balancing, 48–49, 95–96
cost of, 18–20
defining, 88–89
healing and, 94–95
honoring, 90–91
losses and, 89–90
triggers in, 91–94
Grief counseling, ii
Grocery shopping, 271
Growing, 47–48
Growth hormones, 260, 261
Gynecological cancer, 227
GyniGirls Support Group, vi, 60–62, 153, 230, 236, 249, 250–251, 362

H
Habit, making affirmations a constant, 163
Hablitzel, William E., vi, 358–360
Hanh, Thich Nhat, 155, 197, 203
Happiness, 42–43, 180, 246
Harmony, 38
in healing, 38–39
Harvey, Amy, 3, 8, 230
Hawkes, Joyce, 5
Hawkins, David R., 5, 6, 44–45, 148, 366
Healers, passing on knowledge of, 311–364
Healing
as absent in medical education, iii
affirmations of, 160–161
angels in bringing, 144–146
as an inside job, i
aspects of, 39, 65

balance and, 39
caring for whole person, 314
choosing your own form of, 39–40
Eden Energy Medicine and, 314–316
emotional, 74–76
going out of the box to help patients, 316–317
grief and, 94–95
harnessing power of positive affirmations, 161–164
holistic view of, 75–76
information and support as key in, 312–314
lessons of, 76–79
meaning of, 73–85
mental, 74
mind, 65
options in, 339–340
physical, 20, 39, 47, 76, 198, 210
positive energy in promoting, 8–13
psychological, 69
recovery versus, 338
relationships in, 236–237
shamanic, 322
spiritual, xi, 20, 47, 69, 74, 75, 76, 78, 79–81
stories of selfless, 246–247
taking back power in, 226–227
tools for, 103–122
wholeness and harmony in, 38–39
Healing and Feeling: Stress, Support, and Breast Cancer
    (Spiegel), 218
"A Healing Prayer from God to Michael," 150
Healing, self, 254
Healing the Gerson Way: Defeating Cancer and Other Chronic
    Diseases (Gerson), 275
Health, using Law of Attraction to affirm better, 155–164
Heart, listening with your, 222–223

HeartMath, 322
Help, need for, 142
Herbal remedies, 329, 362
Herbs in diet, 263–264
The Hidden Messages in Water (Emoto), 269
Higher power, connecting with, 139–154
Hippocrates, 257
Hirshberg, Caryle, 173, 288
Hoffman, Alice, 235, 242
Holistic medicine, 75–76, 319–320
Holmes, Ernest, 32–33
Honesty, 46
    writing with, 242–243
Hope, looking for, 142–143
Hormones, 17, 48, 163, 199, 247, 287
    stress, 292
Hospices, 134–135
Human experience, miracles as part of the, 206–207
Humor, 291
    immune system and, 291
    use of, 300
Hydration, adequate, 353

I
Image, self, 239
Imagination, 44, 345
Immune system
    balance and, 24
    functioning of, 293
    healthy, 41, 353–354
    humor and, 291
    impact of thoughts and feelings on, 16
    mindfulness and, 120–121
    stress and, 220–221

Immunologic stress, 354
Infection, bone, 10–11
Inhalation breath, 151
Inner guidance system, tuning into via meditation, 151–152
Inside out, transforming life from, 157–159
Integrative medicine, 305–310, 314, 316, 319–320, 331, 341–342, 361
Integrative psychology, 40
The Intention Experiment: Using Your Thoughts to Change Your Life and the World (McTaggart), 6
Intentions, 163, 202
    in inviting a miracle, 147–148
    putting in writing, 82–84, 210–211
    in release of pain, 97–98
Internet, using the, 240
Intimacy
    affirming greater, 240
    cancer and, 234
    defined, 235–236
    fostering, 237–242
    healing value of, 233–243
Intuition, 44, 200
    in choosing medical team, 306–308
    in guidance, ii
    trusting your, 272, 343
Isoflavones, 262

J
Job, inability to quit, 182–185
Journal
    gratitude, 285
    synchronicity, 209–210
Journaling, 92, 176, 194. *See also* Writing
Joy, 180

expressing, 293
Joy Zone, taking regular shortcuts to the, 290–292
Judgment, self, 32
Juicing, 276–277

K
Kabat-Zinn, Jon, 120–122
Katie, Byron, 139
Katra, Jane, 286
Katz, Lewis, 245
Keep It Simple (KIS), 239, 260, 309–310
Keller, Helen, ix
Kelley, Patricia, 129
Kelp in diet, 262
Kidney beans, 262
Kindness, 46
    focusing on small acts of, 253
    gift of unexpected, 61
Kocubinski, Tom, 367, 368
Kübler-Ross, Elisabeth, ix, 123, 128, 136
Kushi Institute, 274
Kushner, Harold, 87

L
Labels, being wary of, 271
Ladies Who Inspire (radio show), 127
Lang, Judy, 293–297
Lasley, Janet, 315, 316
Law of Attraction, 7, 228, 287
    in affirming better health, 155–164
LDLs, 266
Legumes in diet, 262–263
Leiomyosarcoma, 315
Lentinian, 263

LeShan, Lawrence, 5
Letting go, art of, 32–33
Leukemia & Lymphoma Society, 65
Life. *See also* Living
	cancer gifting you with, 215–216
	spiritual aspects of your, 325
	transforming, from inside out, 157–159
Life After Loss: Conquering Grief and Finding Hope (Moody),
	128
Lifestyle
	changes to combat or prevent cancer, 352–357
	coaching, 13
	examining your, 324
	monastic, 26–27
	truth about changes in, 337
	wake-up call on, 58
Like energy, 44–45, 85
Lipsenthal, Lee, 318
Lipton, Bruce, 5, 6, 37
Listening
	for answers, 202
	with your heart, 222–223
*The Little Book of Energy Medicine: The Essential Guide to
	Balancing Your Body's Energies* (Eden), 112
Liver cancer, 299
Living. *See also* Life
	in alignment, 179–195
	fully, 137–138
	passionately, 293
Lombardi, Vince, 49
Long-term alignment, rating levels of, 189–191
Losses, grief and, 89–90
The Lost Mode of Prayer (Braden), 149
Love, 6, 64

connecting with, 175–176
kinds of, 41–42
self, 29–31, 42, 66–67, 74, 189, 191, 289–290
signs of forever, 132–133
unconditional, 41, 166–168, 169, 193, 207–208
Love, Medicine & Miracles (Siegel), 342
Loving support, 58–59
Low vibrations, 15–21, 128, 157
cancer and, 16
cost of grief and, 18–20
science of negativity and, 17–18, 21
Loyalty, 46
Lung cancer, 19

M
Macrobiotic diet, 274, 279
Macronutrients, 273
Macrophage cells, 21
Massage, 13, 341, 362
McTaggart, Lynne, 6
Meals. *See also* Diet; Nutrition
eating small, 272
Medical education, 321–322, 359–360
healing as absent in, iii
Medical team, creating your, 305–310
Meditation, 100, 163, 176, 198, 200, 279, 316, 328, 341,
360, 362
tuning into inner guidance via, 151–152
Meditative breath, 151
Mehl-Madrona, Lewis, 255
Memorial Sloan Kettering Hospital (New York City), cancer
treatment at, 8, 278–279
Mental healing, 74
Messages from Water (Emoto), 6

Micronutrients, 273
Mind, 5–6
    feeding with spiritual food, 152–153
    purposefully caring for your, 284–301
Mind-body connection, 16, 17, 21
Mindfulness, 120–121, 152
    immune system and, 120–121
Mindfulness-Based Stress Reduction Program, 120
Mind healing, 65
Mint, 263–264
Miracles, 126
    cancer and, 207–208
    existence of, 143–144
    inviting, into your life, 208–211
    opening yourself to, 205–216
    as part of the human experience, 206–207
    prayer and intention in inviting, 147–148
Miracles of Mind: Exploring Nonlocal Consciousness and
    Spiritual Healing (Katra and Targ), 286
Miso, 262
Molecules of Emotion: The Science Behind Mind-Body
    Medicine (Pert), 17
Moment-by-moment alignment, 187–188
Monastic lifestyle, 26–27
Moody, Raymond A., Jr., 128
Moorjani, Anita, 15, 128, 175, 179, 288
Morse, Melvin, 128, 129
Mother
    healing presence of, 212–213
    spending time with your, 59
Movement, 356
Multiple sclerosis, 227
Mushrooms in diet, 263
Music, 191, 200, 344

filling journey with, 292–293

Myself, time with, 59

N

Native American Medicine, 40

Natural killer cells, 21, 262

Nature

connecting with the divine in, 150–151

disconnection from, 29

healing properties of, 151

immersing yourself in, 288–289

Naturopathy, 279

"Navigating Metastatic Breast Cancer and Beyond" (Feit), 369

NDEs (near-death experiences), 41, 136, 140, 166, 175

books dealing with, 128–129

Needs, asking others for your, 229

Negative emotions

cost of, 18

properties of, 17–18

Negative energy

replacing with positive energy, 186

unblocking, 117

Negative experiences, Law of Attraction in creating, 156–157

Negative thoughts, 21, 88

committing to make significant changes in, 209

pain from, 105

Negativity, 228, 355

science of, 17–18

Neuro-emotional technique, 327

Neuropeptides, 17, 163

Neurotransmitters, 17

The No-Dairy Breast Cancer Prevention Program (Plant), 261, 267, 269, 270

No, learning to say, 188–189

Non-Hodgkin lymphoma, 50–53, 307
Norepinephrine, 247
Nutmeg, 355
Nutrition, 257–281, 316, 326, 354. *See also* Diet; Meals
  principles of healing, cancer-fighting diet and, 260–271
  quality, 354–355
  significance of, in fighting cancer, 258–260
Nutrition counseling, 13
Nutritionist, 326

O

O'Keeffe, Amy Harvey, vi, 360–364
Olive oil in diet, 265–266
Omega 3 fatty acids, 266
Omega 6 fats, 265
One-on-one counseling, ii
"One Year Later: A Cancer Survivor" (Lang), 295–296
On Life after Death (Kübler-Ross), 128
Operating room environment, 344
Oregano, 263–264
Organic foods in diet, 261
Others
  asking for your needs, 229
  connecting with, 229–230
  forgiveness for, 170–172
  helping, 251–255
Out-of-alignment life, symptoms of, 180
Ovarian cancer, 18

P

Pain
  breathing out your, 110, 186
  intentional release of, 97–98
  negative thoughts and, 105

Pancreatitis, 299

Parting Visions: Uses and Meanings of Pre-Death, Psychic and Spiritual Experiences (Morse and Perry), 129

Past, detachment from, 65

Paxdieta, 276

Peace, 198

    breaking into life, 183

    Energy Medicine in providing, 134

    making with death, 137–138

    sense of, 19

Peace diet, 275–276

Peace plan, 15-minute, 199–203

Peale, Norman Vincent, 164

Pennsylvania, University of, cancer treatment at, 10

Peptides, 17

Permission, giving yourself, to be open to extraordinary experiences, 208

Perry, Paul, 128, 129

Personal growth, 48

Perspective

    gift of, 59–60

    shifting gears of, 46–47

Pert, Candace, 5, 17

Peters, Cash, 365

Pets, developing loving relationship with, 241–242, 289

Pew Forum on Religion, 206

Pheochromocytoma, 58, 216

Phillips, Peter, 10

Phosphate additives, 260

Physical healing, 20, 39, 47, 76, 195, 210

Physical wellness, 74

Physics, quantum, 4–5, 7

Phytochemicals, 261

Phytoestrogens, 262

Pity, self, 195, 228
Plant, Jane, 261, 267, 268–269, 270, 273
Plastic containers, being wary of, 272
Platelet count, chemotherapy and, 11
Platelet transfusions, 11–12
Poetry, writing, 293–297
Polyphenols, 263
Polysaccharides, 263
Positive affirmations, harnessing the healing power of, 161–164
Positive changes, 30
Positive energy
    in promoting healing, 8–13
    replacing negative energy with, 186
Positive experiences, Law of Attraction in creating, 156–157
Positive thoughts, 16, 51, 355
Positivity, 42
    practicing, 228
Potential, 346–347
Power
    of choice, 65
    finding alignment through reclaiming, 191–195
    gift of taking, 60–61
    in managing treatment, 133
    of purpose, 297–301
    taking back in healing, 226–227
Power vs. Force (Hawkins), 6
A Practical Guide to Vibrational Medicine: Energy Healing
    and Spiritual Transformation (Gerber), 6
Practicality, 46
Prayer, 11, 148–150, 163, 198, 360, 362
    affirmation and, 253–255
    healing, from God to Michael, 150
    in inviting a miracle, 147–148
    with loved ones, 240–241

Preciousness of time, 68–69
Presence, 46
Primary biliary cirrhosis, 299
Primary relationships, 27
Priorities
    cancer in shifting your, 141
    gift of clear, 61
    re-ordering, 30
Processed foods and drinks, including ready-made, in diet, 260
Proof of Heaven (Alexander), 128
Prostate cancer, 269, 270
Protease inhibitors, 262
Proteins in diet, 267–268
Psychological healing, 69
Psychology
    energy, 100, 117
    integrative, 40
Psychoneuroimmunology, 16
Psychotherapist, 326–328
Pumpkin, 265
Purpose, power of, 297–301

Q
Qi, 325, 329
Qigong, 48, 95, 309, 322, 328
Quantum physics, 4–5, 7
Quiet time, need for, 26–27
Quillin, Patrick, 257, 268, 278

R
Radical remission, 305
Radical Remission: Surviving Cancer Against All Odds (Turner),
    269, 272–273, 288
Radin, Dean, 5

Rainbow, creating on plate, 265
Ready-made processed foods and drinks in diet, 260
Receiving, gift of asking and, 214–215
Recovery versus healing, 338
Reflection, 360
Reflections on Life After Life (Moody), 128
Re-forgiveness, 177
Reiki, 11, 13, 40, 48, 113, 134, 192, 212–213, 309, 322, 341, 355, 362
Reinventing Medicine: Beyond Mind-Body to a New Era of Healing (Dossey), 6
Relationships, 67
   asking universe for needed, 228
   attracting healthy, 228–229
   developing loving, with pet, 241–242
   falling away of nonworking, 224
   in healing, 236–237
   identifying nonworking, 221–223
   valuing your, 67
   visualizing better, 228
Relaxation Response, 198
The Relaxation Response (Benson), 198–199
Relaxing breaths, 183–184
Remarkable Recovery: What Extraordinary Healings Tell Us About Getting Well and Staying Well (Hirshberg and Barasch), 173, 288
Remen, Rachel Naomi, 23, 73, 139, 152, 205, 245, 247
Renal cancer, 236
Repressing feelings, 106–107
Resilience, 77
Resistance, 70–71
Responsibility, claiming, 68
Rhythmic breathing, 199, 202
Rosemary, 263–264, 355

Roseto Effect, 219
Roseto, Pennsylvania, story of, 219–221

S
Sage, 264
Salt in diet, 268
The Saving of Gordon: Lifelines to W-I-N Against Cancer
    (Aldrich), 127
Saxon, Jamie, 314
Scarlett, William L., vi, 334–335
Schickel, Sarto, 275
Schlitz, Marilyn, 5
Schrödinger, 5
Science
    of breath, 198–199
    on energy, 4–6
Seasonings in diet, 263–264
Seaweed in diet, 262
Second opinion, need for, 10, 309
Sedentary lifestyle, 25–26
See/feel technique, 241
Selenium, 267
Self-actualization, 29
Self-anger, 167
Self-confidence, 239
Self-criticism, 32
Self-esteem, 352
Self-forgiveness, 168–169
    moving forward with tool for, 169–170
Self-healing, 254
Self-image, 239
Selfishness, 189
Self-judgment, 32
Selflessness, 245–255

healing power of, 246–247
    helping others and, 251–255
    service and, 247–248
    stories of healing and, 246–247
Self-love, 42, 66–67, 74, 189, 191, 289–290
    lack of, 29–31
Self-pity, 195, 228
Servan-Schreiber, David, 260, 262–263, 264, 270
Service, selflessness and, 247–248
Shamanic healing, 322
Sheldrake, Rupert, 5
"She Let Go" (Holmes), 32–33
Shore, Dinah, 217
Siegel, Bernie, vi, x, 85, 342–347
Significant changes, committing to make in negative
    thoughts, feelings and beliefs, 209
Sklarz, Andrew (Andy) R., 62–66
Sleep, adequate, 356
Sloan Kettering Cancer Center, 8, 278–279
Social networks, 27–28
Social support system, 218, 324
Soriano, Scarlet, vi, 332–334
Sorrow, expressing, 293
Soul, purposefully caring for your, 284–301
Source, 107, 140
    connecting to your, 40
Soy, 262
Soybeans, 262
Soy milk, 262
Spices in diet, 263–264
Spiegel, David, 218
Spirit, nourishing your, with uplifting stories, 288
Spiritual food, feeding mind with, 152–153
Spiritual foundation, nourishing, 148–154

Spiritual growth, 51–52, 64, 65, 139–154, 366
    adversity as opportunity for, iii
    cancer as catalyst in, 141–144
    gift of, 61–62
Spiritual healing, xi, 20, 47, 69, 74, 75, 76, 78, 79–81
Spirituality, 28, 140, 153
    rediscovering, 208
Stem cell transplants, 9
Stories
    Alicia's, 132–133
    Allie's, 130–131
    Amanda's, 99–101
    Andy's, 62–66
    Barry's, 146–147
    Bea's, 113–115
    in coming to terms with fears, 128–129
    Daniel's, 96–99
    Darlene's, 226–227
    Diane's, 224–226, 278–280
    Eileen's, 297–301
    Elena's, 191–195
    Hanna's, 147–148
    immersing yourself in, of the miraculous, 211
    Jean's, 249–251
    Jennifer's, 157–159
    Josey's, 76–79
    Julia's, 115–117
    Lauren's, 8–13
    Linda's, 144–146
    Malika's, 131–132
    Mary Ellen's, 50–53
    Maya's, 18–20
    nourishing your spirit with uplifting, 288
    of Roseto, Pennsylvania, 219–221

Selena's, 236–237
of selfless healing, 246–247
Tom's, 175–176
uplifting, 288
Stress, 16, 111
immune system and, 220–221
immunologic, 354
Stress hormones, 292
Stronger Than Death: When Suicide Touches Your Life
(Chance), 173–175
Strong, silent, solitary types, 217–231
Sugar, avoiding refined, in diet, 266
Suicide, 173–175, 250
Sun Hee, 275, 278
Support groups, 153, 219, 230, 240, 339. *See also* GyniGirls
Support Group
Supportive community, connecting with, 153–154
Suppressed emotions, 103
Survival Lessons (Hoffman), 235, 242
Survivorship care plan, ii
Synchronicities, 62, 125, 126–127, 128, 143, 206
willingness to open oneself to, 126
Synchronicity journal, 209–210

T
Tagore, Rabindranath, 310
Tai chi, 48, 95, 113, 309, 322, 328, 362
Tapping, 13, 90, 111, 117–120, 152, 158
gamut in, 118, 119
The Tapping Cure (Temes), 117
Targ, Russell, 5, 286
Taxol, 263
T-cells, 21
Teaching, 253

Temes, Roberta, 117
Tempeh, 262
Temple, nourishing your, 289–290
Therapeutic Touch, 40, 113, 309
Therapy. *See also* Chemotherapy
    art, 339–340, 345
    energy, 20
    Gerson, 274–275
    radiation, 10, 270, 318–319
        responding to patient not comfortable with traditional,
            318–319
    Thought Field, 117
Third party, sharing thoughts and feelings with a, 238
Thought Field Therapy, 117
Thought habits, 21
Thoughts
    choosing, 110, 186–187
    embracing your, 106–107
    facing your, 106
    feel-good, 7
    impact on immune system, 16
    negative, 21, 88, 105, 209
    positive, 16, 51, 365
    replacing your, 108–109
Thrivership care plan, ii
Thyme, 263–264
Thyroiditis, 299
Time
    with myself, 59
    preciousness of, 68–69
    spending with mother, 59
Tofu, 262
Tomatoes in diet, 264–265
Touched by the Extraordinary, 129, 137, 146

Touched by the Extraordinary, Book One, 366
Touched by the Extraordinary, Book Two, 129, 211, 213, 366
*Touched by the Extraordinary: Healing Stories of Love, Loss,
    and Hope,* 129
Tough-to-forgive, forgiveness for the, 172–173
Toxins, cleansing body of, 272–273
Transcendental Meditation, 198
Transformed by the Light (Morse and Perry), 129
Transfusion, platelet, 11–12
Transition, death as a, 124–125
Transplants, stem cell, 9
Treasures (Kocubinski), 367, 368
Treatment
    choosing right, 308–309, 335–336
    having the power to manage your, 133
Triggers, grief and, 91–94
Trust, 290, 343
Tumors. *See also* Cancer
    adrenal, 58
    brain, 8–9
Turmeric, 264, 355
Turner, Kelly A, 269, 272–273, 288, 305
Twain, Mark, 311

U

Unconditional love, 41, 140, 166–169, 193, 207–208, 289
Unhealthful foods in diet, 25
Universe, asking for needed relationship, 228

V

Values
    alignment with, 46
    getting clear on, 221–222
Van Gogh, Vincent, 231

Vegetables, in diet, 261
Vibrational energy, 6, 7, 28, 40–41, 44, 48, 104, 106, 156
Vibrations, 149. *See also* Low vibrations
Virtue, Doreen, 214, 215
Visualization, 64, 98, 106, 108–109, 200–202, 228, 241, 300
    alignment, 187
Volunteer activities, 190, 253

W
Wake-up call on lifestyle, 58
Walter, Jess, 195
Warner, Wendy, vi, 317–322
Warren, Diana, vi–vii, 115, 315
Water in diet, 269–270
Waters, Meghan, v
Weight gain, 319
Well-being
    achieving sense of, 183, 192
    balance and, 24
    blessings of peace, love, and, viii
    challenge of breast cancer and, vii
    control and, 70
    creating sense of, 160, 246
    decision making and, 30
    denial of, 167
    emotional, 221
    energy and, 95, 198, 315
    feelings of warmth and, 198
    as foundation, 233
    happiness and, 285
    healing and, 38, 64, 194, 203, 206, 223, 267
    health and, 307, 327
    herbal remedies and, 329
    as higher level, 110, 112

implications concerning, 159
integrative medicine and, 331
intentions and, 210
love, peacefulness and, 45
motivations and, 227
needs and, 82
of others, 68, 81, 220, 228
power and, 63
returning to sense of, 109, 309
sacrificing own, 78
sense of peace and, 106, 108
universal, 285
vibrational energy and, 96
Wellness, physical, 74
Western medicine, 39–40, 308, 320, 331, 358, 359
White, Geoff, 315
Whole foods, relying on, 273
Whole grains in diet, 267
Wholeness in healing, 38–39
Williamson, Marianne, 290
Will to live, tapping into, 49
Wisdom, 6, 46
Wolf, Stewart, 219
Wooden, John, 245
Words, said to self, 159–160
Workday, building breaks into, 184
Work ethic, 19
Work-life balance, 68
Wrazen, Linda, 92–93
Writing. *See also* Journaling
    automatic, 93–94
    down your affirmations, 82–84, 163, 194
    down your blessings, 285
    down your intentions, 82–84, 210–211

with honesty, 242–243
poetry, 293–296, 297
workshops for, 340

Y
Yang, Jingduan, vi, 322–332
Yi, Peter, vi, 312–317
Yoga, 100, 184, 279, 316, 341, 362
Yogurt, 268, 269
Your Life in Your Hands: Understanding, Preventing, and Overcoming Breast Cancer (Plant), 269

Z
Zinc, 267

Book Susan Apollon to Speak to Your Organization or Group.

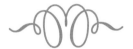

Susan Apollon speaks joyfully and passionately to hospital staffs and patients, medical students, college students, and other organizations and groups about everyone's ability to live full, satisfying lives, be happy, create their own miracles, and heal themselves. Often, she is honored to be asked to serve as a keynote speaker.

In addition, Susan conducts a rich variety of workshops and seminars that provide a blend of her contagious enthusiasm with her tried and true methods and interventions for energetic, physical, psychological and spiritual healing, empowerment, and creating a joyful and healthy life.

Susan is happy to speak and conduct interactive sessions on a variety of topics ranging from cancer, grief, integrative medicine, healing, love, near-death experiences, angels, prayers, and miracles. For a complete list of topics please visit www.AnInsideJob-ForHealingCancer.com. Or call (215) 493-8434 for more information.